CMSRN Exam Study Guide

All-in-One CMSRN Review + 600 Med Surg Certification Questions with In-Depth Answer Explanations for the Certified Medical-Surgical Registered Nurse Exam (Includes 4 Full Length Practice Tests)

Margaret Jenkins
Emma L. Lyons
© 2024-2025
Printed in USA.

Disclaimer:

Contents

Why do you need to be CMSRN Certified?

➤ Firstly, being CMSRN certified validates your expertise in emergency nursing, enabling you to stand out among your peers and gain professional recognition. It showcases your commitment to continuous learning and staying updated with the latest advancements in the field.

➤ Additionally, the CMSRN certification signifies your ability to deliver safe and high-quality care to patients in emergency situations. This can enhance patient trust and satisfaction, and lead to improved patient outcomes.

➤ Furthermore, the CMSRN certification sets you apart in the job market, making you a sought-after candidate for positions in emergency departments, trauma centers, and critical care units. Many employers prioritize hiring CMSRN certified nurses due to the added confidence in their skills and knowledge.

➤ Lastly, obtaining the CMSRN certification can open up opportunities for career advancement and higher salaries. Many healthcare organizations value the expertise and dedication of CMSRN certified nurses and may offer increased responsibilities and compensation packages accordingly.

<u>Willing to Join Our Author Panel?</u>

Dear,

We would like to invite you to join our 'Panel of Authors'.
First of all, Thank you for your hard work and dedication to your patients. We know that the hours are long and the workload is demanding, but you do it with grace and dignity. Your compassion is evident in the way you treat your patients, and we are grateful for all that you do.
We believe that your expertise and experience will be a valuable contribution to our books. Our goal is to provide valuable content that helps our readers to step forward in their career development. This is a unique opportunity to share your expertise with others in need and help shape their future.

The requirements for joining our panel of authors are as follows:
- A minimum experience of 8 year
- Proper certification from a renowned organization
- Good writing and teaching skills
- Enthusiasm in sharing knowledge
If you meet these requirements and are interested in joining our panel, please send us your resume along with a writing sample for our review to propublisher@zohomail.com.
We would be happy to have you on board!
We are happy that our panel of authors can provide the best content because they are experienced and passionate in their own field. We would love for you to join our panel of authors and help us continue to provide quality content for our readers. You will also be able to connect with other experts in your domain from around the world and build a network of support. Undoubtedly, this will be a great opportunity for you to make a difference in your profession.

Thank You.

Why is this book the right choice for you to clear the CMSRN Exam?

Latest Study Guide:

If you are looking for an up-to-date study guide for the CMSRN Exam, then look no further than this book. This book provides everything you need to know to ace the exam with tons of practice questions to help you prepare. This book is also constantly updated to ensure that it always covers the latest information on the exam as per the content outline.

CMSRN® TEST CONTENT OUTLINE

1. Gastrointestinal System
2. Respiratory System
3. Hematological System
4. Integumentary Systems
5. Cardiovascular System & Shock
6. Endocrine System & Diabetes
7. Renal & Urological Systems
8. Musculoskeletal & Neurologic Systems
9. Pain, Cancer, Per-op, Nutrition
10. Nursing Practice Roles

Experienced Set of Authors:

There are many reasons to choose this book over others, but one of the most important is that it is written by experienced authors who are CMSRN Certified. The authors of this book have a wealth of experience in taking and passing exams, and we have used our knowledge to create a study guide that is comprehensive and easy to follow.

With our experienced authors and comprehensive coverage, our book is the best way to prepare for this important test.

Detailed rationale for the answer:

We provide an in-depth explanation for each question, so you can understand not only the correct answer but also why it is correct. This book also gives you an ample amount of practice to help you feel confident on exam day.

Similar Question Format as that in the actual exam:

One of the most important features of this book is that the questions and answers follow the same pattern as the actual exam. This is extremely important because you need to be familiar with the format of the exam to do well on it.

Fine Tunes your thinking:

Going through the questions, answers and explanations repeatedly will sharpen your thinking and understanding ability. This will help you to understand the root of the question in the CMSRN Exam and make the right selection of the answer.

Clear and Concise:

This CMSRN Prep is written in simple language and is not overly technical. This sets this book apart from other study materials because when you are studying for the CMSRN Exam, you need to be able to understand the material without getting bogged down in details. This book will help you do just that. This combination of easy-to-understand language and practical testing will help you be successful on the CMSRN exam.

Magical Steps to Pass the CMSRN Exam with Ease:

1. Belief: You must believe that you can pass the CMSRN exam with ease. This belief will help you stay focused and motivated throughout your studies. We help build your confidence by giving you the feel of attending virtual exams in our book, making you familiar with the type of questions that will be asked in the exam, and giving you a thorough idea about all the topics covered in the exam.

2. Visualization: Visualize yourself passing the CMSRN exam with flying colors. This will help you stay positive and focused on your goal. Taking multiple tests and solving various questions will help improve your positivity and confidence. We try our best to improve your positivity.

3. Study: Make sure to study all the material thoroughly. Quality Learning is more important than Quantity Learning. Time yourself when you take tests and try to complete them within the stipulated time.

4. Practice: The more you practice the more is the chance of passing the exam. By doing this, you will get a feel for the types of questions that will be asked and how to best answer them. We have an abundant number of questions for you to practice.

5. Relax: On the day of the exam, make sure to relax and stay calm. This will help you think more clearly and perform at your best.

Smart Learning with Trust in Yourself will make Success knock at your door!
All the Best!

CMSRN

Guide

1 Patient/Care Management

The topic of 'Patient/Care Management' in medical-surgical nursing involves assessing, planning, implementing, and evaluating patient care. Effective communication, collaboration with interdisciplinary teams, patient education, and ensuring patient safety and quality outcomes are crucial. Medical-surgical nurses play a key role in coordinating care, advocating for patients, and utilizing evidence-based practice. By focusing on these aspects, nurses can provide comprehensive care, promote positive patient outcomes, and enhance the overall quality of care delivery.

1.1 Patient Safety

The topic of 'Patient Safety' in 'Patient/Care Management' is crucial for CMSRNs. Effective communication among healthcare team members is vital to ensure patient well-being. Medication safety plays a key role in preventing adverse events. Infection control practices are essential in reducing healthcare-associated infections. Implementing fall prevention strategies helps minimize patient falls. Proper patient identification procedures are necessary to prevent errors in treatment. These aspects are integral to providing safe and high-quality care to patients.

1.1.1 Nursing process - assessment, diagnosis, planning, implementation, evaluation

The nursing process, encompassing assessment, diagnosis, planning, implementation, and evaluation, is vital for ensuring patient safety and effective care management. Assessment gathers crucial patient data, diagnosis identifies needs, planning creates comprehensive care plans, implementation applies evidence-based interventions, and evaluation assesses outcomes. This process enhances care quality, promotes safety, and optimizes patient outcomes across healthcare settings. Thorough assessment, accurate diagnosis, comprehensive planning, evidence-based implementation, and outcome evaluation are key steps in providing high-quality patient care and achieving positive patient outcomes.

1.1.2 Patient safety protocols

Patient safety protocols are vital in ensuring safe patient care. These protocols outline procedures to prevent errors and promote patient well-being. Common protocols include hand hygiene, medication administration checks, and fall prevention measures. Healthcare providers play a crucial role in implementing these protocols to minimize risks and enhance outcomes. Adherence to protocols is key in reducing adverse events and improving quality of care. Patient safety protocols significantly impact patient outcomes by reducing complications and promoting a culture of safety within healthcare settings. Prioritizing adherence to these protocols is essential for ensuring patient safety and delivering high-quality care.

1.1.2.1 Skin

Skin assessment plays a vital role in patient safety and care management. The skin acts as a crucial barrier against infections and injuries, highlighting the importance of its integrity for overall patient well-being. Common skin conditions like pressure ulcers, dermatitis, and wounds can compromise patient safety. Nursing interventions such as regular skin assessments, proper documentation, and collaboration with the healthcare team are essential for preventing and managing skin issues effectively. By prioritizing skin health, nurses can ensure optimal patient safety and contribute to comprehensive care management.

1.1.2.2 Falls

Falls in patient safety protocols involve identifying risk factors like age, mobility issues, and medication side effects. Strategies for prevention include keeping pathways clear, using bed alarms, and providing mobility aids. Assessment tools like Morse Fall Scale help evaluate fall risk. Interventions include frequent rounding, patient education, and using non-slip socks. Falls can lead to injuries, longer hospital stays, and decreased quality of life. Healthcare providers play a crucial role in preventing falls by implementing safety measures, conducting regular assessments, and educating patients and families.

1.1.2.3 Restraints

Restraints in patient safety protocols are tools used to prevent harm to patients or healthcare providers. Medical surgical nurses must understand the rationale, types, risks, and benefits of restraint use. Common types include physical and chemical restraints. Legal and ethical considerations are crucial, as restraints can infringe on patient autonomy. Proper application and continuous monitoring are essential to prevent complications. Alternative strategies like de-escalation techniques and patient-centered care prioritize a therapeutic environment. By being knowledgeable about restraints and exploring alternatives, nurses can ensure patient safety while promoting holistic care.

1.1.2.4 Rounding

Rounding in healthcare involves regular checks on patients to ensure safety and well-being. Types include hourly rounding, purposeful rounding, and bedside shift report. It aids in proactive monitoring, early issue identification, and timely intervention. Nurses play a crucial role in conducting rounds, communicating with patients, and collaborating with the team for optimal care. Effective rounding improves patient outcomes, satisfaction, and care quality. Tools and technologies support rounding processes and enhance communication. Documentation and follow-up actions post-rounding observations ensure care continuity and accountability in patient management.

1.1.2.5 Suicide

Suicide in patient safety protocols involves recognizing risk factors, warning signs, and using assessment tools for prevention. Medical-surgical nurses play a crucial role in identifying at-risk patients, implementing safety measures, and collaborating with teams for support. Thorough assessments, individualized care plans, close monitoring, and referrals to mental health professionals are essential. Legal and ethical considerations in documentation and reporting are paramount. Suicide impacts patients, families, healthcare providers, and the system. Nurses must provide emotional support, promote a safe environment, and prioritize patient well-being.

1.1.3 Risk factors

In the realm of patient safety and care management, risk factors encompass elements that predispose patients to potential harm or adverse outcomes. Identifying and addressing these risk factors is crucial to safeguarding patients' well-being. Common risk factors in medical-surgical settings include medication errors, falls, infections, and communication breakdowns. Medical surgical nurses play a pivotal role in mitigating these risks by adhering to best practices, conducting thorough assessments, promoting effective communication among healthcare team members, and implementing preventive measures. By proactively managing risk factors, nurses can uphold high-quality care standards and enhance positive patient outcomes.

1.1.3.1   Pharmacological

Pharmacological principles in medical-surgical nursing are crucial for managing patient conditions and ensuring safety. Medications play a vital role in treatment but also pose risks. Nurses must understand drug actions, interactions, and side effects to prevent errors. Patient safety is paramount when administering medications; double-checking, verifying, and educating patients are key strategies. Pharmacological management impacts patient outcomes and care quality significantly. Common interventions include pain management with analgesics, infection control with antibiotics, and chronic disease management with various medications. Nurses must be vigilant, knowledgeable, and proactive in pharmacological care to optimize patient well-being.

1.1.3.2   Environment

In medical-surgical nursing, the environment encompasses physical surroundings, equipment, and organizational factors. It serves as a crucial risk factor affecting patient safety and care management. Environmental conditions in healthcare settings can impact patient outcomes by contributing to complications and influencing care quality. Examples of environmental risk factors include noise levels, infection control practices, and ergonomic considerations. Strategies to enhance patient safety include proper lighting, clutter-free spaces, and infection prevention measures. Considering the environment in care planning is vital for optimizing patient well-being and treatment effectiveness.

1.1.3.3   Equipment

In the realm of medical-surgical nursing, equipment plays a pivotal role in ensuring patient safety and effective care management. Proper maintenance, calibration, and inspection of equipment are crucial in averting adverse events and upholding patient well-being. Equipment aids in identifying and managing risk factors, thereby enhancing patient outcomes. Medical-surgical nurses bear the responsibility of vigilantly monitoring and utilizing equipment to prevent failures that could compromise patient care. Common equipment like infusion pumps, cardiac monitors, and ventilators are indispensable in delivering quality care and managing patients effectively. Regular checks and adherence to protocols are essential for seamless equipment functionality.

1.1.3.4   Demographics

In medical-surgical nursing, demographics play a crucial role in understanding patients' risk factors, ensuring patient safety, and effective care management. Demographics encompass age, gender, ethnicity, socioeconomic status, and geographic location, all influencing patients' risk profiles. By considering demographics, nurses can tailor care plans to meet diverse patient needs, enhancing safety measures. Demographics also shed light on healthcare disparities, resource distribution, and access to quality care, guiding nurses in addressing inequities. Understanding how demographics impact patient care is essential for providing effective and equitable medical-surgical nursing services.

1.1.4   Patient safety culture

Patient safety culture in Patient Safety and Patient/Care Management refers to the shared values, beliefs, and attitudes that shape staff behaviors regarding patient safety in healthcare settings. Key aspects include defining a culture of safety, its critical importance in preventing errors and harm, components like communication, teamwork, and learning from mistakes. Strategies to enhance this culture involve open communication, reporting incidents, and continuous training. A positive safety culture improves patient outcomes by reducing errors and promoting a safe environment. Healthcare providers play a vital role in fostering this culture through leadership, support, and accountability. Initiatives like TeamSTEPPS and Just Culture promote safety culture in healthcare.

1.1.4.1   Near miss reporting

Near miss reporting is vital for patient safety culture. It involves documenting incidents with potential harm. Key aspects include importance of reporting for risk identification, confidentiality to ensure safe reporting, learning opportunities for system improvement, communication among staff for shared learning, detailed documentation for trend tracking, and feedback mechanisms for transparency. Near miss reporting enhances patient safety by proactively addressing risks, improving processes, and fostering a culture of continuous quality improvement in healthcare.

1.1.4.2   "Just culture"

In healthcare, a just culture fosters fairness, accountability, and learning. It promotes open communication, transparency, and trust among providers, patients, and organizations. Balancing individual accountability with system factors is crucial for reporting errors without fear of retribution. Leadership plays a vital role in nurturing a just culture , improving patient outcomes, enhancing care quality, and preventing medical errors. Key aspects include fairness, accountability, and learning. This culture supports error reporting and emphasizes the importance of addressing system issues to enhance patient safety and care management.

1.1.4.3   "Speak up"

In the context of Patient safety culture, Patient Safety, and Patient/Care Management, 'speak up' refers to healthcare providers voicing safety concerns. It is crucial for patient outcomes as it enhances error prevention and promotes a culture of safety. Effective communication fosters better patient care and reduces adverse events. Encouraging open communication involves active listening, non-punitive responses, and team collaboration. Assertiveness plays a vital role in advocating for patient safety by addressing issues promptly and ensuring patient well-being. Healthcare providers must prioritize speaking up to create a safe and effective care environment.

1.1.4.4   High accountable organizations

High accountable organizations in healthcare prioritize patient safety culture, ensuring optimal patient outcomes. Key aspects include fostering a culture of safety, implementing effective policies, and managing care efficiently. These organizations demonstrate accountability and transparency through robust practices, leading to improved patient results and enhanced quality of care. Their impact on patient safety and excellence in care is significant, highlighting the crucial role they play in promoting a culture of safety and quality within healthcare settings.

1.1.5   Care bundles

Care bundles in patient safety and care management are sets of evidence-based practices designed to improve patient outcomes and reduce healthcare-associated infections. They consist of multiple interventions that, when implemented together, have a synergistic effect on patient care. Common components include hand hygiene, timely antibiotic administration, and daily assessment of readiness for extubation. These bundles are crucial in standardizing care delivery, ensuring consistency and quality. Medical-surgical nurses play a vital role in implementing and monitoring care bundles, promoting adherence to best practices and ultimately enhancing patient safety and quality of care.

1.1.5.1   Checklist

In medical-surgical nursing, checklists within care bundles are vital tools for ensuring adherence to best practices and guidelines, enhancing patient safety and management. Checklists streamline processes, reduce errors, and improve communication among healthcare team members. Examples include medication administration, surgical site preparation, and discharge planning checklists. They promote a systematic approach to care delivery, foster a culture of safety, and support evidence-based practice. By utilizing checklists, healthcare professionals can standardize care, minimize risks, and ultimately improve patient outcomes.

1.1.5.2   Algorithms

Algorithms in healthcare, specifically within care bundles, patient safety, and care management, play a crucial role in optimizing patient care. By streamlining clinical decision-making, standardizing care practices, and promoting evidence-based care delivery, algorithms enhance adherence to protocols, reduce medical errors, and improve patient outcomes. They also contribute to healthcare quality, efficiency, and cost-effectiveness in medical-surgical nursing practice. Algorithms are essential tools that support healthcare professionals in providing consistent, high-quality care, ultimately leading to better patient safety and management.

1.1.6   Patient safety assessments and reporting

Patient safety assessments and reporting are crucial in patient care management. Key components include identifying risks, implementing preventive measures, and evaluating outcomes. Certified Medical Surgical Registered Nurses (CMSRNs) play a vital role in ensuring patient safety through regular assessments and incident reporting. Effective communication and collaboration among healthcare team members are essential for promoting a safety culture. Utilizing evidence-based practices and quality improvement initiatives is important for enhancing patient safety outcomes. Healthcare providers must prioritize patient safety to deliver high-quality care.

1.1.6.1   Abuse

Abuse in patient care encompasses physical, emotional, sexual, and financial harm. Signs of abuse include unexplained injuries, changes in behavior, fear, and financial exploitation. Reporting suspected abuse is crucial for patient safety and involves ethical considerations. Healthcare professionals play a vital role in preventing and addressing abuse to ensure patient well-being. Understanding the types of abuse, recognizing signs, and reporting appropriately are essential in maintaining a safe medical-surgical environment.

1.1.6.2   Human trafficking

Human trafficking in patient safety assessments involves identifying individuals coerced into exploitation for profit. Prevalent globally, risk factors include poverty and vulnerability. Signs include unexplained injuries, fearfulness, and inconsistent stories. Impact on healthcare includes physical and psychological trauma. Legal considerations involve mandatory reporting laws. Healthcare providers play a crucial role in recognizing and reporting human trafficking cases to safeguard patient well-being.

1.1.6.3   Social determinants

In patient safety assessments and reporting, social determinants encompass factors like socioeconomic status, education level, healthcare access, living conditions, and social support networks. Understanding these influences is crucial for enhancing patient safety outcomes and care management. Social determinants significantly impact a patient's health, healthcare utilization, treatment adherence, and overall well-being. Healthcare providers can address these factors by tailoring care plans, connecting patients with community resources, and advocating for policies that promote health equity. By recognizing and addressing social determinants, healthcare professionals can optimize patient safety, care quality, and health outcomes.

1.1.7   Risk assessment methods

In patient safety and care management, risk assessment methods are crucial for preventing adverse events and enhancing patient outcomes. Medical surgical nurses utilize various tools and scales to identify risks, including the Braden Scale for predicting pressure sore risk and the Morse Fall Scale for fall risk assessment. The risk assessment process involves identifying, analyzing, evaluating risks, and implementing mitigation strategies. Effective communication of findings to healthcare teams ensures comprehensive patient safety. Regular risk assessments are essential in healthcare settings to proactively address potential hazards and ensure high-quality care delivery.

1.1.7.1   Root Cause Analysis [RCA]

Root Cause Analysis (RCA) is a vital tool in healthcare for identifying underlying causes of adverse events, errors, or near misses. It involves steps like data collection, analysis, identifying contributing factors, and developing action plans to prevent recurrence. RCA promotes a culture of safety, quality improvement, and proactive risk management in medical-surgical nursing. By utilizing RCA, healthcare organizations can enhance patient outcomes, reduce medical errors, and improve overall care quality. RCA plays a crucial role in patient safety, care management, and risk assessment methods within healthcare settings.

1.1.7.2   Failure Mode and Effects Analysis [FMEA]

Failure Mode and Effects Analysis (FMEA) is a crucial risk assessment tool in medical-surgical nursing. It helps in identifying potential failure modes, assessing their impact on patient outcomes, and devising strategies to mitigate risks. Steps include identifying failure modes, determining causes/effects, assigning risk priority numbers, and creating action plans. FMEA plays a vital role in enhancing patient safety, improving care quality, and optimizing management processes. In clinical practice, FMEA can prevent adverse events, reduce errors, and foster a culture of continuous quality improvement. Its application ensures proactive risk management and fosters a safer healthcare environment.

1.1.7.3 Safety rounds

Safety rounds in medical-surgical nursing involve systematic assessments to identify and mitigate risks, enhance patient safety, and optimize care management. These rounds are crucial for preventing adverse events and ensuring patient well-being. Conducted regularly by a multidisciplinary team, including nurses, physicians, and other healthcare professionals, safety rounds focus on areas like infection control, medication safety, and fall prevention. By facilitating risk identification, promoting team communication, and improving care quality, safety rounds play a vital role in enhancing patient outcomes. Medical surgical nurses lead these rounds, implementing interventions to address safety concerns promptly and effectively.

1.1.7.4 Safety huddles

Safety huddles are brief, regular meetings among healthcare team members to discuss potential risks, patient safety issues, and care management strategies. They promote a culture of safety by enhancing communication, situational awareness, and risk identification. Effective huddles involve frequent sessions with key participants, structured agendas, and clear follow-up actions. These huddles play a vital role in proactive risk management and quality improvement in medical-surgical nursing practice. By fostering open dialogue and collaboration, safety huddles empower teams to address challenges promptly and ensure optimal patient outcomes.

1.2 Infection Prevention

Infection prevention in patient/care management involves implementing strategies to reduce the spread of infections in healthcare settings. Medical surgical nurses play a crucial role in this by ensuring proper hand hygiene, using personal protective equipment, and maintaining clean environments. Key principles include breaking the chain of infection, recognizing infectious diseases, and applying isolation precautions. Healthcare-associated infections can negatively impact patient outcomes and increase healthcare costs. It is essential for nurses to be vigilant in following infection control protocols to safeguard patients and maintain a safe healthcare environment.

1.2.1 Universal and transmission-based precautions

The Certified Medical Surgical Registered Nurse (CMSRN) exam covers Universal and Transmission-Based Precautions in infection prevention. Universal precautions involve standard practices like hand hygiene and PPE to prevent infection spread. Transmission-based precautions are extra measures for known/suspected infections spread through contact, droplet, or airborne routes. They include specific PPE, patient isolation, and environmental controls. Understanding and applying both precautions are vital for nurses to safeguard themselves and patients from infections. By adhering to these protocols, nurses create a safe healthcare environment.

1.2.2 Infection control practices and standards

Infection control practices are crucial in healthcare to prevent infections. Standard precautions, like hand hygiene and PPE use, are fundamental. Transmission-based precautions target specific pathogens. Environmental cleaning is vital to reduce contamination. Preventing healthcare-associated infections is a priority. Medical surgical nurses play a key role in ensuring adherence to these practices. By promoting proper infection control measures, nurses contribute to patient safety and quality care. Adhering to standards in infection prevention and patient/care management is essential for a safe healthcare environment.

1.2.3 Current evidence-based practice for infection control and prevention procedures

As a CMSRN, staying updated on evidence-based infection control practices is vital. Key aspects include hand hygiene, proper PPE use, and environmental cleaning. CDC and WHO guidelines emphasize isolation precautions, antimicrobial stewardship, and vaccination. Implementing these practices reduces healthcare-associated infections and enhances patient safety.

1.2.4 Antimicrobial stewardship

Antimicrobial stewardship in infection prevention and patient/care management involves optimizing patient outcomes, reducing resistance, and minimizing adverse effects. Key principles include appropriate selection, dosing, and duration of antimicrobials, along with de-escalation and discontinuation strategies. Healthcare providers, including medical surgical nurses, play a crucial role in implementing stewardship practices to ensure safe and effective antimicrobial use. By adhering to these principles, healthcare professionals can combat antimicrobial resistance, improve patient safety, and enhance overall quality of care.

1.2.4.1 Surgical scrub

In the realm of surgical scrub, antimicrobial stewardship, infection prevention, and patient/care management are paramount. Surgical scrub plays a crucial role in reducing the risk of surgical site infections by eliminating pathogens. The proper technique involves thorough hand and forearm washing with antimicrobial soap for at least 2-5 minutes. Common antimicrobial agents include chlorhexidine and povidone-iodine. Effective surgical scrub practices not only enhance patient outcomes but also contribute to cost savings by preventing complications. Medical surgical nurses play a vital role in advocating and ensuring adherence to proper surgical scrub protocols for optimal patient safety and care.

1.2.4.2 Antibiotics

Antibiotics play a crucial role in antimicrobial stewardship, infection prevention, and patient/care management. Proper antibiotic selection, dosing, and duration are vital to combat antibiotic resistance. Healthcare providers, including medical surgical nurses, educate patients on appropriate antibiotic use. Interdisciplinary collaboration is key in implementing antimicrobial stewardship programs for optimal patient outcomes and reducing healthcare-associated infections. Monitoring antibiotic therapy effectiveness and managing adverse reactions are essential. Together, we can promote responsible antibiotic use, enhance patient care, and combat the spread of infections through comprehensive strategies and teamwork.

1.2.4.3 Probiotics

In the realm of medical-surgical nursing, probiotics play a crucial role in antimicrobial stewardship, infection prevention, and patient care management. Probiotics help maintain gut health by restoring the balance of good bacteria, potentially reducing the need for antibiotics and supporting immune function. By incorporating probiotics into care plans, healthcare-associated infections can be prevented, leading to improved patient outcomes. However, it's essential to consider the benefits and risks of probiotic use in medical-surgical practice to ensure safe and effective implementation.

1.3 Medication Management

Medication Management in Patient/Care Management involves overseeing the entire medication process to ensure safe and effective treatment. This includes medication reconciliation, administration, monitoring, and patient education. Medical Surgical Nurses play a crucial role in medication management by verifying prescriptions, administering medications accurately, monitoring patient responses, and educating patients on proper usage. Common medication errors include wrong dosage or medication, administration errors, and drug interactions. Strategies to prevent these errors include double-checking medications, using technology for accuracy, and thorough patient assessment. Interdisciplinary collaboration is vital for comprehensive care, and medication adherence significantly impacts patient outcomes.

1.3.1 Safe medication administration practices

Safe medication administration practices are crucial in ensuring patient safety and optimal outcomes. Verifying the five rights (patient, medication, dose, route, time) is essential. Administer medications using proper techniques for various routes. Prevent errors and adverse reactions through vigilant checks. Medication reconciliation aids in safe administration. Accurate documentation is key. Educate patients on medications and side effects. Promote adherence with tailored strategies. Interdisciplinary collaboration enhances safety. Utilize technology for efficiency. Consider cultural competence and health literacy. These aspects collectively contribute to effective medication management and patient care.

1.3.1.1 Interaction

In the realm of safe medication administration practices, medication management, and patient/care management, interaction refers to the effects when two or more substances interact with each other. Recognizing and managing drug interactions, such as drug-drug, drug-food, and drug-supplement interactions, is crucial to prevent adverse outcomes. Healthcare providers, including medical surgical nurses, can identify potential interactions through thorough medication reconciliation, assess their impact on patient outcomes by monitoring for signs/symptoms, and take appropriate actions like adjusting dosages or choosing alternative medications. Effective communication, interdisciplinary collaboration, and patient education play vital roles in addressing medication interactions for safe and effective care delivery.

1.3.1.2 Adverse reaction

Adverse reactions in medication administration refer to unexpected, harmful responses to drugs. Types include allergic reactions, side effects, and drug interactions. Signs like rash, nausea, or difficulty breathing may indicate adverse reactions. Prompt recognition and management are crucial to prevent complications. Strategies to prevent include thorough patient assessment and medication reconciliation. Nurses play a key role in identifying and addressing adverse reactions promptly. These reactions can impact patient outcomes and care management significantly. Collaboration with the healthcare team is essential for effective management and ensuring patient safety.

1.3.1.3 Intravenous therapy

Intravenous therapy plays a crucial role in safe medication administration, medication management, and patient/care management by delivering medications, fluids, and blood products directly into the bloodstream. Key considerations for safe administration include proper insertion techniques, monitoring for complications, and maintaining aseptic technique. Medical surgical nurses are responsible for vein selection, calculating drip rates, and identifying infiltration or phlebitis. Accurate documentation and communication are vital for patient safety and continuity of care. Vein selection, drip rate calculation, complication recognition, and documentation are essential aspects of managing intravenous therapy effectively.

1.3.2 Patient medication education

Patient medication education in medication and patient/care management is crucial for adherence, error prevention, and health outcomes. Key components include clear medication information, administration instructions, side effects, and adherence importance. Nurses play a vital role by assessing learning needs, providing tailored education, and evaluating understanding. Effective communication, health literacy, and cultural competence are essential for successful patient medication education.

1.3.3 Polypharmacy

Polypharmacy in Medication Management and Patient Care involves the use of multiple medications by a patient. Risks include drug interactions, adverse effects, and non-adherence, while benefits include better disease management. Polypharmacy can impact patient outcomes negatively, affecting adherence and overall health. Strategies to prevent polypharmacy include medication reconciliation, deprescribing unnecessary medications, and collaborating with healthcare teams. Medical surgical nurses play a crucial role in managing polypharmacy by assessing medication regimens, educating patients, and promoting safe medication practices to enhance patient well-being.

1.3.4 Safe drug management and disposal

Safe drug management and disposal is crucial in medication and patient care. Proper storage maintains medication efficacy and safety. Improper management poses risks like errors, accidental ingestion, and diversion. Administering drugs safely involves dosage accuracy, patient verification, and adverse reaction monitoring. Improper disposal harms the environment, stressing adherence to disposal guidelines. Healthcare providers educate patients on safe practices and disposal. Facilities must follow regulatory guidelines for safe handling, administration, and disposal to ensure patient safety and legal compliance.

1.3.4.1 Stewardship

Stewardship in medical-surgical nursing involves responsible management of medications, emphasizing safe drug handling, proper disposal, and patient-centered care. It plays a crucial role in preventing errors, ensuring patient safety, and reducing environmental impact. Key principles include rational prescribing, adherence to guidelines, monitoring for side effects, and appropriate disposal. Medical-surgical nurses are vital in promoting stewardship by advocating for best practices, educating patients on medication use, and collaborating with healthcare teams to enhance outcomes and sustainability. By championing stewardship initiatives, nurses contribute significantly to optimizing patient care and overall healthcare quality.

1.3.4.2 Home medication management

Home medication management encompasses safe drug handling, storage, and disposal, vital for patient safety. Key aspects include promoting medication adherence, ensuring proper storage conditions, and educating patients on administration techniques. Disposal of expired medications is crucial to prevent misuse. Medication reconciliation aids in tracking patient drug regimens accurately. Educating patients on potential drug interactions and monitoring for side effects are essential. Healthcare providers play a pivotal role in supporting patients with medication management at home, ensuring optimal therapeutic outcomes and patient well-being.

1.3.5 Advanced access devices

Advanced access devices, like central venous catheters, PICCs, and implantable ports, play a crucial role in medication management and patient care. These devices enhance medication administration accuracy, lower complication risks, and boost patient comfort. Nurses must adhere to best practices for device maintenance to prevent infections and ensure optimal functionality. Understanding the types and benefits of advanced access devices is essential for medical-surgical nurses to provide safe and effective care.

1.3.5.1 Ports

Ports in medical-surgical nursing play a crucial role in advanced access devices, medication management, and patient care. These devices facilitate intravenous therapy, blood draws, and medication administration. Common types include implanted ports and tunneled ports, each with specific features and indications. Nursing care involves proper maintenance, flushing, and infection prevention. Educating patients on port care and complications is essential. Interdisciplinary collaboration with healthcare providers and pharmacists optimizes patient safety and outcomes. Understanding ports is vital for Medical Surgical Nurses to provide comprehensive care.

1.3.5.2 Central lines

Central lines are essential for long-term venous access in medication management, fluids, blood products, and nutrition. Types include PICCs, tunneled catheters, and implanted ports. Insertion and maintenance require strict sterile technique, dressing changes, and flushing protocols. Complications like infection, thrombosis, and mechanical issues can arise, necessitating vigilant nursing interventions. Medical-surgical nurses play a crucial role in assessing, monitoring, and caring for patients with central lines to ensure safe and effective treatment.

1.3.5.3 Epidurals

Epidurals are commonly used in medical-surgical settings for pain management. When considering advanced access devices, epidurals are administered through a catheter placed in the epidural space. Medications like local anesthetics and opioids are often used in epidurals to provide pain relief. While epidurals offer effective pain control, they come with risks such as hypotension and nerve damage. Proper patient assessment is crucial before administering an epidural to ensure safety and efficacy. Medical-surgical nurses play a vital role in monitoring patients with epidurals, assessing for complications, managing side effects, and providing education to patients and their families.

1.3.6 Financial implications to patients

Financial implications greatly impact patients in managing medications and healthcare needs. Firstly, the cost of medications and treatments can be a significant burden, especially for those with chronic conditions. Insurance coverage plays a crucial role, but out-of-pocket expenses can still be high. Medication adherence is vital to avoid increased healthcare costs due to complications. Access to affordable healthcare services is essential for overall well-being. To help patients manage financial burdens, healthcare providers can offer resources, such as patient assistance programs and generic medication options, to alleviate costs and ensure optimal care.

1.4 Pain Management

The topic of 'Pain Management' in 'Patient/Care Management' is crucial for CMSRNs. Assessing pain is vital to provide optimal care. Types of pain include acute, chronic, nociceptive, neuropathic, and breakthrough pain. Pharmacological options include analgesics, while non-pharmacological strategies encompass physical therapy and relaxation techniques. The healthcare team collaborates to create individualized pain management plans. Barriers like communication issues or opioid misuse can hinder effective pain control. Patient education on pain assessment, treatment options, and potential side effects is key for successful pain management outcomes.

1.4.1 Chronic and/or acute pain management

Chronic and acute pain management is crucial in patient care. Chronic pain persists over time, often due to conditions like arthritis, while acute pain is sudden and usually signals injury. Pharmacological treatments for chronic pain include NSAIDs, while opioids are more common for acute pain. Non-pharmacological options like physical therapy can also help. Accurate pain assessment is key, ensuring proper treatment. Medical surgical nurses play a vital role in advocating for effective pain management, collaborating with the healthcare team to enhance patient outcomes.

1.4.1.1 Pharmacological

Pharmacological management in chronic and/or acute pain involves various medication classes. Nonsteroidal anti-inflammatory drugs (NSAIDs) reduce inflammation and pain. Opioids act on the central nervous system to alleviate pain but carry a risk of dependence. Adjuvant medications like antidepressants and anticonvulsants enhance pain relief. Non-opioid analgesics such as acetaminophen provide mild to moderate pain control. Monitoring for side effects like gastrointestinal upset, sedation, and respiratory depression is crucial. Individualized treatment plans, multimodal approaches, and patient education on adherence, risks, and alternative strategies are vital for effective pain management.

1.4.1.2 Nonpharmacological

The 'Certified Medical Surgical Registered Nurse(CMSRN)' exam covers nonpharmacological interventions in pain management. Nonpharmacological techniques include cognitive-behavioral therapy, acupuncture, and physical therapy. These interventions are effective in managing chronic and acute pain by reducing reliance on medications. For example, relaxation techniques and guided imagery can help patients cope with pain. Nonpharmacological approaches play a crucial role in holistic patient care by addressing the physical, emotional, and psychological aspects of pain. Understanding these interventions is essential for providing comprehensive care to patients experiencing pain.

1.4.1.3 Multimodal

In the context of pain management, 'multimodal' refers to utilizing a combination of techniques and interventions to address pain comprehensively. This approach is crucial in both chronic and acute pain scenarios to enhance relief, improve patient outcomes, and mitigate opioid-related risks. Key components include integrating pharmacological and non-pharmacological therapies, fostering interprofessional collaboration, and tailoring treatment plans to individual patient needs. Evidence supports the efficacy of multimodal strategies across diverse patient populations and clinical settings, highlighting its significance in optimizing pain management and promoting holistic care.

1.4.2 Patient pain management expectations

In the context of Pain Management and Patient/Care Management, understanding and addressing patient pain management expectations is crucial. Factors influencing these expectations include cultural background, previous experiences, and communication. Common patient expectations include timely pain relief, personalized care, and active involvement in decision-making. Healthcare providers play a key role in managing and meeting these expectations through effective communication, holistic assessment, and individualized treatment plans. Unmet expectations can lead to decreased patient satisfaction, noncompliance, and negative outcomes. It is essential to prioritize patient-centered care to optimize pain management and overall patient well-being.

1.4.3 Patient advocacy

Patient advocacy in pain management and patient/care management is crucial for ensuring optimal outcomes. Medical surgical nurses play a vital role in advocating for patients' rights, preferences, and effective pain management interventions. Empowering patients to participate in decision-making, advocating for their needs, fostering transparent communication, and ensuring appropriate pain relief are key aspects. By advocating for patients' best interests and providing support throughout the pain management process, nurses contribute significantly to enhancing patient care quality and satisfaction. Patient advocacy is a cornerstone of compassionate and effective medical-surgical nursing practice.

1.5 NonPharmacological Interventions

Nonpharmacological interventions in patient/care management encompass non-drug therapies to enhance patient well-being and health outcomes. These interventions, such as relaxation techniques, music therapy, and guided imagery, play a vital role in promoting holistic care. They complement pharmacological treatments by reducing reliance on medications, minimizing side effects, and addressing patient needs comprehensively. Medical-surgical nurses are pivotal in implementing and evaluating the effectiveness of these interventions, tailoring them to individual patient needs and collaborating with interdisciplinary teams to optimize patient care. Their role is crucial in ensuring a holistic approach to patient management.

1.5.1 Non-pharmacological interventions

Non-pharmacological interventions in patient/care management involve treatments that do not require medications. These interventions play a crucial role in managing various health conditions by addressing physical, emotional, and social aspects of care. Examples include therapeutic communication, relaxation techniques, and physical therapy. When combined with pharmacological treatments, non-pharmacological interventions can improve patient outcomes by reducing symptoms, enhancing overall well-being, and promoting faster recovery. Medical-surgical nurses are instrumental in implementing and evaluating these interventions to ensure personalized care plans and optimal patient responses. Their role is vital in promoting holistic patient care and achieving positive health outcomes.

1.5.1.1 Repositioning

Repositioning is a vital non-pharmacological intervention in patient care, aimed at preventing pressure ulcers and maintaining skin integrity. Regular repositioning helps reduce the risk of skin breakdown by relieving pressure on vulnerable areas. Recommended frequency is every 2 hours while techniques include using pillows, foam wedges, and specialized beds. Repositioning enhances patient comfort, circulation, and overall well-being. Improper repositioning can lead to skin damage and discomfort. Best practices involve assessing patient needs, using proper body mechanics, and involving interdisciplinary teams for optimal outcomes in medical-surgical settings.

1.5.1.2 Heat or cold

Heat and cold therapy are non-pharmacological interventions used in patient care management. Heat therapy increases blood flow, relaxes muscles, and reduces pain and stiffness. It is indicated for chronic conditions like arthritis. Cold therapy decreases inflammation, numbs the area, and reduces swelling. It is indicated for acute injuries like sprains. Contraindications for heat therapy include acute injuries, while contraindications for cold therapy include conditions like Raynaud's disease. Best practices include using a barrier between the skin and the heat/cold source, limiting application time, and monitoring skin for adverse reactions. Patient education should focus on proper application techniques and potential risks like burns or frostbite.

1.5.2 Complementary and alternative therapies

Complementary and alternative therapies play a vital role in non-pharmacological interventions and patient/care management in medical-surgical nursing. Common therapies include acupuncture, chiropractic care, herbal supplements, massage therapy, meditation, and yoga. These therapies offer benefits such as pain relief, stress reduction, and improved well-being. However, risks like potential interactions with conventional treatments exist. Medical-surgical nurses can integrate these therapies by assessing patient needs, collaborating with healthcare team, and ensuring safety through proper training and monitoring. Incorporating complementary and alternative therapies enhances holistic patient care, promoting overall health outcomes.

1.5.2.1 Acupuncture

Acupuncture, a key component of complementary and alternative therapies, involves the insertion of thin needles into specific points on the body to promote healing and alleviate symptoms. Rooted in traditional Chinese medicine, acupuncture operates on the principles of restoring the flow of energy or Qi along meridians. Techniques include manual stimulation or electrical impulses. Benefits may include pain relief, stress reduction, and improved overall well-being. Evidence supports its efficacy in various conditions. Safety considerations encompass proper training and sterile needle use. Integration into patient care plans involves collaboration with healthcare providers to enhance holistic treatment approaches.

1.5.2.2 Aromatherapy

Aromatherapy involves using essential oils to promote healing and well-being. In medical-surgical settings, it complements traditional treatments by aiding in stress reduction, pain management, and improved sleep. Nurses must consider safety and contraindications when incorporating aromatherapy into patient care plans. Evidence-based research supports its efficacy in enhancing patient outcomes. Nurses play a crucial role in educating patients about aromatherapy and integrating it into their care plans. Following guidelines and best practices ensures safe and effective use of aromatherapy in medical-surgical settings.

1.6 Surgical/Procedural Nursing Management

The topic of Surgical/Procedural Nursing Management in Patient/Care Management encompasses various crucial elements. Preoperative assessment involves gathering patient data, preparing them for surgery, and obtaining informed consent. Intraoperative care focuses on maintaining patient safety, monitoring vital signs, and assisting the surgical team. Postoperative monitoring includes assessing for complications, managing pain, and promoting wound healing. Effective wound care and patient education are essential for recovery. Discharge planning ensures a smooth transition post-surgery. Collaboration with the healthcare team optimizes patient outcomes. Medical Surgical Nurses play a vital role in providing comprehensive care and ensuring patient well-being throughout the surgical process.

1.6.1 Pre- and post-procedural unit standards

In Surgical/Procedural Nursing Management, pre- and post-procedural unit standards are crucial for optimal patient outcomes. Pre-procedural care involves thorough patient assessment, medication administration adherence, and infection control measures. Patient education is key. Post-procedural care focuses on monitoring, pain management, and complication prevention. Interdisciplinary collaboration ensures comprehensive care. Medical-surgical nurses play a vital role in implementing and monitoring these standards, ensuring high-quality care and patient safety throughout the surgical/procedural journey. Adhering to these standards is essential for successful patient outcomes and overall healthcare quality.

1.6.1.1 Consent

In the context of pre- and post-procedural unit standards, surgical/procedural nursing management, and patient/care management, consent plays a crucial role. Informed consent is vital before any surgical or procedural intervention. Key elements include ensuring the patient understands the procedure, associated risks, potential benefits, alternative options, and the right to refuse treatment. Medical-surgical nurses are responsible for ensuring patients provide voluntary and informed consent, considering legal and ethical implications. Documentation requirements in healthcare settings are essential for accurate record-keeping. Maintaining precise records is crucial for legal and ethical reasons.

1.6.1.2 Timeout

Timeout in surgical and procedural nursing management is a crucial safety practice. It involves a pause before a procedure to verify patient identity, procedure, and surgical site. Team members, including the surgeon, anesthesiologist, and nurses, participate. Steps include confirming patient details, procedure type, and site marking. Medical surgical nurses play a key role in coordinating timeouts and fostering a safety culture. Failure to adhere to timeout protocols can lead to wrong-site surgery, patient harm, and compromised care quality. Adherence to timeouts is vital for patient safety and error prevention in pre- and post-procedural care.

1.6.1.3 Frequent monitoring

In the perioperative setting, frequent monitoring is vital for ensuring patient safety and optimal outcomes. Medical surgical nurses play a crucial role in conducting and documenting this monitoring. Key aspects include tracking vital signs like blood pressure, heart rate, respiratory rate, and temperature regularly. During pre-procedural, intraoperative, and post-procedural phases, monitoring frequency varies. Inadequate monitoring can lead to complications, delayed interventions, and compromised patient recovery. Therefore, meticulous and timely monitoring by nurses is essential for early detection of any deviations from baseline, facilitating prompt interventions and promoting positive patient outcomes.

1.6.2 Pertinent potential complications and management

In Surgical/Procedural Nursing Management and Patient/Care Management, nurses must be vigilant for potential complications. Common issues include surgical site infections, hemorrhage, deep vein thrombosis, respiratory complications, and adverse reactions to anesthesia. Recognizing signs like fever, increased pain, swelling, or abnormal bleeding is crucial. Immediate interventions such as wound care, monitoring vital signs, administering medications, and promoting mobility are essential. Early detection and proactive management are key to preventing complications from worsening and ensuring positive patient outcomes. Regular assessment and communication with the healthcare team are vital for comprehensive care.

1.6.3 Scope of practice related to procedures

In the realm of surgical/procedural nursing management, Certified Medical Surgical Registered Nurses (CMSRNs) play a vital role in performing, assisting, and overseeing various procedures. They must adhere to legal and ethical standards, ensuring patient safety and privacy. Following evidence-based practice guidelines is crucial for optimal patient outcomes. Collaboration with interdisciplinary team members is essential to guarantee comprehensive care and effective procedural outcomes. CMSRNs must communicate effectively, coordinate care, and advocate for patients throughout the procedure process. By upholding these standards, CMSRNs contribute significantly to the quality and safety of patient care in surgical/procedural settings.

1.6.3.1 Moderate/procedural sedation

Moderate/procedural sedation involves administering medications to induce a depressed level of consciousness while maintaining the patient's ability to independently maintain their airway and respond to physical or verbal stimuli. In the perioperative setting, the purpose of moderate/procedural sedation is to ensure patient comfort, reduce anxiety, and facilitate the completion of procedures. Criteria for selecting patients include assessing their medical history, current health status, and the complexity of the procedure. Nursing responsibilities include continuous monitoring of vital signs, airway patency, and sedation level. Complications may include respiratory depression, hypotension, and allergic reactions. Nurses must be prepared to intervene promptly and collaborate with the interprofessional team. Legal and ethical considerations emphasize patient autonomy, confidentiality, and ensuring informed consent. Patient education is crucial to ensure understanding of the procedure, risks, and benefits.

1.6.4 Supplies, instruments, and equipment

In Surgical/Procedural Nursing Management, proper selection, maintenance, and utilization of supplies, instruments, and equipment are crucial. Ensuring safety protocols and infection control measures are followed is paramount for patient care. Medical-surgical nurses play a vital role in maintaining the availability, functionality, and sterility of these items. They must optimize patient outcomes by guaranteeing the readiness of supplies, instruments, and equipment. By adhering to best practices, nurses contribute to a safe healthcare environment, promoting effective care delivery and positive patient experiences.

1.7 Nutrition

Nutrition in patient/care management is vital for optimal health outcomes. A balanced diet supports recovery and overall well-being. Malnutrition can significantly impact patient outcomes, emphasizing the need to assess nutritional status. Medical-surgical nurses play a crucial role in educating patients on proper nutrition, collaborating with dietitians for personalized plans, and monitoring intake and responses. Addressing nutritional needs is essential across various patient populations, especially those with chronic illnesses, undergoing surgery, or managing acute conditions. Understanding and implementing effective nutrition strategies are key aspects of comprehensive patient care.

1.7.1 Individualized nutritional needs

In patient care management, individualized nutritional needs are crucial. Assessing factors like age, gender, medical history, dietary preferences, and cultural aspects is vital. Healthcare providers tailor nutrition plans to meet each patient's unique requirements and health goals. Medical-surgical nurses collaborate with dietitians, physicians, and the healthcare team to create personalized nutrition interventions. Ongoing monitoring and evaluation ensure patients receive adequate nutrition for optimal health outcomes. This approach enhances patient care and promotes better health results.

1.7.1.1 Malnutrition

Malnutrition refers to inadequate or excess intake of nutrients leading to health issues. Causes include poor diet, illness, or socioeconomic factors. Risk factors include age, chronic diseases, and low income. Signs: weight loss, fatigue. Complications: impaired wound healing, increased infection risk. Assessment: nutritional screening tools. Management: dietary modifications, supplements. Impact on outcomes: delays healing, prolongs hospital stay. Nurse's role: assess, educate, collaborate with dietitians. Preventing and managing malnutrition is crucial for improving patient outcomes and quality of life.

1.7.1.2 Disease processes

In the realm of disease processes, understanding individualized nutritional needs is crucial for optimal patient care. Various diseases can significantly impact nutritional requirements and the body's ability to metabolize nutrients. For instance, conditions like diabetes, cancer, and gastrointestinal disorders can alter nutrient absorption and utilization. It's essential to tailor nutrition plans to each patient's specific health challenges. Strategies may include dietary modifications, supplements, or specialized feeding methods. By comprehending disease processes and their effects on nutrition, healthcare providers can devise personalized nutrition interventions to enhance patient outcomes and overall well-being.

1.7.1.3 Complications

In the realm of individualized nutritional needs and patient/care management, complications can pose significant challenges. These complications encompass a range of potential risks and adverse outcomes, impacting patient well-being. Healthcare providers play a crucial role in identifying and addressing these issues promptly. Common complications include malnutrition, dehydration, electrolyte imbalances, and tube feeding-related problems. Proactive monitoring and intervention are vital to optimize patient health. Strategies for prevention involve thorough assessment, tailored nutritional plans, close observation, and prompt intervention when complications arise. By prioritizing vigilance and proactive care, healthcare professionals can enhance patient outcomes and ensure effective management of individualized nutritional needs.

1.7.1.4 Cultural

Cultural considerations in individualized nutritional needs and patient/care management involve understanding how cultural beliefs, practices, and preferences impact dietary choices. Cultural competence is crucial for improving patient outcomes. Healthcare providers must respect diverse cultural backgrounds to provide effective care. Strategies for culturally sensitive care include acknowledging cultural dietary restrictions, involving patients in care decisions, and providing educational resources in multiple languages. By recognizing and respecting cultural differences, healthcare professionals can enhance patient trust, satisfaction, and overall health outcomes.

1.7.2 Nutrition administration modalities

Nutrition Administration Modalities encompass various methods to deliver essential nutrients to patients. Enteral nutrition involves feeding through the gastrointestinal tract, commonly via feeding tubes. Parenteral nutrition delivers nutrients intravenously when the digestive system is compromised. Oral supplements provide additional nutrients in liquid or pill form. These modalities are crucial in ensuring patients receive adequate nutrition for recovery and overall health. Proper administration plays a vital role in supporting patient well-being and enhancing their response to treatment. Understanding these modalities is essential for Medical Surgical Nurses to optimize patient care.

1.7.2.1 Enteral

Enteral nutrition administration involves delivering nutrients directly into the gastrointestinal tract. It is crucial in providing adequate nutrition for patients who cannot consume food orally. Indications include impaired swallowing, malnutrition, and gastrointestinal disorders. Contraindications may include bowel obstruction or severe gastrointestinal bleeding. Types of enteral feeding tubes include nasogastric, nasojejunal, and gastrostomy tubes. Proper administration techniques involve verifying tube placement, flushing before and after feedings, and monitoring residuals. Complications can include aspiration, tube dislodgement, and diarrhea. Nursing considerations include assessing tolerance, maintaining tube patency, and providing patient education.

1.7.2.2   Parenteral

Parenteral nutrition refers to the delivery of nutrients intravenously when the digestive system is unable to function adequately. It plays a crucial role in patient care management by providing essential nutrients directly into the bloodstream. Key aspects include various administration methods such as total parenteral nutrition (TPN), indications like malnutrition or bowel rest, contraindications such as intact gastrointestinal function, monitoring parameters like blood glucose levels, and potential complications like infections or metabolic imbalances. Medical-surgical nurses are pivotal in assessing patients' nutritional needs, implementing parenteral nutrition therapy, and evaluating its effectiveness to ensure optimal patient outcomes.

1.7.3   Resources for alternate nutrition administration

In the realm of alternate nutrition administration, medical-surgical nurses play a crucial role in ensuring optimal patient care. Enteral and parenteral nutrition are common methods used when oral intake is not feasible. Understanding the equipment and supplies needed for each method is essential. Proper training for healthcare providers and patients is vital to prevent complications. Nurses must coordinate and oversee the administration of alternate nutrition effectively. Challenges may arise, but with strategies in place, patient safety and well-being can be maintained.

1.7.3.1   Speech consultation

Speech consultation plays a vital role in assessing patients needing alternate nutrition like enteral or parenteral feeding. Speech-language pathologists evaluate swallowing function, oral motor skills, and communication abilities to ensure safe nutrition intake. They identify swallowing issues, aspiration risks, and factors affecting nutrition and health. Collaboration among speech-language pathologists, dietitians, nurses, and other healthcare professionals is crucial in developing comprehensive care plans for complex nutrition needs. This teamwork enhances patient outcomes, improves care quality, and optimizes nutrition management in medical-surgical settings.

1.7.3.2   Dietary consultation

In the realm of dietary consultation for patients requiring alternate nutrition administration, a medical surgical nurse plays a vital role. Collaborating with dietitians, the nurse helps create personalized nutrition plans by assessing needs, considering restrictions, and promoting healthy eating habits. This collaboration ensures optimal nutrition, supporting patient recovery and well-being. Ongoing monitoring and adjustments are key in maintaining effectiveness. By facilitating dietary consultations, nurses contribute significantly to patient care management, emphasizing the importance of tailored nutrition interventions for improved outcomes.

1.7.4   Indications for alternate nutrition administration

Indications for alternate nutrition administration are crucial in patient care. Various situations necessitate alternate routes like dysphagia, GI disorders, post-op complications, or malnutrition. Factors such as oral intake tolerance, specific nutrient needs, and overall nutrition support goals must be considered. Methods like enteral feeding, parenteral nutrition, or total parenteral nutrition can be tailored to individual patient needs. Understanding when to utilize alternate nutrition routes and how to customize them ensures optimal patient outcomes. It's essential to assess each patient's condition carefully to determine the most appropriate nutrition administration method.

2   Holistic Patient Care

In medical-surgical nursing, 'Holistic Patient Care' focuses on addressing the physical, emotional, social, and spiritual needs of patients. It involves treating the patient as a whole person to promote healing and overall health. Medical-surgical nurses play a crucial role in providing holistic care by considering all aspects of a patient's well-being. By incorporating holistic approaches, nurses can positively impact patient outcomes, leading to improved recovery and well-being. Prioritizing holistic patient care ensures comprehensive support for patients, enhancing their overall quality of life during their healthcare journey.

2.1   Patient-Centered Care

The 'Certified Medical Surgical Registered Nurse (CMSRN)' exam covers 'Patient-Centered Care' in the context of 'Holistic Patient Care'. This approach emphasizes communication, respecting patient preferences, coordinating care, providing emotional support, ensuring physical comfort, involving family and friends, and promoting patient autonomy and empowerment. Effective communication fosters trust and understanding. Respecting patient preferences acknowledges individuality. Coordinating care ensures comprehensive treatment. Emotional support aids in healing. Providing physical comfort enhances well-being. Involving family and friends creates a supportive environment. Promoting patient autonomy empowers individuals in their healthcare decisions.

2.1.1   Patient-centered care

Patient-centered care in holistic patient care emphasizes communication, empathy, respect for patient preferences, shared decision-making, and individualized care plans. Building a therapeutic relationship with patients, involving them in their care, and addressing their physical, emotional, and spiritual needs are crucial. Patient-centered care empowers patients, enhances health outcomes, and improves the overall patient experience. It focuses on collaboration, dignity, and understanding the patient as a whole. By prioritizing the patient's values and preferences, healthcare providers can deliver more effective and personalized care.

2.1.1.1   Active listening

Active listening in patient-centered care involves truly understanding patients' emotions, concerns, and needs. It goes beyond hearing words to building therapeutic relationships. Key components include eye contact, open body language, paraphrasing, and asking clarifying questions. This approach helps nurses gather vital information, offer emotional support, and engage patients in decision-making. By fostering trust, empathy, and collaboration, active listening enhances patient outcomes and satisfaction. It plays a crucial role in holistic patient care, promoting a deeper connection between healthcare providers and patients for more effective, personalized treatment.

2.1.1.2 Communication preferences

In the context of patient-centered care, understanding and respecting patients' communication preferences are crucial. This includes being attuned to verbal and non-verbal cues, addressing language barriers, acknowledging cultural differences, and adapting to individual communication styles. Effective communication tailored to these preferences enhances care quality, improves outcomes, and fosters strong nurse-patient relationships. Active listening, empathy, and clear communication play vital roles in meeting patients' needs and promoting a patient-centered approach to care. By prioritizing communication preferences, nurses can provide holistic and personalized care that truly meets the individual needs of each patient.

2.1.1.3 Family involvement

In the context of patient-centered care, family involvement plays a crucial role in ensuring holistic patient well-being. Engaging family members in care plans and decision-making processes enhances communication, support, and overall outcomes. Collaborating with healthcare providers, patients, and families promotes a patient-centered approach, fostering a comprehensive care experience. Family involvement not only provides emotional support but also contributes to a more personalized and effective care plan. By valuing the input and involvement of family members, healthcare teams can create a more inclusive and patient-focused care environment.

2.1.1.4 Health goals

In patient-centered and holistic care, health goals are personalized objectives that patients and healthcare providers collaboratively set to enhance well-being. Establishing health goals is crucial for tailoring care plans and improving outcomes. Medical surgical nurses play a vital role in guiding patients through this process, considering their preferences, values, and lifestyle. Setting realistic and achievable goals is key, fostering patient engagement and empowerment. Monitoring and reassessing goals over time are essential for adapting care plans and promoting sustained patient involvement in their healthcare journey.

2.1.2 Resources for patient-centered care

Patient-centered care emphasizes the importance of providing holistic care that meets the diverse needs of patients. Adequate resources, such as access to healthcare professionals, educational materials, support groups, and community resources, play a crucial role in supporting patient-centered care initiatives. These resources contribute to improving patient outcomes, enhancing satisfaction, and fostering a collaborative healthcare approach. Technology and innovative tools further enhance resource availability. Healthcare organizations must ensure these resources are accessible to effectively address patients' needs and promote a patient-centered care environment.

2.1.3 Patient advocacy

Patient advocacy in patient-centered care involves empowering patients, respecting their rights, preferences, and collaborating with the healthcare team. Key aspects include informed decision-making, upholding patient rights, respecting values, and addressing barriers. Nurses provide support, promote communication, and advocate for policies ensuring patient safety and quality care. Advocacy enhances patient experiences, improves outcomes, and aligns with holistic care principles. As a medical-surgical nurse, advocating for patients is vital for positive impacts on their healthcare journey.

2.1.4 Patient satisfaction management

Patient satisfaction management in patient-centered and holistic care involves prioritizing patient needs, preferences, and well-being. It is crucial for improving patient outcomes, care quality, and overall experience. Effective strategies include enhancing communication, addressing concerns promptly, encouraging patient engagement, and creating a supportive care environment. Medical surgical nurses play a vital role in ensuring high levels of patient satisfaction by delivering compassionate, personalized care and promoting a patient-centered approach. By focusing on patient satisfaction, healthcare providers can enhance care delivery and foster positive relationships with patients, ultimately leading to better health outcomes.

2.1.4.1 Grievances

In the realm of patient care, grievances refer to concerns or complaints expressed by patients regarding their healthcare experience. Addressing grievances is crucial in patient satisfaction management, patient-centered care, and holistic patient care. By resolving grievances promptly, healthcare providers can enhance patient outcomes and the overall quality of care. Common sources of grievances include communication breakdowns, long wait times, and perceived lack of empathy. Strategies for managing grievances involve active listening, prompt resolution, and continuous improvement. Medical Surgical Nurses play a vital role in addressing grievances, ensuring a patient-centered and holistic approach to care.

2.1.4.2 Concerns regarding practices

In the context of Patient satisfaction management, Patient-Centered Care, and Holistic Patient Care, healthcare providers may face challenges such as communication barriers, time constraints, and lack of resources. These issues can impact patient outcomes by affecting care coordination, treatment adherence, and overall patient experience. Addressing concerns regarding practices is crucial to ensure effective delivery of patient-centered and holistic care, leading to enhanced patient satisfaction and improved quality of care. By prioritizing communication, collaboration, and individualized care plans, healthcare providers can overcome challenges and promote positive patient outcomes.

2.1.4.3 Second opinion

In healthcare, a second opinion plays a crucial role in patient satisfaction management, patient-centered care, and holistic patient care. Seeking a second opinion is vital for making well-informed decisions about treatment plans, leading to increased confidence, improved patient satisfaction, and higher quality of care. By considering multiple perspectives and treatment options, second opinions promote a patient-centered approach, empowering patients to actively participate in their healthcare journey. This process supports holistic patient care by ensuring comprehensive evaluation and personalized treatment strategies, ultimately enhancing patient outcomes and overall well-being.

2.1.4.4 Service recovery

Service recovery in healthcare refers to the process of addressing and resolving patient concerns to enhance satisfaction. It plays a vital role in patient-centered and holistic care by improving outcomes and experiences. Key strategies include active listening, prompt resolution, and empathy. Medical surgical nurses are crucial in service recovery efforts, fostering trust and loyalty. By implementing effective techniques, such as apology and follow-up, nurses can positively impact patient satisfaction and overall quality of care. Service recovery is essential for building strong patient relationships and ensuring optimal healthcare delivery.

2.2 Diversity and Inclusion

In holistic patient care, diversity and inclusion play a vital role. Understanding social determinants of health, respecting cultural beliefs, and effective communication are key. Cultural competence and advocacy for equitable healthcare policies are essential. Embracing diversity enhances patient satisfaction and improves health outcomes. By fostering an inclusive environment, medical surgical nurses contribute to a more equitable healthcare system.

2.2.1 Cultural and linguistic needs

In the context of diversity and inclusion, addressing cultural and linguistic needs is vital for providing holistic patient care. Cultural beliefs greatly influence healthcare decisions, emphasizing the importance of cultural competence among healthcare providers. Language barriers can hinder effective patient-provider communication, impacting care quality. Strategies to promote cultural competence include cultural sensitivity training and utilizing interpreters. Respecting and valuing diverse cultural backgrounds is key to delivering patient-centered care, fostering trust and improving health outcomes. Prioritizing cultural and linguistic needs enhances the overall quality of care provided to patients.

2.2.1.1 Sign

In the realm of cultural and linguistic needs, diversity, and holistic patient care, the concept of 'sign' holds significant importance. Signs and signals can vary based on cultural backgrounds and languages, emphasizing the need to recognize and address these differences. Understanding and respecting diverse signs can greatly enhance communication and foster inclusivity in healthcare settings. By considering signs in a holistic manner, healthcare professionals can adopt a more comprehensive approach to patient care that respects individual cultural beliefs, values, and preferences. This approach ultimately leads to improved patient outcomes and a deeper level of care.

2.2.1.2 Oral

In providing oral care to diverse patient populations, understanding cultural and linguistic needs is crucial. Language barriers, cultural practices, and beliefs significantly impact oral health management. By incorporating diversity and inclusion principles, patient outcomes and satisfaction can improve. Holistic patient care recognizes oral health as integral to overall well-being. Medical surgical nurses can ensure comprehensive and culturally competent oral care by implementing strategies such as offering multilingual education materials, respecting cultural preferences for oral hygiene practices, and collaborating with interpreters or cultural liaisons.

2.2.1.3 Written languages

In the context of cultural and linguistic needs, diversity, and inclusion, written languages are pivotal in healthcare. They bridge communication gaps, ensure accurate documentation, and aid in patient education. Addressing language barriers improves patient outcomes, while providing materials in multiple languages caters to diverse populations. Health literacy, empowered through written languages, enables informed decision-making. Understanding cultural nuances in written communication fosters trust with patients from varied backgrounds. Integrating written languages into holistic care elevates quality and fosters inclusivity in healthcare environments.

2.2.2 Cultural and linguistic resources

In the context of diversity and inclusion, cultural and linguistic resources play a vital role in providing holistic patient care. Understanding and respecting patients' cultural backgrounds, beliefs, and languages are essential for effective healthcare delivery. These resources help bridge communication gaps, build trust, and improve health outcomes for diverse patient populations. Cultural competence, language access services, interpretation services, and culturally sensitive care practices create a welcoming healthcare environment. Healthcare providers can utilize these resources to enhance patient-centered care by tailoring interventions to meet the unique needs of multicultural patients.

2.2.2.1 Translated materials

In healthcare, providing translated materials is crucial for effective communication and understanding among diverse patient populations. By offering medical information, consent forms, and educational resources in multiple languages, healthcare providers promote cultural competence, reduce disparities, and enhance patient outcomes. Challenges in developing and implementing translated materials include ensuring accuracy, maintaining updated content, and addressing varying literacy levels. Best practices involve utilizing professional translators, incorporating patient feedback, and integrating translated materials into routine care processes. Ultimately, the availability of translated resources supports holistic patient care by fostering inclusivity and improving patient-provider interactions.

2.2.2.2 Interpreter services

In healthcare, interpreter services play a crucial role in providing culturally and linguistically appropriate care, fostering diversity, inclusion, and holistic patient care. Professional interpreters bridge communication gaps between healthcare providers and patients with limited English proficiency or diverse cultural backgrounds, ensuring accurate transmission of medical information, informed consent, and patient autonomy. Challenges such as availability, quality, and confidentiality must be addressed. Best practices include using trained interpreters, promoting cultural competence, and respecting patient preferences. Effective interpreter services enhance patient outcomes and satisfaction by promoting understanding, trust, and collaboration in healthcare settings.

2.2.3 Implicit bias

In the context of diversity and inclusion, implicit bias plays a significant role in shaping healthcare interactions. Medical Surgical Nurses must recognize and address their unconscious biases to provide equitable and patient-centered care. Implicit biases, such as racial or gender biases, can lead to disparities in healthcare outcomes. By actively mitigating these biases, nurses can create a more inclusive environment that respects patients' diverse backgrounds. This approach fosters improved patient satisfaction, treatment adherence, and overall health outcomes. Understanding and addressing implicit bias is essential for delivering high-quality, patient-centered care that promotes diversity and inclusion in healthcare settings.

2.3 Education of Patients and Families

In holistic patient care, educating patients and families is vital for optimal outcomes. Medical surgical nurses play a crucial role in providing tailored education. Clear communication, cultural sensitivity, and individualized teaching strategies are key. By promoting understanding and engagement, nurses enhance treatment adherence, self-care management, and overall health outcomes. Patient and family education empower individuals to actively participate in their care, leading to improved well-being. Effective education fosters a collaborative approach, ensuring patients and families are equipped with the knowledge and skills necessary for holistic healing.

2.3.1 Health maintenance and disease prevention

In holistic patient care, health maintenance and disease prevention play vital roles. Educating patients and families empowers them to make informed decisions. Lifestyle modifications, regular screenings, vaccinations, and early detection are key in promoting overall well-being. Patient education fosters healthy behaviors and reduces illness risks. Medical surgical nurses promote preventive care practices by collaborating with patients. Strategies include personalized wellness plans, community outreach programs, and culturally sensitive education materials. By emphasizing prevention, healthcare providers enhance patient-centered care and support individuals in taking control of their health.

2.3.2 Health literacy

Health literacy is the ability to understand, interpret, and navigate the healthcare system, enabling patients to make informed decisions about their health. It plays a crucial role in patient education and holistic care, empowering individuals to comprehend medical information and communicate effectively with healthcare providers. Low health literacy can lead to poor patient outcomes and healthcare disparities. Medical surgical nurses can promote health literacy by simplifying complex medical jargon, using visual aids, and encouraging open dialogue. By enhancing health literacy among patients and families, nurses can improve care quality and foster positive health outcomes.

2.3.3 Teaching methods

In the context of holistic patient care, utilizing effective teaching methods is crucial for promoting patient understanding, compliance, and overall health outcomes. Various approaches such as verbal instructions, visual aids, demonstrations, interactive sessions, and technology-based tools play a vital role in patient education. Tailoring teaching methods to individual patient needs, preferences, and cultural backgrounds enhances learning and retention. Medical-surgical nurses play a key role in selecting appropriate teaching methods, assessing learning outcomes, and empowering patients through education. By employing diverse and personalized teaching strategies, nurses can empower patients to actively participate in their care journey.

2.4 Health Promotion

In the context of holistic patient care, 'Health Promotion' focuses on preventive care, patient education, lifestyle modifications, and community resources to enhance overall well-being and prevent illness. Empowering patients through health promotion strategies enables them to make informed decisions, improving their quality of life. Medical surgical nurses play a vital role in promoting health and wellness by implementing holistic approaches, advocating for patients, and providing comprehensive care that addresses physical, emotional, and social aspects of health. By emphasizing health promotion, nurses contribute to better patient outcomes and a healthier community.

2.4.1 Health promotion goals

In the context of holistic patient care, health promotion goals play a vital role in enhancing overall well-being. Setting SMART goals - specific, measurable, achievable, relevant, and time-bound - is crucial for effective health promotion. Common examples of health promotion goals in medical-surgical settings include improving mobility post-surgery, managing pain levels, and promoting wound healing. Medical-surgical nurses collaborate with patients to identify, plan, and achieve these goals, considering social determinants of health and cultural factors. Addressing these aspects ensures tailored and effective health promotion strategies for diverse patient populations.

2.4.2 Resources available for patient/family

In the realm of health promotion and holistic patient care, a plethora of resources exist to support patients and their families. Community resources offer access to local health programs and services. Support groups provide emotional assistance and shared experiences. Educational materials empower individuals with knowledge. Financial assistance programs alleviate burdens. Counseling services address mental health needs. These resources collectively contribute to the overall well-being of patients by addressing their physical, emotional, and social needs comprehensively. By utilizing these resources, patients and families can enhance their health outcomes and experience a more holistic approach to care.

2.4.3 Health information to meet patient needs

In the realm of health promotion and holistic patient care, providing tailored health information is paramount. Healthcare professionals must adeptly communicate with patients of diverse backgrounds, cultures, and health literacy levels. Strategies include utilizing clear communication, culturally sensitive patient education materials, and technology for enhanced understanding. Overcoming language barriers and addressing limited health literacy are crucial. Individual preferences should guide the delivery of information. Interdisciplinary collaboration ensures comprehensive and patient-centered care. By prioritizing effective communication and education, healthcare providers can empower patients to comprehend and act upon health information, fostering improved health outcomes.

2.5 Palliative/End-ofLife Care

Palliative/End-of-Life Care in the context of Holistic Patient Care focuses on enhancing the quality of life for patients with serious illnesses. It addresses physical, emotional, social, and spiritual needs. Key aspects include principles, goals, and interventions to provide comprehensive care to patients nearing the end of life. Medical surgical nurses play a crucial role in delivering Palliative/End-of-

Life Care by ensuring effective communication, symptom management, and family support. Their focus is on promoting comfort, dignity, and respect for patients during this sensitive phase of care.

2.5.1 Palliative or end-of-life patient/caregiver resources

The topic of 'Palliative or end-of-life patient/caregiver resources' in Palliative/End-of-Life Care and Holistic Patient Care is crucial. Resources include counseling, support groups, and educational materials. Healthcare providers play a key role in connecting patients and caregivers to these resources. Addressing emotional and spiritual needs is vital for comprehensive care. Access to such resources enhances the quality of care provided to patients at the end of life, promoting comfort and dignity. By integrating these resources, healthcare professionals can ensure holistic support for patients and their families during challenging times.

2.5.1.1 Hospice

In the context of Palliative or end-of-life care, hospice focuses on providing compassionate and holistic care to patients and their families. The philosophy of hospice care centers around enhancing quality of life and ensuring comfort. Services in hospice settings include pain management, emotional support, and spiritual care. An interdisciplinary team comprising nurses, doctors, social workers, and counselors collaborates to meet the physical, emotional, and spiritual needs of patients. The goals of hospice care are to alleviate suffering, promote dignity, and support patients in their end-of-life journey. Eligibility criteria for hospice services typically involve a prognosis of six months or less. Family members play a crucial role in hospice care by providing comfort and participating in decision-making. Benefits of hospice care include improved quality of life, symptom management, and emotional support for both patients and their families.

2.5.1.2 Spiritual

In palliative or end-of-life care, spirituality encompasses beliefs, values, and practices that provide meaning and purpose. Addressing spiritual needs is crucial for patients with life-limiting illnesses, offering comfort and support. Cultural and religious considerations play a significant role in meeting these needs. Integrating spiritual practices into care plans can enhance holistic patient care, promoting emotional and psychological well-being. Spiritual well-being impacts patient outcomes and quality of life in palliative settings, emphasizing the importance of a comprehensive approach. Recognizing and supporting spirituality in patients and families fosters a more compassionate and effective end-of-life journey.

2.5.1.3 Cultural

In the context of Palliative/End-of-Life Care, understanding cultural beliefs, practices, and values is crucial. Cultural competence ensures respectful care delivery, considering diverse backgrounds. Cultural sensitivity promotes effective communication and trust with patients and families. Awareness of cultural traditions helps tailor care plans to meet individual needs. Holistic patient care in end-of-life settings requires acknowledging and respecting cultural differences. Providing culturally competent care enhances patient-centered outcomes and fosters a supportive environment for individuals facing end-of-life situations. Cultural awareness is essential for delivering compassionate and holistic care in Palliative/End-of-Life settings.

2.5.1.4 Physical

In palliative or end-of-life care, addressing physical needs is crucial for patient comfort. Key aspects include pain management, symptom control (nausea, fatigue), mobility, nutrition, skin care, and end-of-life interventions (mouth care, positioning). Proper pain management enhances quality of life, while symptom control and mobility maintenance prevent complications. Nutrition and hydration support physical strength, and skin care prevents breakdown. End-of-life interventions like mouth care and positioning ensure comfort. Integrating these aspects into care approaches is vital for comprehensive support in palliative or end-of-life settings.

2.5.2 End-of-life preferences

In the context of palliative and end-of-life care, addressing end-of-life preferences is crucial for providing holistic patient-centered care. End-of-life preferences refer to the individual's desires regarding their care, treatment, and quality of life as they approach the end of life. Respecting and honoring these preferences is essential to uphold patient autonomy and dignity. Factors influencing preferences include personal values, beliefs, past experiences, and cultural backgrounds. Nurses play a vital role in eliciting, documenting, and advocating for patients' preferences. Collaboration with interdisciplinary teams ensures comprehensive care aligned with patients' wishes. Cultural, spiritual, and religious beliefs significantly impact end-of-life decisions, requiring sensitivity and respect. Emotional support for patients and families navigating these preferences is paramount.

2.5.2.1 Advance directives

Advance directives are crucial in honoring patients' end-of-life preferences, ensuring holistic care. They encompass living wills and durable power of attorney for healthcare, guiding decisions when patients can't communicate. Advance directives uphold patient autonomy, dignity, and quality of life, promoting informed decision-making. Healthcare providers must discuss advance care planning to navigate ethical and legal considerations effectively. By respecting patients' wishes, advance directives play a vital role in delivering patient-centered care, especially in palliative and end-of-life settings.

2.5.2.2 Code status

In the context of end-of-life care, 'code status' refers to a patient's preferences for resuscitation in the event of cardiac or respiratory arrest. It is crucial to discuss code status with patients and families to ensure their wishes are respected. Code status options include 'full code' (all resuscitative measures), 'do not resuscitate' (no CPR), 'do not intubate' (no artificial ventilation), and 'comfort care' (focus on symptom management). Healthcare providers play a vital role in honoring these preferences, which greatly impact end-of-life decision-making and care delivery.

2.5.3 Post-mortem care

Post-mortem care in Palliative/End-of-Life Care involves crucial aspects. Procedures include confirming death, preparing the body respectfully, and documenting. Emotional support for the family is vital, offering empathy and guidance. Cultural considerations respect diverse beliefs and practices. The healthcare team plays a key role in providing compassionate care, ensuring dignity for the deceased.

Holistic Patient Care emphasizes physical, emotional, and spiritual support during this sensitive time. Understanding these elements is essential for CMSRN exam readiness.

2.5.4 Organ donation process

In palliative care, discussing organ donation is vital for honoring patients' wishes and providing comfort. Ethical dilemmas arise regarding end-of-life decisions, requiring sensitive communication and shared decision-making. Medical-surgical nurses play a crucial role in guiding patients and families, offering emotional support and education throughout the donation process. A holistic approach considers physical, emotional, and spiritual aspects, ensuring comprehensive care. Collaboration with healthcare teams, procurement organizations, and transplant centers ensures a seamless and respectful process. Understanding and respecting cultural and religious beliefs is essential for facilitating informed decisions in palliative care settings.

2.5.5 Regulatory requirements for reporting death

In the context of Palliative/End-of-Life Care and Holistic Patient Care, medical surgical nurses must adhere to specific regulatory requirements when reporting a patient's death. Legal obligations mandate accurate and timely reporting, detailed documentation, and clear communication with the healthcare team and family members. Nurses should follow established procedures for end-of-life care situations, considering ethical implications. Ensuring proper reporting of death is crucial for maintaining holistic patient care standards. Compliance with regulatory guidelines is essential to uphold professionalism and respect for the deceased and their loved ones.

2.5.5.1 Coroner's case

In medical-surgical nursing, a coroner's case involves investigating deaths to determine cause. Nurses must adhere to regulatory requirements for reporting deaths, ensuring legal compliance. Understanding the coroner's role is crucial, considering legal and ethical implications. Collaboration with coroners is vital for comprehensive patient care. Effective communication, thorough documentation, and interdisciplinary teamwork are key in managing coroner's cases. Nurses play a significant role in providing holistic care, especially in palliative/end-of-life situations. Compassion and empathy are essential when supporting patients and families through these challenging times.

3   Elements of Interprofessional Care

In medical-surgical nursing, 'Elements of Interprofessional Care' focus on effective communication, collaboration, mutual respect, and shared decision-making among healthcare team members. These aspects are crucial in providing comprehensive patient care. Interprofessional care enhances patient outcomes, improves safety, and promotes a holistic approach to healthcare delivery. By working together, healthcare professionals can address patients' needs more effectively, leading to better overall health outcomes. Effective interprofessional care ensures that patients receive well-coordinated and patient-centered care, ultimately improving the quality of healthcare services provided.

3.1   Nursing Process/Clinical Judgement Measurement Model

The Nursing Process/Clinical Judgement Measurement Model is vital for effective interprofessional care. It involves assessment, diagnosis, planning, implementation, and evaluation. Clinical judgement plays a key role in decision-making, ensuring optimal patient outcomes. Measurement models help evaluate care quality and patient progress. By utilizing this model, healthcare teams enhance patient care, foster teamwork, and achieve better health outcomes. This approach promotes collaboration among healthcare professionals, leading to comprehensive and patient-centered care delivery.

3.1.1 Nursing process - assessment, diagnosis, planning, implementation, evaluation

The nursing process, integral to CMSRN exam, comprises assessment, diagnosis, planning, implementation, and evaluation. Assessment involves gathering patient data. Diagnosis is identifying health issues. Planning includes setting goals. Implementation is executing interventions. Evaluation assesses outcomes. In the Nursing Process/Clinical Judgement Measurement Model, thorough assessment ensures accurate diagnosis. Individualized planning tailors care. Effective implementation of interventions promotes patient well-being. Comprehensive evaluation measures success. These stages enhance clinical judgement, foster interprofessional collaboration, and deliver patient-centered care, emphasizing optimal outcomes.

3.1.2 Strategies to individualize care

To individualize care effectively, nurses must integrate the Nursing Process/Clinical Judgement Measurement Model. This involves assessing patients holistically, considering their cultural beliefs, preferences, and health literacy levels. By tailoring care plans to meet these unique needs, nurses can enhance patient outcomes significantly. Collaboration with other healthcare professionals is crucial in developing personalized care strategies. Through interprofessional teamwork, nurses can leverage diverse expertise to create comprehensive and patient-centered interventions. Evidence-based practice serves as a guiding principle, ensuring that care plans are based on the latest research and continuously evaluated for effectiveness.

3.2   Interprofessional Collaboration

In the context of the Certified Medical Surgical Registered Nurse (CMSRN) exam, 'Interprofessional Collaboration' focuses on effective communication, mutual respect, shared decision-making, and teamwork among healthcare professionals. This collaboration is vital for providing high-quality patient care. By working together, different disciplines can improve patient outcomes, enhance safety, and increase satisfaction. CMSRNs play a crucial role in promoting interprofessional collaboration within the medical-surgical team, ensuring seamless coordination and holistic patient care.

3.2.1 Role within the interdisciplinary team

In the interdisciplinary team, Medical Surgical Nurses play a vital role in promoting holistic patient care through effective communication, collaboration, and teamwork. They contribute to care coordination, advocate for patients, and enhance positive outcomes. Respecting and valuing the expertise of other healthcare professionals is crucial for optimal patient care. Medical Surgical Nurses foster a collaborative approach by working closely with physicians, pharmacists, physical therapists, and social workers. Their key responsibilities include promoting patient-centered care, sharing knowledge, and ensuring a cohesive team effort for the well-being of patients.

3.2.1.1 Teamwork

Teamwork within the interdisciplinary team is crucial for providing holistic patient care. It involves effective collaboration among healthcare professionals from various disciplines, promoting communication and enhancing patient outcomes. Key aspects include mutual respect, trust, shared decision-making, and accountability. Effective teamwork ensures a positive work environment, coordinated care, and patient-centered approach. It contributes to high-quality, safe, and efficient healthcare services. Challenges include communication barriers and role confusion. Strategies to promote teamwork include fostering open communication, clarifying roles, and promoting a culture of collaboration in healthcare settings.

3.2.1.2 Communication skills

Effective communication skills are vital in the interdisciplinary team and interprofessional collaboration in healthcare. Essential elements include active listening, clear messaging, empathy, and cultural competence. Strong communication enhances teamwork, patient outcomes, and overall healthcare delivery. Barriers like hierarchy, language differences, and lack of trust can impede effective communication. Strategies to overcome these challenges include fostering open dialogue, promoting mutual respect, and utilizing standardized communication tools. By prioritizing effective communication, healthcare professionals can ensure seamless coordination and delivery of patient-centered care in a multidisciplinary setting.

3.2.2 Interprofessional rounding

Interprofessional rounding involves healthcare team members from various disciplines coming together to discuss patient care. The purpose is to enhance communication, collaboration, and decision-making. Key members include nurses, physicians, pharmacists, and therapists. Benefits include improved patient outcomes and satisfaction. Strategies for effective rounding include setting clear goals and fostering open communication. Challenges may include time constraints and hierarchy issues. Effective communication and teamwork are crucial. Medical surgical nurses play a vital role in providing insights and coordinating care. Best practices include active participation, respect for all team members, and a patient-centered approach.

3.2.3 Care coordination

Care coordination in interprofessional collaboration involves synchronizing efforts among healthcare team members to deliver seamless care. It encompasses communication, patient advocacy, continuity of care, and shared decision-making. Effective care coordination enhances patient outcomes, satisfaction, and optimizes resource utilization. Communication ensures information exchange, advocacy supports patient needs, continuity of care promotes consistent treatment, and collaboration aids in comprehensive decision-making. Together, these elements streamline healthcare delivery, improve patient experiences, and maximize the efficiency of the healthcare system.

3.2.4 Collaborative problem solving

In healthcare, collaborative problem solving is vital for effective interprofessional collaboration. It fosters teamwork and communication among diverse healthcare professionals. Key elements include active listening, mutual respect, shared decision-making, and conflict resolution. For example, when a nurse, physician, and pharmacist work together to address a patient's complex medication regimen, collaborative problem solving ensures comprehensive care. This approach leads to improved patient outcomes, enhanced quality of care, and increased job satisfaction. By valuing each team member's expertise and input, healthcare professionals can collectively provide optimal patient-centered care.

3.3 Care Coordination and Transition Management

The topic of 'Care Coordination and Transition Management' within the context of 'Elements of Interprofessional Care' is crucial for ensuring seamless transitions for patients across healthcare settings. Medical surgical nurses play a vital role in facilitating communication among healthcare team members, patients, and families to enhance patient outcomes. Key strategies for promoting care coordination include comprehensive care planning, medication reconciliation, and patient education. Transition management is essential for supporting patients during care transitions, encompassing discharge planning, post-discharge follow-up, and coordination of community resources. Effective care coordination and transition management are fundamental aspects of providing high-quality patient care.

3.3.1 Community resources

In care coordination and transition management, community resources play a vital role in supporting patients across healthcare settings. These resources, such as local support groups, home health services, transportation assistance, and financial aid programs, help ensure seamless transitions of care. Medical-surgical nurses can collaborate with these resources to enhance patient outcomes, improve access to care, and promote continuity of care. Community resources address social determinants of health, provide patient education, and empower individuals to manage their health effectively outside clinical settings. By leveraging these resources, nurses can better support patients in their healthcare journey.

3.3.2 Interdisciplinary collaboration integration methods

In the realm of interprofessional care, effective interdisciplinary collaboration is crucial for improving patient outcomes, enhancing communication, and ensuring seamless transitions of care. Key methods include regular team meetings, care planning sessions, shared electronic health records, and standardized communication protocols. Leadership plays a vital role in fostering a collaborative environment and overcoming teamwork barriers. Continuous education and training are essential for healthcare professionals to enhance their collaboration skills and deliver high-quality, patient-centered care.

3.3.2.1 Discharge planning

Discharge planning involves coordinating post-discharge care to ensure smooth transitions for patients. It includes assessing patient needs, medication reconciliation, education, and follow-up arrangements. Interdisciplinary collaboration is crucial in this process to optimize patient outcomes and prevent readmissions. Medical surgical nurses play a key role in discharge planning by working with the healthcare team to address patient needs comprehensively. Care coordination and transition management are essential elements in facilitating a successful transition from the hospital to home or other healthcare settings. Effective discharge planning enhances patient safety and continuity of care.

3.3.2.2 Mobility

Mobility in healthcare involves promoting movement and independence in patients. It is crucial for overall well-being and quality of life. Various healthcare professionals, such as physical therapists and nurses, play key roles in enhancing mobility through tailored interventions. Strategies for improving mobility include exercise programs and assistive devices. Limited mobility can negatively impact patient outcomes. Interdisciplinary collaboration optimizes mobility interventions, while care coordination ensures seamless mobility care. Transition management facilitates continuity of care across different settings. Effective interprofessional care enhances mobility outcomes and improves patient well-being.

3.3.2.3 Physical therapy

Physical therapy plays a crucial role in interdisciplinary collaboration by providing specialized interventions to improve patient mobility and function. Within care coordination and transition management, physical therapists work alongside other healthcare professionals to create individualized treatment plans and facilitate smooth transitions between care settings. Key aspects include setting functional goals, utilizing interventions like therapeutic exercises and manual therapy, and measuring outcomes to enhance patient recovery. Effective communication and coordination among team members are essential for optimizing patient care, highlighting the significance of physical therapy in promoting holistic and comprehensive healthcare delivery.

3.3.3 Health history assessment from multiple sources

Conducting a health history assessment from multiple sources is crucial in care coordination and transition management. Gathering information from patients, family, records, and healthcare providers ensures comprehensive data for continuity of care, accurate diagnosis, and effective treatment planning. However, challenges like data discrepancies and privacy concerns may arise. Synthesizing information from various sources provides a holistic view of the patient's health status, facilitating collaborative interprofessional care. This process enhances care quality, patient outcomes, and promotes a patient-centered approach in medical-surgical nursing practice.

3.3.4 Discharge procedures

In the context of care coordination and transition management, effective communication among healthcare team members is crucial during the discharge process. Steps for preparing a patient for discharge include medication reconciliation, patient education, and follow-up care instructions. Medical surgical nurses play a vital role in ensuring a smooth transition for patients from the hospital to home or another care setting. Assessing the patient's understanding of the discharge plan and addressing concerns is essential. Collaboration with case managers, social workers, and pharmacists is key to facilitating a comprehensive and coordinated discharge process.

3.3.4.1 Medication reconciliation

Medication reconciliation is vital in discharge procedures, care coordination, and transition management. It involves comparing a patient's medications to ensure accuracy and safety, preventing errors and improving outcomes. Interprofessional collaboration among nurses, pharmacists, physicians, and other providers is crucial for comprehensive medication lists. Challenges include clear communication, standardized processes, and patient involvement. Best practices emphasize the need for accurate reconciliation to enhance patient safety during transitions of care.

3.3.5 Patient/family centered care

In the context of Care Coordination and Transition Management, Elements of Interprofessional Care, Patient/Family Centered Care is crucial. Involving patients and families in decision-making, promoting open communication, respecting cultural beliefs, and providing education and support are vital aspects. Collaboration among healthcare professionals ensures holistic, individualized care. Medical surgical nurses play a key role in advocating for patients and families, facilitating shared decision-making, and promoting a patient-centered approach to care delivery. This approach enhances outcomes and fosters a supportive environment for patients and their families.

3.3.6 Care coordination and transition

Care coordination and transition in Care Coordination and Transition Management are vital for Medical Surgical Nurses. Seamless transitions between healthcare settings, effective communication among providers, patient education, and interdisciplinary collaboration are key. Nurses play a crucial role in ensuring continuity of care. Coordination improves outcomes, enhances safety, reduces costs, and promotes patient-centered care. Challenges include fragmented systems and communication gaps. Strategies like standardized protocols, technology integration, and patient engagement can overcome these barriers. Understanding and implementing care coordination are essential for Medical Surgical Nurses to provide high-quality, holistic care.

3.3.7 Interprofessional roles and responsibilities

In the realm of care coordination and transition management, interprofessional collaboration plays a pivotal role in ensuring seamless patient care. Effective communication, collaboration, and teamwork among healthcare professionals are essential for optimal outcomes. Medical surgical nurses are key advocates, sharing expertise, and engaging in care planning. Interprofessional teamwork enhances patient outcomes, improves care quality, and facilitates smooth transitions between healthcare settings. Successful examples include multidisciplinary rounds, where diverse perspectives converge to address patient needs comprehensively. Such collaborative efforts underscore the significance of interprofessional roles in delivering holistic and patient-centered care.

3.3.8 Continuum of care

The 'Continuum of care' in 'Care Coordination and Transition Management' focuses on seamless transitions and collaboration among healthcare providers. Elements of Interprofessional Care emphasize a patient-centered approach. Medical surgical nurses play a crucial role in ensuring continuity of care across various healthcare settings. They coordinate with multidisciplinary teams, advocate for patients, and provide holistic care. By facilitating effective communication and care coordination, medical surgical nurses enhance patient outcomes and promote a smooth transition between different levels of care. Their dedication to patient-centered care is fundamental in achieving optimal health outcomes and improving the overall healthcare experience.

3.3.9 Patients at risk for readmissions

In the context of Care Coordination and Transition Management, Patients at risk for readmissions are those vulnerable to hospital readmission due to factors like chronic conditions, lack of social support, medication non-adherence, and inadequate discharge planning. Identifying these patients early is crucial to implement targeted interventions and prevent readmissions. Interprofessional care teams play a vital role in assessing, monitoring, and managing at-risk patients, leading to improved outcomes and reduced healthcare costs. Effective collaboration among healthcare professionals is key to providing comprehensive care and support to these patients.

3.3.10 Social determinants of health

In the context of Care Coordination and Transition Management, Elements of Interprofessional Care, social determinants of health refer to factors influencing individuals' well-being. Key aspects include socioeconomic status, education level, access to healthcare, housing stability, and social support networks. These determinants significantly impact health outcomes, highlighting the importance of addressing them in care coordination and interprofessional care. By recognizing and addressing social determinants, healthcare professionals can better support patients in achieving optimal health and well-being.

3.3.11 Quality patient outcome measures

In medical-surgical nursing, quality patient outcome measures are vital in evaluating care coordination and transition management. These measures assess the effectiveness of interprofessional care delivery. Examples include readmission rates, patient satisfaction scores, and adherence to care plans. Interprofessional collaboration plays a key role in implementing and measuring these outcomes, enhancing patient care and healthcare delivery. By utilizing these measures, nurses can ensure seamless transitions, improve patient outcomes, and enhance overall quality of care. Effective interprofessional teamwork is essential in achieving optimal patient outcomes and promoting excellence in medical-surgical nursing practice.

3.4 Documentation

Documentation is vital in interprofessional care for effective communication and collaboration. Accurate and timely documentation ensures patient safety, care continuity, and legal compliance. Thorough documentation supports care coordination, interdisciplinary communication, and optimal patient outcomes. Various types of documentation include electronic health records, progress notes, care plans, and handoff reports. Medical-surgical nurses play a crucial role in maintaining precise documentation to enhance care quality and promote a patient-centered approach within the healthcare team.

3.4.1 Documentation of patient care

In the medical-surgical nursing setting, documentation of patient care is crucial for ensuring continuity and quality of care. Key elements include accurate recording of assessments, interventions, and outcomes in a timely manner. Clear and concise documentation facilitates effective communication among interprofessional team members, promoting coordinated care delivery. Nurses must be vigilant in avoiding errors in documentation due to the legal and ethical implications involved. Comprehensive and detailed documentation by the medical-surgical nurse plays a vital role in safeguarding patient safety and promoting optimal outcomes.

3.4.2 Electronic health records

Electronic Health Records (EHRs) play a crucial role in enhancing communication and collaboration among healthcare team members. With features like digital charting, real-time updates, and accessibility, EHRs improve patient safety, care coordination, and healthcare efficiency. However, challenges such as EHR implementation, data security, and interoperability exist. Despite these challenges, EHRs promote evidence-based practice and elevate the quality of patient care in multidisciplinary healthcare settings.

3.4.3 Downtime procedures

Downtime procedures are crucial for Medical Surgical Nurses during system outages. Proper documentation is vital to ensure patient data accuracy and care continuity. Interprofessional collaboration is key, involving effective communication with team members to coordinate care seamlessly. Following established procedures is essential to uphold patient safety and prevent errors. During downtime, nurses must prioritize patient needs, communicate effectively with the healthcare team, and document all care provided meticulously. By adhering to downtime protocols, Medical Surgical Nurses can maintain quality care delivery and ensure patient well-being.

3.4.4 Coaching for documentation performance improvement

Coaching for documentation performance improvement in the context of interprofessional care is crucial for enhancing accuracy, completeness, and timeliness of documentation in the medical-surgical setting. Effective coaching involves providing constructive feedback, setting achievable goals, and offering support and resources for improvement. Medical-surgical nurses play a vital role in coaching their peers to improve documentation practices, leading to improved patient outcomes, increased efficiency in care delivery, and reduced risk of errors or omissions. Implementing a coaching program can significantly benefit the healthcare team and ultimately enhance the quality of patient care.

3.5 Technology

In the realm of interprofessional care, technology plays a pivotal role in enhancing collaboration and communication among healthcare teams. Electronic health records (EHR) streamline information sharing, while telemedicine enables remote consultations, fostering teamwork across distances. Communication platforms like secure messaging systems facilitate real-time interaction, ensuring prompt decision-making. Despite these benefits, challenges such as data security and interoperability exist. Commonly used tools include Epic for EHR, Zoom for telemedicine, and Slack for team communication. Integrating technology effectively empowers healthcare professionals to deliver comprehensive, patient-centered care through seamless interprofessional collaboration.

3.5.1 Technology, equipment use, and troubleshooting

In the realm of interprofessional care, technology, equipment use, and troubleshooting play pivotal roles in enhancing patient outcomes. Medical surgical nurses are key players in leveraging various technologies and equipment to deliver high-quality care. Common tools include IV pumps, patient monitors, and electronic health records. Challenges such as equipment malfunctions require adept troubleshooting skills to ensure uninterrupted care delivery. Proficiency in troubleshooting is essential for maintaining the functionality of critical equipment, ultimately safeguarding patient safety and treatment efficacy.

3.5.2 Technology trends in health care

In the realm of health care, technology trends are revolutionizing interprofessional care. Telemedicine enables remote care and consultations, enhancing accessibility. Electronic Health Records (EHR) systems facilitate seamless information sharing among healthcare providers. Wearable health technology monitors patient health beyond clinical settings. Artificial Intelligence (AI) aids in predictive analytics and personalized treatment plans. Robotics in surgery offer benefits and challenges in medical procedures. Virtual reality (VR) and augmented reality (AR) aid in training and patient education. Internet of Things (IoT) devices and blockchain technology ensure secure data management. 3D printing creates personalized medical devices. Ethical considerations and barriers must be addressed for successful adoption.

3.5.3 Nursing informatics

Nursing informatics leverages technology to enhance interprofessional care, improving patient outcomes and communication. It integrates nursing, computer, and information sciences to support evidence-based practice. Key components include EHR, clinical decision support systems, telehealth, and health information exchange. Data management, IT security, and ethical considerations are crucial. Nursing informatics plays a vital role in decision-making, promoting efficient care delivery.

4 Professional Concepts

Professional Concepts in medical-surgical nursing encompass key principles, ethical considerations, legal regulations, and professional standards guiding nurses in providing optimal patient care. Upholding ethical values, adhering to legal mandates, and following professional standards are vital. Continuous professional development, embracing lifelong learning, fostering interdisciplinary collaboration, and advocating for patients are integral components. Nurses must prioritize ongoing education, engage in teamwork, and advocate for patients' rights to enhance healthcare outcomes. Embracing these professional concepts ensures medical-surgical nurses deliver safe, effective, and compassionate care within a dynamic healthcare landscape.

4.1 Communication

Communication in professional concepts for CMSRNs is vital for optimal patient care. Effective communication enhances patient outcomes, interdisciplinary collaboration, and patient safety. Nurses utilize verbal, non-verbal, written, and electronic communication. Key principles of therapeutic communication, like active listening and empathy, strengthen nurse-patient relationships. Challenges in communication include language barriers and distractions. Strategies to overcome these barriers include using clear language, active listening, and utilizing communication tools. Mastering communication skills is essential for CMSRNs to provide high-quality care and promote positive patient outcomes.

4.1.1 Chain of command

In healthcare settings, the Chain of Command is vital for effective communication and professional concepts among Medical Surgical Nurses. It establishes a clear hierarchy, aiding in decision-making, care coordination, and conflict resolution. The typical hierarchy includes staff nurses, charge nurses, nurse managers, and ultimately, the Chief Nursing Officer. Each level has specific roles and responsibilities, ensuring smooth operations and patient safety. Bypassing the chain of command can lead to confusion, errors, and compromised patient care. Adherence to the chain of command is crucial in resolving conflicts promptly, addressing concerns efficiently, and delivering high-quality patient care.

4.1.2 Communication skills

Communication skills in the medical-surgical nursing setting are crucial for effective patient care. These skills encompass conveying information clearly, active listening, utilizing nonverbal cues, demonstrating empathy, practicing cultural competence, and employing therapeutic communication techniques. Strong communication abilities are essential for establishing rapport with patients, collaborating with healthcare team members, delivering patient education, and ultimately, achieving optimal patient outcomes. By honing these skills, Certified Medical Surgical Registered Nurses can enhance patient experiences, promote interdisciplinary teamwork, and ensure comprehensive care delivery.

4.1.2.1 Active listening

Active listening is a vital communication skill for Certified Medical Surgical Registered Nurses (CMSRNs). It involves fully concentrating, understanding, responding, and remembering what a patient is saying. This technique is crucial in establishing trust, fostering relationships, and improving patient outcomes. Key components include interpreting nonverbal cues, summarizing patient statements accurately, and showing empathy. By actively listening, nurses can enhance patient satisfaction, compliance, and overall quality of care. Barriers to active listening may include distractions, biases, and time constraints. Strategies to overcome these barriers include maintaining eye contact, asking clarifying questions, and practicing mindfulness.

4.1.2.2 Verbal

Verbal communication is vital in healthcare for effective patient care and collaboration. Medical-surgical nurses must convey information clearly, listen actively, and show empathy. Clear communication enhances patient education, ensuring understanding of treatment plans and promoting safety. Collaboration with the healthcare team is improved, leading to better outcomes. Essential skills include active listening, using simple language, and non-verbal cues. Challenges like language barriers or complex medical terms can hinder communication. Nurses should adapt communication to suit individual needs, use interpreters when necessary, and provide written materials. Overcoming these barriers ensures effective communication in healthcare settings.

4.1.2.3 Non-verbal

Non-verbal communication, a vital aspect of communication skills, encompasses body language, facial expressions, gestures, eye contact, and tone of voice. These cues complement verbal messages, enhancing or detracting from communication effectiveness. Understanding cultural variations in non-verbal communication is crucial for interactions with diverse individuals. In the medical-surgical nursing field, non-verbal communication plays a key role in building rapport, establishing trust, and fostering positive relationships with patients, colleagues, and healthcare professionals. Mastering non-verbal cues is essential for successful professional interactions and ensuring effective communication in a healthcare setting.

4.1.2.4 Written

Written communication in healthcare is crucial for medical surgical nurses. Accurate documentation, proper charting, and electronic health records are vital for patient safety and care continuity. Clear, concise, and professional writing ensures effective interdisciplinary collaboration. Errors in written communication can have legal and ethical implications. Nurses must prioritize clarity and accuracy in their documentation to prevent misunderstandings and ensure quality care. By mastering written communication skills, medical surgical nurses can enhance patient outcomes and contribute to a safer healthcare environment.

4.1.2.5   Conflict resolution

Conflict resolution in medical-surgical nursing involves effectively managing disagreements to maintain a positive work environment. It is crucial for fostering teamwork, enhancing patient care, and upholding professional standards. Key principles include active listening, empathy, and open communication. Strategies encompass mediation, compromise, and seeking common ground. Unresolved conflicts can lead to errors in patient care, decreased staff morale, and compromised patient safety. Common sources of conflicts include miscommunication, differing priorities, and personality clashes. Addressing conflicts promptly through respectful dialogue and conflict resolution techniques is essential for promoting a harmonious and efficient medical-surgical unit.

4.1.2.6   Mediation

Mediation in healthcare involves resolving conflicts, promoting effective communication, and fostering positive relationships. Medical surgical nurses play a crucial role in utilizing mediation techniques to address conflicts among patients, families, and healthcare team members. Key skills include active listening, empathy, neutrality, and problem-solving. Maintaining confidentiality, impartiality, and respect for diverse perspectives is essential. Mediation enhances patient care outcomes, improves teamwork, and cultivates a culture of collaboration and mutual understanding in medical-surgical nursing practice.

4.1.3   Information sharing

Information sharing in healthcare involves the exchange of relevant data among healthcare professionals to ensure effective communication and collaboration. For medical-surgical nurses, accurate information sharing is crucial for patient safety and continuity of care. Methods such as electronic health records, handoff communication, team meetings, and patient education facilitate this process. Upholding patient confidentiality, adhering to HIPAA regulations, and safeguarding patient information are ethical and legal responsibilities of nurses. Timely and precise information sharing enhances care coordination, promotes interdisciplinary teamwork, and ultimately improves patient outcomes.

4.1.3.1   Situation

In medical-surgical nursing, 'Situation' refers to understanding patient conditions, sharing information, and effective communication. Recognizing and assessing situations is crucial for patient care, involving gathering pertinent data, and collaborating with the healthcare team. Situational awareness and communication enhance patient outcomes and interdisciplinary teamwork. Nurses play a vital role in managing complex scenarios, making critical decisions, and advocating for patients. By prioritizing situational awareness, effective communication, and proactive decision-making, medical-surgical nurses can ensure optimal patient care and promote positive outcomes through interdisciplinary collaboration.

4.1.3.2   Background

In healthcare, 'Background' refers to understanding the context of a situation or individual, including cultural, medical, and social factors. Recognizing background enhances communication and information sharing among healthcare professionals, leading to improved patient care. For example, knowing a patient's cultural beliefs can guide treatment decisions. Understanding medical history aids in providing tailored care. Social determinants of health influence patient needs. Respecting diverse backgrounds fosters patient-centered care. As a CMSRN, valuing background information enhances interdisciplinary collaboration, resulting in better patient outcomes and overall care quality.

4.1.3.3   Assessment

Assessment in medical-surgical nursing involves gathering comprehensive health history, performing physical exams, interpreting diagnostic tests, and applying critical thinking skills. Effective communication ensures accurate information exchange among healthcare team, patients, and families. Using evidence-based tools is crucial for informed decision-making. Ethical considerations like patient confidentiality and informed consent are paramount. Ongoing assessment monitors treatment responses, identifies complications, and enhances positive health outcomes.

4.1.3.4   Recommendation [SBAR]

In healthcare, utilizing the SBAR (Situation, Background, Assessment, Recommendation) framework is crucial for effective communication among healthcare providers. This technique enhances patient safety, improves teamwork, and ensures clear exchange of critical information. Medical surgical nurses can apply SBAR by succinctly presenting the patient's situation, providing relevant background information, offering their assessment of the issue, and making clear recommendations for further action. For example, when handing over patient care during shift change, using SBAR helps in conveying important details accurately and efficiently, leading to better outcomes and streamlined decision-making processes.

4.1.3.5   Hand-off

In the medical-surgical setting, a 'hand-off' refers to the transfer of patient care responsibility from one healthcare provider to another. Effective hand-offs are crucial for patient safety, continuity of care, and teamwork among providers. Key elements include accurate patient information transfer, maintaining care continuity, and promoting effective communication. CMSRNs play a vital role in ensuring successful hand-offs by utilizing standardized protocols, clear communication, and upholding ethical and legal standards. It is essential to prioritize patient confidentiality, document exchanged information, and utilize tools to facilitate seamless transitions of care.

4.1.3.6   Closed-loop

Closed-loop communication in medical-surgical nursing is vital for effective information exchange among healthcare team members. It ensures clear message transmission, active listening, and feedback acknowledgment. Key aspects include promoting clear communication, verifying information, and preventing errors. Nurses must engage in closed-loop communication during handoffs, collaborations, and care transitions. Strategies to enhance this practice include active listening and seeking feedback. Implementing closed-loop communication fosters patient safety and quality care delivery.

4.1.3.7 Check- back

In healthcare, check-back is a vital communication technique where the receiver repeats and confirms information back to the sender. It ensures accurate understanding, reduces errors, and enhances patient safety. Check-backs promote teamwork, collaboration, and trust among healthcare providers. For instance, in medical-surgical nursing, using check-backs during handoffs, medication administration, and critical procedures can prevent misunderstandings and improve patient outcomes. By incorporating check-backs into daily practice, nurses can foster a culture of clear communication, leading to better care coordination and ultimately, enhanced patient care quality.

4.1.3.8 Read-back

In the medical-surgical setting, read-back is a crucial communication practice where the receiver repeats back information received to confirm understanding. This process enhances patient safety by reducing errors, improving teamwork, and ensuring accurate data transmission. For instance, during handoffs, nurses can use read-back to verify medication orders, lab results, and treatment plans. Implementing read-back protocols involves clear articulation, active listening, and mutual respect among team members. By fostering a culture of accountability and safety, read-back promotes effective communication, minimizes misunderstandings, and ultimately enhances patient outcomes in healthcare settings.

4.1.3.9 Huddle

In the healthcare setting, a 'huddle' refers to a brief and regular meeting where team members come together to share information, communicate effectively, and discuss patient care. Huddles play a crucial role in promoting collaboration, enhancing patient safety, and improving the overall quality of care. Key components of a huddle include its purpose of sharing important updates, structured format, participants from various disciplines, regular frequency, and use of clear communication methods. Benefits of huddles include promoting teamwork, fostering open communication, and addressing barriers to effective information sharing.

4.1.3.10 Verbal orders

Verbal orders play a crucial role in medical-surgical nursing by facilitating prompt patient care. Clear and accurate communication is vital to prevent errors and ensure patient safety. Nurses must verify orders with the provider and document them accurately. Risks of verbal orders include miscommunication and potential errors. To mitigate these risks, nurses should repeat and clarify orders, use read-backs, and seek written confirmation whenever possible. Legal and ethical considerations mandate obtaining verbal orders from authorized providers and documenting them appropriately. Upholding professional responsibilities in giving and receiving verbal orders is essential for safe and effective patient care.

4.1.3.11 Bedside report

Bedside report in medical-surgical nursing is a vital practice that enhances information sharing, communication, and professional concepts. It serves to ensure continuity of care, promote patient safety, and facilitate interdisciplinary collaboration. Nurses play a key role in conducting bedside reports by exchanging essential patient information, discussing care plans, and addressing any concerns. The purpose of bedside report is to provide a comprehensive handover, including patient condition, treatment updates, and upcoming interventions. By prioritizing bedside report, healthcare teams can deliver patient-centered care, improve outcomes, and uphold professional standards in nursing practice.

4.1.3.12 Interdisciplinary

Interdisciplinary collaboration in healthcare involves professionals from various disciplines working together to share information, communicate effectively, and uphold professional standards. This collaboration is vital for enhancing patient care outcomes, improving communication among team members, and fostering mutual respect. Interdisciplinary teams play a crucial role in providing holistic care, addressing complex patient needs, and boosting satisfaction. Challenges like differing perspectives and communication breakdowns can hinder collaboration. Strategies to overcome these barriers include promoting open communication, respecting each other's expertise, and establishing clear roles. Successful interdisciplinary relationships are key to delivering high-quality care in medical-surgical nursing practice.

4.1.4 Communication barriers

Communication barriers in healthcare refer to obstacles that hinder effective exchange of information. In medical-surgical nursing, barriers like language differences, cultural nuances, physical limitations, emotional distress, and technological challenges can impede communication. These barriers can strain nurse-patient relationships, lead to misunderstandings affecting patient outcomes, and reduce care quality. Nurses can overcome these barriers by using interpreters, respecting cultural practices, providing written materials, offering emotional support, and utilizing communication aids. By addressing these barriers proactively, nurses can enhance communication and provide optimal care.

4.1.4.1 Need for interpreter/translator

In healthcare settings, interpreters/translators play a crucial role in bridging communication gaps between healthcare providers and patients who speak different languages. Language barriers can lead to misunderstandings, errors in diagnosis, and compromised patient safety. Utilizing interpreters/translators enhances patient outcomes by ensuring accurate transmission of medical information, improving patient satisfaction, and fostering effective communication. Ethical considerations and professional responsibilities include respecting patient confidentiality and cultural sensitivity. Situations where interpreters/translators are vital include obtaining informed consent, discussing treatment plans, and conveying critical information during emergencies.

4.1.4.2 Physical and cognitive limitations

In the context of Communication barriers, Communication, and Professional Concepts, understanding physical and cognitive limitations is crucial for effective patient care. Healthcare providers face challenges in comprehending and meeting the needs of patients with such limitations. Utilizing appropriate communication strategies and tools is vital to overcome these barriers. Demonstrating empathy, patience, and cultural competence when interacting with these patients is key. By acknowledging and addressing physical and cognitive limitations, healthcare professionals can enhance communication, provide optimal care, and foster positive patient outcomes.

4.1.5   De-escalation techniques

In the healthcare setting, mastering de-escalation techniques is vital for Medical Surgical Nurses. These techniques focus on active listening, empathy, maintaining a calm demeanor, setting boundaries, and using non-confrontational language. Recognizing early signs of escalating behavior is crucial to prevent further escalation. Implementing de-escalation strategies enhances patient outcomes, fosters teamwork, and cultivates a culture of safety. Practice, patience, and effective communication are key to successfully utilizing these techniques. By honing these skills, nurses can navigate challenging situations with confidence and promote a harmonious environment in healthcare settings.

4.1.5.1   Verbal intervention

Verbal intervention in de-escalation techniques, communication, and professional concepts involves using words to manage challenging situations in healthcare. As a Medical Surgical Nurse, mastering verbal intervention is crucial for preventing conflicts, ensuring patient safety, and maintaining a therapeutic environment. Effective techniques include active listening, empathy, clear communication, and de-escalation language. Ethical considerations and cultural sensitivity are vital when employing verbal intervention. These skills enable nurses to communicate effectively with patients, families, and the healthcare team in diverse clinical scenarios. Mastering verbal intervention is essential for providing quality care and fostering positive relationships in healthcare settings.

4.1.5.2   Calm communication

In the context of de-escalation techniques, communication, and professional concepts, calm communication is vital for medical-surgical nurses. Maintaining a composed demeanor when dealing with agitated patients is crucial for fostering trust and diffusing tense situations. Key components include using a soothing tone, active listening, showing empathy, and utilizing non-verbal cues effectively. By employing calm communication strategies, nurses can enhance patient outcomes and improve the overall quality of care. For instance, by actively listening to a distressed patient, acknowledging their concerns, and responding with empathy, nurses can establish a supportive environment that promotes healing and trust.

4.2   Critical Thinking

In the context of 'Professional Concepts' for Certified Medical Surgical Registered Nurses (CMSRNs), 'Critical Thinking' is a vital skill that plays a crucial role in clinical decision-making, problem-solving, and providing quality patient care. Nurses with strong critical thinking skills can analyze complex situations, consider multiple perspectives, and make sound judgments. This ability is essential in promoting evidence-based practice, improving patient outcomes, and enhancing overall nursing practice. By applying critical thinking, nurses can navigate challenging scenarios effectively, leading to better patient care and a higher standard of practice.

4.2.1   Time management and prioritization of care

In the dynamic role of a Medical Surgical Nurse, mastering time management and prioritization of care is crucial for optimizing patient outcomes. Efficient time allocation enhances care quality by ensuring timely interventions and treatments. Common tasks like medication administration, wound care, and patient assessments demand precise prioritization based on acuity levels and available resources. Nurses can employ strategies such as the ABCDE prioritization method and the use of clinical judgment to make informed decisions swiftly. Developing critical thinking skills is paramount in navigating complex patient needs and ethical dilemmas that may arise. Continuous practice and reflection are key to honing these essential skills as a Certified Medical Surgical Registered Nurse (CMSRN).

4.2.2   Crisis situations and resources

In medical-surgical nursing, crisis situations demand swift action and critical thinking. Nurses encounter rapid patient deterioration, life-threatening emergencies, and unexpected complications. Critical thinking is vital for effective crisis management. Nurses utilize resources like medical equipment, medications, interdisciplinary team support, and evidence-based guidelines. By leveraging these resources, nurses can deliver timely and appropriate care during crises, ensuring optimal patient outcomes. Understanding crisis characteristics, applying critical thinking, and utilizing available resources are key for medical-surgical nurses in managing challenging situations effectively.

4.2.2.1   Rapid response team

In medical-surgical nursing, a rapid response team is a specialized group of healthcare professionals who are summoned to manage critical situations promptly. These teams play a vital role in assessing and stabilizing patients during emergencies, ensuring timely interventions to prevent adverse outcomes. Critical thinking skills are crucial for rapid response team members to analyze complex situations, prioritize actions, and deliver effective care under pressure. Professional concepts such as teamwork, communication, and evidence-based practice guide their decision-making process. Ethical considerations, including patient autonomy and beneficence, shape their actions when responding to medical crises.

4.2.2.2   Deteriorating patients

In medical-surgical nursing, deteriorating patients refer to individuals whose condition is worsening and requires immediate attention. Key indicators include changes in vital signs, altered mental status, and increased pain. Nurses must promptly assess, notify the healthcare team, and initiate appropriate interventions. Critical thinking is vital in recognizing subtle changes and making timely decisions. Nurses play a crucial role in managing deteriorating patients by utilizing resources effectively, communicating efficiently with the team, and implementing evidence-based practices. Ethical considerations include advocating for patients, providing patient-centered care, and collaborating to ensure optimal outcomes in crisis situations.

4.2.2.3   Early warning systems

Early warning systems in medical-surgical nursing are vital tools for timely identification and response to deteriorating patient conditions. These systems play a crucial role in improving patient outcomes and safety by enabling early intervention. Key components include monitoring vital signs, clinical indicators, and using standardized assessment tools. Critical thinking is essential in interpreting data from these systems to make informed clinical decisions promptly. Medical-surgical nurses have professional responsibilities to implement and adhere to early warning protocols, ensuring patient well-being through proactive monitoring and intervention.

4.2.3   Crisis management

Crisis management in medical-surgical nursing involves the ability to swiftly identify and address critical situations using sound judgment and quick decision-making. Critical thinking skills play a vital role in recognizing and resolving crises effectively. Professional concepts like ethical decision-making, clear communication, and teamwork are integral to crisis management. For instance, during a sudden patient deterioration, nurses must make ethical choices, communicate clearly with the healthcare team, and collaborate to provide timely interventions. These skills are essential for ensuring patient safety and delivering high-quality care in challenging situations.

4.2.4   Critical thinking

Critical thinking in nursing involves analyzing information, evaluating situations, and making sound decisions. For medical-surgical nurses, critical thinking is vital for delivering optimal patient care. It enhances problem-solving skills, clinical judgment, and decision-making processes. Nurses use critical thinking to assess patient conditions, develop care plans, implement interventions, and evaluate outcomes effectively. Reflection, evidence-based practice, and continuous learning play key roles in nurturing critical thinking skills. By applying critical thinking, nurses promote patient safety, improve outcomes, and enhance overall healthcare delivery. It is a cornerstone of professional nursing practice, ensuring quality care and positive patient experiences.

4.2.4.1   Self-regulation

Self-regulation in medical-surgical nursing involves monitoring, evaluating, and adjusting one's thoughts and actions. It is crucial for critical thinking and upholding professional standards. Self-regulation enables nurses to make sound decisions, solve problems effectively, and enhance critical thinking skills in patient care. For instance, a nurse practicing self-regulation may reflect on past experiences to improve future outcomes. This process leads to better patient care, improved outcomes, and fosters continuous professional development. Ultimately, self-regulation empowers nurses to deliver high-quality care and adapt to the dynamic healthcare environment.

4.2.4.2   Problem solving

Problem solving in medical-surgical nursing involves critical thinking and professional skills. It is crucial for nurses to effectively address challenges in patient care. Effective problem solving leads to improved patient outcomes, enhanced interdisciplinary collaboration, and better quality of care. The process includes identifying the issue, gathering data, brainstorming solutions, evaluating options, decision-making, and assessing the chosen solution. Critical thinking aids nurses in analyzing complex scenarios, making informed decisions, and improving clinical judgment. Continuous learning and reflection are vital for honing problem-solving abilities and advancing professional development in medical-surgical nursing.

4.2.4.3   Analysis

Analysis in medical-surgical nursing involves critical thinking and professional concepts. It is crucial for clinical decision-making, problem-solving, and delivering high-quality patient care. Key components include data collection, interpretation, evaluation, and synthesis. Nurses use analysis to assess situations, identify issues, and develop interventions. Critical thinking is essential in this process to ensure effective problem-solving. Incorporating evidence-based practice and current research is vital to make informed decisions. By utilizing analysis, medical-surgical nurses can enhance patient outcomes and provide optimal care based on the best available information.

4.2.4.4   Interpretation

Interpretation in the context of critical thinking is vital for Medical Surgical Nurses. It involves analyzing patient data, interpreting lab results, understanding medical orders, evaluating changes in patient status, and communicating effectively with the healthcare team. By applying critical thinking skills, nurses can interpret complex medical information to make evidence-based decisions. This skill is essential for assessing patient conditions, guiding care through diagnostic tests, and ensuring accurate treatment plans. Interpretation plays a key role in providing safe and effective patient care, highlighting the importance of strong critical thinking abilities in the nursing profession.

4.2.4.5   Inference

For medical-surgical nurses, inference is crucial in decision-making, enabling them to analyze patient data, make clinical judgments, and create effective care plans. By accurately inferring information from assessments, lab results, and patient interactions, nurses can anticipate complications, tailor interventions, and improve outcomes. For example, correctly inferring early signs of sepsis can prompt timely interventions, leading to better patient recovery. Utilizing inference enhances nursing practice by fostering critical thinking skills and promoting evidence-based care delivery.

4.3   Healthy Practice Environment

The topic of 'Healthy Practice Environment' falls under 'Professional Concepts' for the CMSRN exam. A healthy practice environment is crucial for ensuring patient safety, quality care, and nurse well-being. Key aspects include effective communication, interdisciplinary collaboration, safe staffing levels, supportive leadership, a culture of safety, and opportunities for professional growth. Such an environment enhances job satisfaction, reduces burnout, and improves patient outcomes significantly. Nurses in a healthy practice environment feel supported, valued, and empowered to deliver the best possible care, ultimately leading to better overall healthcare outcomes.

4.3.1   Workplace safety

Workplace safety for CMSRNs in medical-surgical units is crucial for maintaining a healthy practice environment. Identifying hazards like slippery floors or heavy lifting is key. Implementing safety protocols, such as proper lifting techniques, reduces risks. Promoting a safety culture among team members fosters collaboration. Adhering to regulatory guidelines ensures compliance. CMSRNs play a vital role in advocating for safety, preventing injuries, and responding to emergencies promptly. Prioritizing workplace safety not only protects healthcare providers but also enhances patient care quality.

4.3.1.1 Physical

In the context of workplace safety, healthy practice environment, and professional concepts, physical well-being is paramount for Certified Medical Surgical Registered Nurses (CMSRNs). Ergonomics, safe patient handling, and injury prevention are crucial components. Maintaining physical health enhances job satisfaction, performance, and patient care quality. Nurses must prioritize their own well-being to deliver optimal care. Physical health directly impacts workplace safety, productivity, and overall job satisfaction. By focusing on ergonomics, safe patient handling, and injury prevention, nurses create a healthier practice environment, leading to improved outcomes for both themselves and their patients.

4.3.1.2 Emotional

In the context of Workplace Safety, Healthy Practice Environment, and Professional Concepts, emotional well-being plays a crucial role. Emotions impact safety, teamwork, and patient care significantly. Emotional intelligence is key to fostering a healthy work environment and enhancing professional relationships. Stress, burnout, and compassion fatigue can adversely affect emotional health and job performance in medical-surgical nursing. Strategies for managing emotions effectively, fostering resilience, and seeking support when needed are essential for maintaining emotional well-being in the workplace. Prioritizing emotional health is vital for overall success in the medical-surgical nursing setting.

4.3.1.3 Environmental

Environmental considerations in healthcare encompass workplace safety, healthy practice environments, and professional concepts. Prioritizing environmental factors is crucial for enhancing patient outcomes, staff well-being, and overall care quality. Healthcare professionals play a vital role in promoting sustainability, waste reduction, and carbon footprint minimization. Adhering to environmental regulations ensures a safe work environment for all. Integrating environmental awareness into nursing practice elevates patient safety and healthcare system efficiency. Embracing environmental responsibility is key to fostering a culture of safety and excellence in medical-surgical nursing.

4.3.2 Nurse resiliency and well-being

Nurse Resiliency and Well-being are vital in maintaining high-quality patient care and job satisfaction. Strategies include self-care practices, recognizing burnout signs, seeking support, and utilizing mental health resources. These aspects contribute to a positive work environment, improved patient outcomes, and long-term career satisfaction in medical-surgical nursing. Prioritizing nurse well-being enhances overall healthcare delivery and fosters a culture of resilience and excellence. Self-care and support systems play a crucial role in sustaining nurses' mental and emotional health, ultimately benefiting both the healthcare team and patients.

4.3.3 Unintended consequences

Unintended consequences in a Healthy Practice Environment and Professional Concepts for Medical Surgical Nurses refer to unexpected outcomes resulting from changes in practice. Awareness is crucial as these consequences can impact patient care, safety, and outcomes. Nurses play a vital role in identifying and mitigating such consequences. Examples include medication errors due to new protocols or increased workload leading to fatigue-related mistakes. Understanding and addressing unintended consequences are essential for maintaining a safe and effective care environment. Nurses must stay vigilant, adapt quickly, and collaborate to minimize risks and enhance patient well-being.

4.3.3.1 Moral distress

Moral distress arises when healthcare professionals feel unable to act in alignment with their ethical beliefs due to various constraints. It can stem from conflicts between patient needs and institutional policies, leading to emotional turmoil and moral dilemmas. To address moral distress, individuals can engage in open communication, seek support from colleagues, practice self-care, and advocate for ethical decision-making. Promoting a healthy practice environment, characterized by transparent communication, ethical leadership, and supportive policies, is crucial in mitigating moral distress and fostering professional well-being. Understanding and managing moral distress is essential for delivering high-quality patient care.

4.3.3.2 Moral injury

Moral injury in medical-surgical nursing refers to the psychological distress resulting from actions that conflict with one's values. Unintended consequences in healthcare, such as medical errors or resource limitations, can lead to moral injury. This can create a challenging practice environment for nurses, causing ethical dilemmas and moral distress. Nurses may experience moral injury when faced with end-of-life decisions, workplace conflicts, or witnessing patient suffering. To address and prevent moral injury, promoting open communication, ethical decision-making frameworks, and self-care strategies are essential in fostering a supportive and healthy workplace for medical-surgical nurses.

4.3.3.3 Compassion fatigue

The topic of compassion fatigue in medical surgical nursing refers to the emotional and physical exhaustion resulting from caring for patients in distress. Causes include high workload, lack of support, and exposure to suffering. Symptoms include apathy, irritability, and decreased empathy. Risk factors include personal history and work environment. Compassion fatigue can lead to burnout, decreased job satisfaction, and compromised patient care quality. Strategies to prevent and manage it include self-care, seeking support, and setting boundaries. A healthy work environment is crucial to support nurses' well-being and prevent compassion fatigue.

4.3.3.4 Burnout

Burnout in medical-surgical nursing refers to emotional exhaustion, depersonalization, and reduced personal accomplishment due to chronic workplace stress. Unintended consequences include decreased job satisfaction, increased errors, and higher turnover rates, impacting both nurses and the healthcare team negatively. Burnout compromises the healthy practice environment by lowering patient care quality, diminishing staff morale, and fostering a negative work culture. Professional concepts like self-care, resilience, and seeking support are crucial in combating burnout. Recognizing signs early and implementing interventions such as mindfulness practices, peer support programs, and workload management are essential in preventing and addressing burnout effectively.

4.3.4 Resource allocation

Resource allocation in healthcare involves distributing staff, equipment, and finances effectively to enhance patient care. Efficient allocation is crucial for optimal outcomes, including patient safety and care quality. Nurses play a vital role in advocating for proper resource distribution to support high-quality, patient-centered care. However, ethical challenges arise when balancing individual patient needs with limited resources. By prioritizing resource allocation, Medical Surgical Nurses can contribute to improved patient outcomes and organizational performance. Effective allocation strategies are essential for creating a healthy practice environment and upholding professional standards in medical-surgical settings.

4.3.4.1 Staffing

Staffing in medical-surgical nursing involves resource allocation, creating a healthy practice environment, and upholding professional concepts. Adequate staffing levels are crucial for ensuring quality patient care and safety. Effective staffing enhances the work environment, boosting job satisfaction and retention among healthcare professionals. Medical-surgical nurses play a vital role in advocating for proper staffing ratios and addressing staffing challenges. Inadequate staffing negatively impacts patient outcomes, leading to nurse burnout and affecting overall healthcare delivery. Strategies like evidence-based staffing models, nurse-to-patient ratios, and interdisciplinary collaboration help optimize staffing levels. Ethical considerations include balancing financial constraints with patient needs and staff well-being, emphasizing continuous monitoring and adjustment of staffing patterns to meet evolving healthcare demands.

4.3.4.2 Equipment

In a medical-surgical setting, equipment is vital for patient care, safety, and outcomes. Effective resource allocation ensures facilities have necessary equipment for high-quality care. Maintaining a healthy practice environment involves proper equipment maintenance, cleaning, and availability. Nurses have a professional responsibility to manage and utilize equipment ethically and legally for optimal patient care. Adhering to standards is crucial.

4.3.5 Peer accountability

Peer accountability in a healthy practice environment for Medical Surgical Nurses is vital. It involves open communication, constructive feedback, and a non-punitive approach to errors. Transparency, recognition of achievements, and collaboration in goal-setting are key. Creating a safe space for voicing concerns without fear of reprisal is crucial. Embracing peer accountability fosters teamwork, collaboration, and better patient outcomes. It promotes excellence, professionalism, and continuous quality improvement in healthcare delivery.

4.4 Scope of Practice and Ethics

In the realm of medical-surgical nursing, the Scope of Practice for CMSRNs delineates the duties and boundaries within which they operate. CMSRNs must uphold ethical principles, ensuring patient welfare and trust. Common ethical dilemmas include end-of-life care decisions and patient confidentiality breaches. To resolve conflicts, CMSRNs can engage in ethical decision-making processes and seek guidance from ethics committees. Upholding professional boundaries fosters ethical practice, safeguarding patient care quality. Ultimately, ethical decision-making profoundly impacts patient outcomes, underscoring the vital role of ethics in the CMSRN profession.

4.4.1 Scope of practice and code of ethics for nurses per local and regional nursing bodies

The scope of practice and code of ethics for nurses, as defined by local and regional nursing bodies, are crucial in ensuring high-quality patient care and upholding professional standards. Nurses must adhere to regulations set by organizations like the Academy of Medical-Surgical Nurses (AMSN) to maintain ethical principles. Violating these standards can lead to severe consequences for both nurses' careers and patient outcomes. It is essential for nurses to follow guidelines on patient confidentiality, informed consent, and professional boundaries to provide safe and effective care. Upholding these standards is paramount for the integrity of the nursing profession.

4.4.1.1 Code of Ethics for Nurses with Interpretive Statements

The Code of Ethics for Nurses with Interpretive Statements plays a crucial role in guiding ethical decision-making in nursing practice. Key principles such as patient advocacy, confidentiality, integrity, and professional boundaries are outlined in the code. It emphasizes promoting a culture of accountability, respect, and excellence in nursing. The code serves as a compass for nurses, ensuring they uphold the highest standards of ethical conduct while providing patient-centered care. By adhering to these principles, nurses can maintain trust, integrity, and professionalism in their interactions with patients, colleagues, and the healthcare system.

4.4.1.2 Standard V of the AMSN Scope and Standards

Standard V of the AMSN Scope and Standards emphasizes the nurse's commitment to maintaining competence and advancing professional practice. This includes engaging in lifelong learning, participating in professional development, and staying updated on evidence-based practices. Nurses are encouraged to seek growth opportunities, pursue advanced certifications, and contribute to the nursing profession through education and mentorship. By adhering to this standard, nurses ensure they provide high-quality care and continuously enhance their skills to meet the evolving healthcare needs.

4.4.1.3 Local governing Scope of Practice

Local governing Scope of Practice in nursing refers to regulations set by local and regional nursing bodies to define the responsibilities and limitations of nurses. These guidelines ensure safe and ethical patient care. Nurses must adhere to specific regulations such as medication administration, treatment protocols, and patient assessment within their defined scope. Understanding and following these rules align with the overall nursing code of ethics, promoting patient well-being. By staying informed about local regulations, nurses can navigate their Scope of Practice effectively, providing high-quality care while upholding professional standards.

4.4.2 Patients' rights and responsibilities

In the 'Patients� rights and responsibilities' topic under 'Scope of Practice and Ethics, Professional Concepts' for the CMSRN exam, understanding informed consent, confidentiality, autonomy, advocacy, and patient education is crucial. Informed consent ensures patients understand treatments; confidentiality protects patient information; autonomy respects patient decisions; advocacy involves speaking up for patients' rights; and patient education empowers patients to make informed choices. These aspects uphold ethical standards, promote patient-centered care, and enhance nurse-patient relationships. Being well-versed in these principles is essential for providing safe, effective, and compassionate medical-surgical care.

4.4.3 Professional reporting and resources

Professional reporting and resources are vital for CMSRNs, ensuring patient safety and interdisciplinary collaboration. Ethical considerations dictate accurate and timely reporting of patient data, emphasizing confidentiality and accountability. CMSRNs utilize electronic health records, standardized forms, and communication tools for effective reporting. These resources facilitate continuity of care and enhance quality through efficient data management. By upholding ethical standards and utilizing available resources, CMSRNs play a crucial role in delivering high-quality patient care.

4.4.3.1 Ethics

In professional nursing practice, ethics play a crucial role in guiding nurses towards providing high-quality care. Ethical principles such as beneficence, non-maleficence, autonomy, and justice are fundamental in decision-making. Maintaining patient confidentiality and privacy is paramount to build trust. Nurses must ethically use resources and report information accurately. Setting professional boundaries and making ethical decisions within the scope of practice ensures patient safety. Upholding professionalism standards through ethical conduct is vital. Nurses may face ethical dilemmas; effective resolution involves ethical reasoning and consultation. Upholding ethical principles is essential for medical-surgical nurses to deliver optimal care.

4.4.3.2 Scope of practice

Scope of practice in nursing refers to the specific duties and responsibilities that a healthcare professional is authorized to perform based on their education, training, and licensure. As a Certified Medical Surgical Registered Nurse (CMSRN), it is crucial to understand and adhere to your scope of practice to ensure safe and effective patient care. Key elements include legal boundaries, professional responsibilities, and ethical considerations. Staying within your scope promotes collaboration, upholds nursing standards, and prevents adverse outcomes. Practicing beyond your scope can lead to legal and ethical consequences. Resources for clarifying and expanding your scope as a CMSRN include continuing education and consultation with supervisors.

4.4.3.3 Unsafe practice

Unsafe practice in medical-surgical nursing refers to actions or behaviors that jeopardize patient safety and well-being. Professional reporting and resources play a crucial role in addressing unsafe practice by providing mechanisms to report incidents and access support. Scope of practice dictates the boundaries within which nurses must work to ensure safe and effective care. Ethics guide nurses in upholding moral principles when faced with unsafe practice situations. Identifying and addressing unsafe practice is a core responsibility of medical-surgical nurses to safeguard patients. Reporting unsafe practice is essential to prevent harm and improve care quality. Resources such as education and support systems aid in addressing and preventing unsafe practice. Professional concepts like accountability, advocacy, and quality improvement are integral in combating unsafe practice and promoting patient safety.

4.4.4 Policies, procedures, regulatory and licensure requirements, standards of practice, and applicable state, federal, and local laws

Understanding and following policies, procedures, regulatory requirements, and laws is crucial in medical-surgical nursing. Compliance ensures safe, ethical, and effective patient care. Violations can harm patients and tarnish a nurse's professional integrity. For instance, breaching confidentiality laws can lead to legal repercussions and loss of trust. Adhering to standards of practice maintains quality care and upholds ethical standards. Non-compliance may result in disciplinary actions, legal penalties, and compromised patient outcomes. Upholding these guidelines is essential for maintaining professionalism and ensuring patient safety in the healthcare setting.

4.5 Quality Management

Quality Management in medical-surgical nursing involves ensuring high-quality patient care through principles like continuous improvement and patient safety. Strategies include risk management and performance improvement. Tools such as audits and checklists aid in monitoring outcomes. CMSRNs play a vital role in implementing Quality Management initiatives, collaborating with teams, and adhering to standards. Evidence-based practice guides decision-making for optimal patient outcomes. By focusing on Quality Management, CMSRNs contribute to enhancing patient care quality and safety in medical-surgical settings.

4.5.1 Evidence-based guidelines for nursing sensitive indicators

Evidence-based guidelines for nursing sensitive indicators play a crucial role in quality management within healthcare settings. These indicators are essential for assessing the quality of nursing care and patient outcomes. Evidence-based practice is key in developing these guidelines, ensuring that interventions are based on the best available research. Commonly used nursing sensitive indicators include pressure ulcers, falls, and hospital-acquired infections. Adherence to these guidelines can lead to improved patient outcomes, enhanced quality of care provided by medical surgical nurses, and overall healthcare quality improvement. It is vital for CMSRNs to understand and implement these guidelines effectively in their practice.

4.5.2 Quality standards and policies

In medical-surgical nursing, quality standards and policies play a crucial role in ensuring optimal patient care. Quality standards are defined benchmarks that guide healthcare practices to achieve excellence. They serve to enhance patient safety, outcomes, and satisfaction. Implementation of these standards involves adherence to protocols, guidelines, and best practices. Quality policies complement standards by outlining specific procedures for compliance and continuous improvement. Aligning these with regulatory requirements and best practices is essential for improving patient outcomes and organizational performance. Examples include infection control protocols, medication administration guidelines, and patient safety initiatives.

4.5.3 Continuous quality and process improvement

Continuous quality and process improvement in healthcare involves ongoing efforts to enhance patient care, operational efficiency, and safety. As a Medical Surgical Nurse, embracing these principles is crucial. By implementing quality improvement tools like root cause analysis and Plan-Do-Study-Act cycles, nurses can pinpoint areas for enhancement and drive positive changes effectively. Analyzing data, monitoring performance metrics, and soliciting feedback are essential in this process. Collaboration, education, and training among healthcare professionals are vital for sustaining a culture of improvement. Ultimately, these initiatives lead to better patient outcomes, streamlined processes, and a safer healthcare environment.

4.5.4 Nursing professional practice model

In the realm of nursing, a Nursing Professional Practice Model serves as a framework that outlines the values, beliefs, and behaviors guiding nursing practice. It encompasses key components such as shared governance, interdisciplinary collaboration, evidence-based practice, and continuous quality improvement. This model plays a vital role in promoting quality patient care, enhancing nursing practice, and improving healthcare outcomes. By fostering a culture of excellence and supporting professional development, it empowers medical surgical nurses to deliver high-quality care. Successful implementation of Nursing Professional Practice Models has shown positive impacts on patient satisfaction, nurse satisfaction, and overall quality of care.

4.5.5 Adverse event reporting

Adverse event reporting in quality management for CMSRNs involves identifying, documenting, and communicating incidents that compromise patient safety. It is crucial in healthcare settings to ensure timely intervention and prevent future occurrences. CMSRNs play a vital role in reporting adverse events, adhering to ethical and legal standards. Reporting impacts patient safety, quality improvement, and regulatory compliance. Common adverse events include medication errors, falls, and pressure ulcers. Understanding and reporting these events are essential for enhancing patient care and maintaining high standards in medical-surgical nursing practice.

4.5.6 Patient customer experience based on data results

Analyzing data results is crucial for enhancing patient customer experience in healthcare. Data-driven insights help improve care quality by identifying areas for enhancement. Key performance indicators (KPIs) like patient satisfaction scores and wait times can be measured to evaluate service quality. Certified Medical Surgical Registered Nurses (CMSRNs) play a vital role in interpreting data to optimize patient experience. Continuous monitoring and adjustment based on data findings are essential for ongoing improvement. By utilizing data effectively, healthcare professionals can ensure high patient satisfaction levels and overall quality of care.

4.5.6.1 Surveys

Surveys play a crucial role in enhancing patient customer experience, quality management, and professional concepts in medical-surgical nursing. They are instrumental in gathering data on patient satisfaction, pinpointing areas for service improvement, and evaluating the effectiveness of quality management strategies. By collecting feedback from patients, surveys help in analyzing healthcare delivery trends and making informed decisions to elevate care quality. Moreover, surveys aid in assessing healthcare professionals' performance, ensuring adherence to professional standards, and fostering continuous learning and development in the field.

4.5.6.2 Value-based purchasing

Value-based purchasing in healthcare emphasizes patient outcomes, quality management, and professional ethics. It aims to improve care quality, reduce costs, and enhance patient satisfaction. Key aspects include defining goals, implementing strategies, and considering implications for providers. Data-driven decisions are crucial, incorporating patient feedback for better outcomes. Aligning with quality management, it promotes high-value care while upholding ethical standards. By focusing on patient experience and cost-effective practices, value-based purchasing drives improvements in care delivery and overall healthcare quality.

4.5.7 Service recovery

Service recovery in healthcare involves addressing and resolving patient concerns to enhance quality care. For Medical Surgical Nurses, service recovery is vital for patient satisfaction and outcomes. Key principles include prompt response, active listening, and empathy. Strategies like apologizing, offering solutions, and following up can improve patient experience. Effective communication, empathy, and problem-solving skills are crucial. Examples of service recovery situations include medication errors, delayed care, or poor communication. By implementing service recovery effectively, nurses can enhance patient trust, satisfaction, and overall quality of care.

4.5.8 Project development

In project development for medical-surgical nursing, key stages include initiation, planning, execution, monitoring, and closure. Setting clear objectives, creating timelines, efficient resource allocation, and effective risk management are crucial. Projects enhance quality outcomes, patient care, and professional growth. Teamwork, communication, and leadership play vital roles in successful project development within healthcare settings. By following these steps and emphasizing collaboration, communication, and leadership, medical-surgical nurses can drive positive change and improve overall patient care quality.

4.6 Evidence-Based Practice and Research

Evidence-Based Practice and Research in nursing involves integrating current research, clinical expertise, and patient values to deliver high-quality care. CMSRNs play a crucial role in promoting evidence-based practice within the healthcare team. By utilizing evidence-based guidelines, nurses can enhance patient outcomes and improve overall care quality in medical-surgical settings. This process involves critically appraising research, applying findings to patient care, and continuously evaluating outcomes to ensure best practices. Embracing evidence-based practice empowers nurses to make informed decisions, leading to better patient outcomes and advancing the standard of care in medical-surgical nursing.

4.6.1 Legislative and licensure requirements

In the realm of medical-surgical nursing, understanding legislative and licensure requirements is crucial for delivering high-quality care. Nurses must comply with laws, such as the Nurse Practice Act, which outline their scope of practice and standards of care. Additionally, staying abreast of professional standards set by organizations like the AMSN is essential. By integrating evidence-based practice into their daily routines, nurses can enhance patient outcomes. This involves utilizing research findings, clinical expertise, and patient preferences to inform decision-making. Upholding these requirements ensures safe and effective patient care.

4.6.2 Evidence-based practice principles

In medical-surgical nursing, evidence-based practice (EBP) is crucial for informed decision-making. Integrating evidence, clinical expertise, and patient preferences ensures high-quality care. The EBP process involves formulating a clinical question, searching for evidence, critically appraising it, and applying findings to practice. Staying updated with research and continuously evaluating practice are key. EBP enhances patient outcomes, promotes safety, and advances the nursing profession. By following EBP principles, medical-surgical nurses can provide optimal care based on the best available evidence, leading to improved patient outcomes and overall healthcare quality.

4.6.3 Research process

In the realm of evidence-based practice and research, medical-surgical nurses play a crucial role in advancing patient care. The research process involves formulating a research question, conducting a thorough literature review, designing a study methodology, collecting and analyzing data, interpreting results, and disseminating findings. Ethical considerations, such as obtaining informed consent, ensuring participant confidentiality, and following research protocols, are paramount. Evidence-based practice guides clinical decision-making, leading to improved patient outcomes. By integrating research findings into their practice, medical-surgical nurses can deliver high-quality, evidence-based care, ultimately enhancing patient well-being.

5   Nursing Teamwork and Collaboration

In medical-surgical nursing, teamwork and collaboration are vital for delivering exceptional patient care. Effective communication, interdisciplinary collaboration, role clarity, mutual respect, and shared decision-making are key aspects. These elements enhance patient outcomes, boost job satisfaction, and create a positive work environment. For instance, a successful scenario could involve nurses, physicians, and therapists working together seamlessly to develop a comprehensive care plan for a post-operative patient, leading to faster recovery and improved overall well-being. Such collaborative efforts showcase the power of teamwork in enhancing patient care in medical-surgical settings.

5.1   Delegation and Supervision

Delegation and supervision are vital in nursing teamwork. Effective delegation ensures safe patient care by following principles like the five rights, clear communication, and accountability. Registered nurses delegate tasks based on scope of practice, competency, and legal considerations. Supervision involves monitoring tasks, providing guidance, and ensuring quality outcomes. Challenges include communication and teamwork issues. Strategies involve open communication, mutual respect, and teamwork. Supervision plays a crucial role in guiding team members and ensuring patient safety. Effective delegation and supervision are essential for efficient teamwork and collaboration in healthcare settings.

5.1.1   Delegation and/or supervision practices

Key aspects of delegation and supervision in nursing teamwork include effective delegation principles, RN's role, legal/ethical considerations, successful strategies, clear communication/feedback importance. Accountability, responsibility, and impact on patient care outcomes are crucial. Challenges like inadequate training, communication issues, and staff resistance can arise. Nurses must prioritize patient safety, competence, and follow organizational policies. Collaboration, trust, and open communication enhance delegation success. Regular feedback, ongoing education, and support promote effective delegation and supervision practices in medical-surgical nursing.

5.1.2   Scope of practice

Scope of Practice in Delegation and Supervision, Nursing Teamwork, and Collaboration is crucial for CMSRNs. It defines the tasks they can perform based on education, training, and experience. Understanding and adhering to this scope ensures safe patient care. Legal and ethical considerations are vital, preventing unauthorized tasks. Delegation expands practice but requires accountability. Effective teamwork maximizes capabilities within the scope. Exceeding one's scope can lead to errors and legal issues. Following guidelines is essential to avoid harm. Collaboration enhances patient outcomes, emphasizing the importance of working within defined boundaries.

5.1.2.1   Licensed and unlicensed team members

In a healthcare setting, licensed team members, such as registered nurses, have advanced education and training, allowing them to assess, diagnose, and treat patients independently within their scope of practice. They can delegate tasks to unlicensed team members, like nursing assistants, who assist with activities of daily living under supervision. Effective communication and collaboration between licensed and unlicensed team members are crucial for patient safety. Clear guidelines and oversight are essential when delegating tasks to unlicensed team members to ensure quality care. Ethical considerations include maintaining patient confidentiality and safety at all times.

5.1.3   Prioritization skills

Prioritization skills are crucial in nursing for effective delegation, supervision, teamwork, and collaboration. Nurses use these skills to manage tasks, make critical decisions, and ensure patient safety. By prioritizing, nurses can delegate tasks to team members based on urgency and complexity, supervise their completion, and foster a collaborative environment. This leads to improved patient outcomes, enhanced interdisciplinary communication, and higher quality of care. For example, prioritizing patient assessments over administrative tasks ensures timely interventions, benefiting overall care delivery.

5.1.3.1   Disease process

In medical-surgical nursing, understanding disease processes is crucial for effective patient care. Nurses must grasp the pathophysiology, progression, and systemic effects of common illnesses. This knowledge enables prioritization of interventions, delegation of tasks based on acuity, and supervision of care delivery. Collaboration with the healthcare team ensures holistic patient management. By comprehending disease processes, nurses can anticipate complications, intervene promptly, and promote positive outcomes. Prioritization skills, delegation, supervision, and teamwork are essential in providing comprehensive and coordinated care to patients with diverse medical conditions.

5.1.4   Budgetary considerations

In the realm of nursing, budgetary considerations play a pivotal role in delegation, supervision, teamwork, and collaboration. Budget constraints directly impact staffing levels, resource allocation, and ultimately, the quality of patient care. Financial limitations can influence decision-making processes regarding task delegation, staff supervision, and fostering effective teamwork among healthcare professionals. Nurse leaders must adeptly manage budgets to ensure optimal patient outcomes while upholding cost-efficiency.

Strategies for balancing budgetary constraints include prioritizing adequate staffing, training, and resources to cultivate a collaborative and efficient healthcare environment.

5.1.4.1 Supplies

In the medical-surgical setting, supplies play a crucial role in patient care. Effective supply management is essential for cost-effectiveness and operational efficiency. Nurses are responsible for delegating tasks related to inventory, ordering, and restocking supplies. Supervision is key to prevent waste and ensure optimal patient outcomes. Collaboration among nursing staff is vital for maintaining adequate supplies. Challenges such as supply shortages can be addressed through teamwork and open communication. By prioritizing supply management, nurses can enhance patient care and streamline healthcare operations.

5.1.4.2 Staffing

Staffing in nursing involves crucial aspects like budgetary considerations, delegation, supervision, and teamwork. Adequate staffing levels are vital for ensuring high-quality patient care, cost management, and fostering a positive work environment. Nurse managers play a pivotal role in making staffing decisions, utilizing strategies to optimize ratios and address budget constraints effectively. Clear communication and accountability are essential for successful delegation and supervision practices. Effective staffing enhances teamwork and collaboration among nursing staff, leading to improved patient outcomes and job satisfaction.

5.1.4.3 Fiscal efficiency

Fiscal efficiency in nursing involves optimizing resource use, cost-effectiveness, and quality care. Nurses play a vital role in managing budgets, delegating tasks, supervising staff, and fostering teamwork. By promoting fiscal efficiency, nurses enhance patient outcomes, organizational sustainability, and healthcare system effectiveness. Budgetary considerations require prudent allocation of funds for essential resources. Delegation and supervision ensure tasks are appropriately assigned and overseen. Nursing teamwork and collaboration facilitate seamless care delivery. Ultimately, prioritizing fiscal efficiency leads to improved patient care, financial stability, and overall healthcare system performance.

5.2 Career Development Relationships

Career Development Relationships in Nursing Teamwork and Collaboration are vital for professional growth. These relationships encompass mentorship, networking, continuing education, and workplace support systems. By fostering strong connections, nurses enhance teamwork, leading to improved patient outcomes and the advancement of the nursing profession. Certified Medical Surgical Registered Nurses (CMSRNs) play a crucial role in promoting these relationships within the medical-surgical specialty, ensuring ongoing learning, collaboration, and excellence in patient care. Through mentorship and networking, CMSRNs contribute to a supportive environment that nurtures career development and elevates the standard of care in medical-surgical nursing.

5.2.1 Professional engagement

Professional engagement in medical-surgical nursing involves active participation in career development relationships, teamwork, and collaboration. It is crucial for creating a positive work environment, improving patient care outcomes, and fostering professional growth. Key aspects include effective communication, interdisciplinary teamwork, continuous learning, and relationship-building. Professional engagement enhances job satisfaction, supports career advancement, and contributes to overall success in the field. By prioritizing engagement, nurses can cultivate strong connections with colleagues and patients, leading to improved teamwork, better patient outcomes, and personal fulfillment in their careers.

5.2.2 Mentoring and coaching resources

In the realm of medical surgical nursing, mentoring and coaching resources play a pivotal role in nurturing career development relationships, fostering nursing teamwork, and promoting collaboration. These resources serve as pillars for professional growth, facilitating knowledge sharing, skill enhancement, and emotional support within the healthcare environment. Effective mentoring and coaching programs not only boost job satisfaction and retention rates but also elevate the overall quality of patient care in the medical surgical unit. By providing guidance, encouragement, and expertise, mentors and coaches empower nurses to excel in their roles, ultimately benefiting both the individual and the healthcare team.

5.2.3 Reflective practice

Reflective practice in career development relationships, nursing teamwork, and collaboration involves self-assessment and learning from experiences. It is crucial for professional growth, enhancing teamwork dynamics, and fostering collaboration in healthcare. By reflecting, nurses identify areas for improvement, enhance critical thinking, and learn from past situations. Engaging in reflective practice improves communication, empathy towards colleagues and patients, leading to better patient outcomes. It promotes continuous learning, self-awareness, and accountability among medical-surgical nurses, creating a culture of excellence and growth.

5.2.4 Roles and responsibilities

In the realm of career development relationships, nursing teamwork, and collaboration, a Medical Surgical Nurse plays a pivotal role. Effective communication, leadership, and accountability are essential in fostering these relationships. Collaborating with healthcare team members ensures optimal patient care. Advocating for patients, creating a safe environment, and upholding ethical standards are key responsibilities. Professional development, continuing education, and lifelong learning enhance the nurse's ability to deliver high-quality care. By embracing these roles and responsibilities, Medical Surgical Nurses contribute significantly to the healthcare team and the well-being of their patients.

5.2.5 Coaching and learning theories

Coaching and learning theories play a vital role in career development, teamwork, and collaboration among medical surgical nurses. Coaching enhances professional growth by providing guidance and support. Learning theories like behaviorism, constructivism, and social learning theory aid in effective coaching and mentorship. They promote continuous learning and improvement. Coaching fosters teamwork, communication, and collaboration within nursing teams. For example, behaviorism focuses on observable behaviors, constructivism emphasizes active learning, and social learning theory highlights the importance of social interactions. Applying these theories can create a culture of learning and development in medical surgical nursing practice.

5.2.6   Professional empowerment

Professional empowerment is vital for career growth, teamwork, and collaboration in medical-surgical nursing. It involves autonomy in decision-making, self-advocacy, and creating a supportive work environment. Nurses benefit from continuous learning, recognizing team contributions, and effective communication with healthcare professionals. Empowerment fosters trust, respect, and a positive culture, enhancing job satisfaction and patient care quality. By empowering nurses, organizations promote professional development and improve overall outcomes.

5.2.7   Orientation planning and preceptor best practices

Orientation planning and preceptor best practices are crucial for fostering career development relationships, nursing teamwork, and collaboration. Preceptors play a vital role in guiding new nurses through orientation, ensuring a smooth transition. Effective orientation planning involves setting clear goals, selecting suitable preceptors, and providing comprehensive training and support. A well-structured orientation program enhances nurse retention, job satisfaction, and ultimately improves patient outcomes. Clear communication, feedback mechanisms, and mentorship are essential components that contribute to the successful integration of new nurses into the healthcare team.

5.2.8   Career development resources

Career development resources play a crucial role in enhancing career growth and job satisfaction for medical-surgical nurses. These resources include continuing education programs, mentorship opportunities, networking events, certification courses, and skill-building workshops. By utilizing these resources, nurses can improve patient outcomes, enhance job performance, and achieve professional success. Moreover, access to career development resources fosters a supportive and collaborative work environment within healthcare teams, promoting effective teamwork and collaboration. Overall, investing in career development resources is essential for nurses to stay current, advance their skills, and contribute positively to the field of medical-surgical nursing.

5.2.8.1   Education

Education is pivotal in nursing career development, nurturing relationships, and fostering teamwork. Continuous learning and formal programs enhance nursing practice, elevating patient care. Professional development opportunities empower nurses to excel, contributing to a knowledgeable workforce. Education improves communication within multidisciplinary teams, promoting collaboration for optimal patient outcomes. By investing in education, nurses build expertise, strengthen relationships, and deliver high-quality, patient-centered care. Prioritizing education is key to advancing in the nursing field, establishing meaningful connections, and cultivating a culture of teamwork and excellence.

5.2.8.2   Training

Training in career development resources, relationships, nursing teamwork, and collaboration is vital for medical-surgical nurses. It enhances skills, knowledge, and competencies, fostering professional growth. Training programs promote effective communication, teamwork, and collaboration among healthcare professionals, leading to optimal patient outcomes. Examples of training initiatives include advanced certification courses, simulation exercises, and interdisciplinary workshops. These opportunities empower nurses to advance their careers, contribute meaningfully to the healthcare team, and deliver high-quality patient care.

5.3   Professional Development

To enhance nursing teamwork and collaboration, prioritize professional development by staying updated on evidence-based practices, actively participating in interdisciplinary team meetings for better communication, pursuing additional education for skill expansion, and engaging in reflective practice for self-improvement. For example, attending workshops on effective communication, completing courses on conflict resolution, and regularly reviewing current literature on teamwork strategies can contribute to improved collaboration within the healthcare team. By continuously investing in professional growth, Medical Surgical Nurses can elevate patient care outcomes and foster a culture of teamwork and collaboration in clinical settings.

5.3.1   Professional nursing practice and individual competencies

Professional nursing practice and individual competencies are vital in professional development, teamwork, and collaboration. Ethical decision-making, evidence-based practice, and quality improvement are key in nursing. Competencies like critical thinking, communication, and cultural sensitivity enhance patient care. Ongoing education boosts nursing practice and fosters teamwork across healthcare disciplines. By honing these skills, nurses can deliver high-quality care, improve patient outcomes, and promote a collaborative healthcare environment.

5.3.2   Professional behaviors

Professional behaviors encompass actions and attitudes that reflect a nurse's commitment to professional development, teamwork, and collaboration. These behaviors are crucial for fostering a positive work environment and improving patient outcomes. Medical-surgical nurses must demonstrate respect, accountability, and effective communication in their practice. By exhibiting professionalism, nurses enhance teamwork, facilitate collaboration, and ensure patient safety. Professional behaviors also play a vital role in maintaining quality care standards and optimizing healthcare delivery. Ultimately, these behaviors contribute to a cohesive healthcare team and promote excellence in patient care.

5.3.2.1   Network

In the realm of medical-surgical nursing, networking plays a pivotal role in fostering professional growth and collaboration. Networking involves establishing and nurturing relationships within the healthcare community to enhance knowledge sharing, career progression, and interdisciplinary teamwork. By attending conferences, joining professional organizations, engaging in online forums, and participating in mentorship programs, nurses can expand their network and stay abreast of industry trends. Effective networking not only cultivates a culture of continuous learning but also contributes to a supportive work environment, improved patient care outcomes, and the advancement of medical-surgical nursing as a whole.

5.3.2.2 Participate in professional organization

Participating in professional organizations like the Academy of Medical-Surgical Nurses (AMSN) is crucial for medical-surgical nurses. It offers networking opportunities, access to continuing education, and advocacy for the nursing profession. Engaging in such organizations enhances professional growth, fosters a sense of community, and advances medical-surgical nursing practice. Moreover, it promotes teamwork and collaboration among nurses, leading to improved patient outcomes and a more cohesive healthcare delivery system. Being actively involved in professional organizations is key to staying updated, connected, and contributing to the betterment of the nursing profession.

5.3.3 Clinical judgement

Clinical judgement in nursing involves the ability to make effective decisions based on critical thinking, evidence-based practice, and patient assessment data. It plays a crucial role in guiding nursing practice within multidisciplinary teams. Nurses rely on their critical thinking skills to interpret complex information, apply evidence-based interventions, and deliver optimal patient care. Effective communication and collaboration among team members are essential for enhancing clinical judgement and achieving positive patient outcomes. Ongoing education, training, and mentorship are vital for developing and refining clinical judgement skills among medical-surgical nurses, ensuring high-quality care delivery in diverse healthcare settings.

5.3.4 Peer review methods

Peer review methods play a crucial role in professional development, nursing teamwork, and collaboration among medical-surgical nurses. Various methods include peer evaluations, feedback, mentoring, and coaching. These methods enhance teamwork by fostering open communication, increasing accountability, and promoting professional growth. Challenges may arise, such as resistance to feedback or lack of standardized processes. Strategies to overcome these challenges include establishing clear evaluation criteria, providing training on giving and receiving feedback, and promoting a culture of continuous learning and improvement. Effective peer review methods ultimately lead to improved patient care outcomes and a more cohesive healthcare team.

5.3.5 Educational needs assessment

Educational needs assessment in professional development involves evaluating learning gaps to enhance nursing teamwork and collaboration. Conducting assessments in healthcare settings is crucial for improving medical-surgical nurses' knowledge and skills. The process includes identifying learning needs, setting objectives, and evaluating program effectiveness. These assessments promote continuous learning, enhance patient outcomes, and foster a collaborative nursing culture. By understanding educational needs, nurses can address skill deficiencies, enhance teamwork, and ultimately provide better patient care. Regular assessments ensure ongoing professional growth and contribute to a positive work environment.

5.4 Leadership

In nursing teamwork and collaboration, leadership involves guiding and inspiring team members towards common goals. Essential aspects include effective communication, decisive decision-making, adept conflict resolution, and the ability to motivate others. Successful nurse leaders enhance patient outcomes, boost team performance, and cultivate a positive work environment. Transformational and servant leadership styles are vital, emphasizing empowerment and service. Continuous professional development and leadership training are crucial for nurses to excel in leading interdisciplinary healthcare teams. Effective leadership in nursing fosters unity, efficiency, and excellence in patient care.

5.4.1 Regulatory and compliance standards

In the realm of healthcare leadership, nursing teamwork, and collaboration, adherence to regulatory and compliance standards is paramount. Regulatory bodies play a crucial role in establishing these standards, ensuring patient safety and quality care. Non-compliance can have detrimental effects on patient outcomes. To maintain adherence, healthcare teams must implement strategies such as regular training and audits. Nurses and leaders bear the responsibility of upholding these standards, with consequences for failure including legal repercussions and compromised patient care. Proactively embracing a culture of compliance fosters a safe environment and enhances patient well-being.

5.4.2 Organizational structure

Organizational structure in healthcare refers to the framework that outlines hierarchical levels, chain of command, communication channels, and decision-making processes. It plays a vital role in promoting effective leadership, enhancing nursing teamwork, and fostering collaboration among healthcare professionals. A well-defined organizational structure contributes to improved patient outcomes, increased staff satisfaction, and overall organizational success. Challenges from ineffective structures can hinder workflow and communication. Best practices for optimal structures include clear roles, open communication, and shared decision-making. Designing and implementing an efficient organizational structure is crucial for healthcare institutions to thrive.

5.4.3 Shared decision-making

Shared decision-making in healthcare leadership, nursing teamwork, and collaboration involves active involvement of all team members to ensure patient-centered care. It promotes effective communication, enhances patient outcomes, and fosters teamwork. Key principles include respecting individual perspectives, open communication, and mutual trust. Involving nurses, physicians, and other professionals in decision-making leads to improved patient satisfaction, increased staff morale, and better quality of care. This approach ensures decisions are made collaboratively, considering the best interest of the patient. Shared decision-making is essential for creating a culture of collaboration and excellence in medical-surgical settings.

5.4.4 Nursing philosophy

Nursing philosophy in leadership, teamwork, and collaboration is vital for guiding medical-surgical nurses. It encompasses core values, beliefs, and principles shaping their practice. A clear philosophy enhances leadership by providing a framework for decision-making. It fosters effective teamwork and collaboration among healthcare professionals, leading to improved patient outcomes. For instance, a philosophy centered on patient-centered care promotes a culture of excellence. By aligning actions with philosophy, nurses can navigate challenges, inspire others, and deliver high-quality care in a medical-surgical setting.

5.4.5 Leadership models

In the realm of medical-surgical nursing, leadership models play a pivotal role in fostering effective teamwork and collaboration among healthcare professionals. Various leadership models, including transformational, situational, servant, and democratic leadership, offer unique approaches to guiding and managing nursing teams. Transformational leadership inspires and motivates team members towards a shared vision. Situational leadership emphasizes adapting leadership styles to suit different situations. Servant leadership focuses on serving others first, while democratic leadership encourages shared decision-making. These models influence job satisfaction, performance, and patient outcomes within medical-surgical units by promoting communication, trust, and empowerment among team members.

5.4.6 Nursing care delivery systems

Nursing care delivery systems are vital in healthcare, emphasizing leadership, teamwork, and collaboration. Types include team nursing, primary nursing, case management, and patient-centered care. Team nursing involves a group of nurses working together, primary nursing assigns one nurse per patient, case management coordinates care across disciplines, and patient-centered care prioritizes individual needs. Each system has unique advantages and challenges. Effective leadership, communication, and teamwork are crucial for successful implementation. These systems enhance patient outcomes, improve care quality, and foster interdisciplinary collaboration, ultimately benefiting both patients and healthcare teams.

5.4.7 Change management

Change management in medical-surgical nursing involves implementing and adapting to organizational changes within a healthcare setting. Effective strategies are crucial for successful transitions. Nursing leaders play a vital role in guiding interdisciplinary teams through change processes, fostering collaboration, and ensuring positive outcomes for patients and staff. Key principles include clear communication, staff involvement, and continuous education. Embracing best practices such as creating a supportive environment, addressing resistance, and promoting a culture of adaptability are essential for delivering high-quality patient care amidst evolving healthcare landscapes.

5.4.7.1 Awareness

In the realm of healthcare, awareness plays a pivotal role in change management, leadership, nursing teamwork, and collaboration. It involves self-awareness, situational awareness, and cultural awareness. Awareness enhances communication, fosters a culture of safety, improves patient outcomes, and facilitates effective decision-making. By being aware of oneself, the surroundings, and diverse cultures, healthcare professionals can create a positive work environment, promote interdisciplinary collaboration, and navigate complex situations adeptly. Ultimately, heightened awareness empowers nurses and healthcare providers to adapt to changes seamlessly and deliver exceptional patient care.

5.4.7.2 Desire

In the realm of change management, leadership, nursing teamwork, and collaboration, desire serves as a powerful motivator for individuals and teams in healthcare settings. It fuels the drive to achieve organizational goals, fosters innovation, and cultivates a positive work environment. Desire plays a crucial role in inspiring healthcare professionals to embrace change, assume leadership responsibilities, and engage in effective teamwork. It significantly impacts employee satisfaction, job performance, and ultimately, patient outcomes in the medical-surgical nursing field. Harnessing the power of desire can lead to enhanced adaptability, leadership development, and successful collaboration within healthcare teams.

5.4.7.3 Knowledge

In the realm of change management, leadership, nursing teamwork, and collaboration, knowledge plays a pivotal role. It enhances decision-making by providing a solid foundation for informed choices. Knowledge fosters innovation, driving improvements in patient care. Effective communication is facilitated by a deep understanding of best practices. Continuous learning and professional development are essential for expanding knowledge, enabling healthcare professionals to adapt to change, inspire others, and cultivate a collaborative culture. The various types of knowledge, including theoretical, practical, evidence-based, and experiential, influence decision-making and problem-solving in the dynamic healthcare setting. Challenges in acquiring, sharing, and applying knowledge exist but present opportunities for growth and improved patient outcomes.

5.4.7.4 Ability

In the realm of medical-surgical nursing, Ability encompasses adaptability, critical thinking, communication, and problem-solving skills. These abilities are crucial for managing change, leading teams, and fostering collaboration. For instance, adaptability allows nurses to adjust to new situations swiftly. Critical thinking aids in making sound clinical judgments. Effective communication ensures clear information exchange, while problem-solving skills help in resolving complex issues. By possessing these abilities, nurses can enhance patient outcomes and team effectiveness. For example, strong communication skills can lead to better patient education and improved interdisciplinary collaboration, ultimately resulting in higher-quality care.

5.4.7.5 Reinforcement [ADKAR])

In change management, leadership, nursing teamwork, and collaboration, reinforcement plays a crucial role in sustaining positive changes. The ADKAR model emphasizes the importance of reinforcement to drive successful change efforts. Effective reinforcement strategies enhance leadership practices by providing continuous support and recognition. They also promote teamwork among nursing staff by reinforcing desired behaviors and fostering a culture of collaboration within healthcare teams. By utilizing the ADKAR model, organizations can ensure long-term sustainability of change initiatives and achieve their organizational goals through consistent reinforcement of new practices and behaviors.

5.4.8 Recruitment and retention

Recruitment and retention are vital in nursing leadership, teamwork, and collaboration. Effective strategies to attract and keep qualified staff are crucial. Leadership plays a key role in creating a positive work environment that enhances retention. Teamwork significantly impacts recruitment success, while collaboration fosters a supportive workplace culture. Challenges in recruiting and retaining nurses exist, but innovative solutions can address these issues. Long-term benefits of successful recruitment and retention practices include staff satisfaction, improved patient outcomes, and enhanced organizational success in healthcare settings.

5.4.9 Employee engagement

Employee engagement is vital in healthcare, especially within nursing teams. Effective leadership fosters engagement, creating a positive work environment. Benefits include increased job satisfaction, better patient outcomes, and enhanced teamwork. Nurse leaders can boost engagement by promoting open communication, recognizing achievements, providing growth opportunities, and fostering a supportive culture. Encouraging collaboration and involving staff in decision-making also enhances engagement levels. Overall, high employee engagement leads to a more motivated workforce, improved patient care, and a positive workplace atmosphere.

5.4.10 Staff advocacy

Staff advocacy in nursing leadership involves advocating for the rights, well-being, and needs of the nursing team. Nurse leaders play a crucial role in creating a positive work environment, enhancing job satisfaction, and improving team performance through effective advocacy. Key strategies include active listening, open communication, and addressing workplace challenges promptly. By fostering a culture of support and empowerment, nurse leaders can boost retention rates and overall team morale. Staff advocacy is essential for promoting collaboration, teamwork, and ensuring the success and resilience of the healthcare professionals within the organization.

5.4.11 Conflict management

Conflict management in medical-surgical nursing involves resolving disagreements effectively to maintain a harmonious work environment. It is crucial for leaders to address conflicts promptly to enhance teamwork and collaboration. Effective strategies include open communication, active listening, and compromise. Nurses can utilize negotiation skills and mediation techniques to find common ground and reach resolutions. Unresolved conflicts can negatively impact patient care quality and team cohesion. By implementing sound conflict resolution practices, medical-surgical nurses can foster a positive atmosphere, improve team dynamics, and ultimately enhance patient outcomes.

5.4.12 Financial stewardship

Financial stewardship in nursing leadership involves budget management, cost containment, revenue generation, and regulatory compliance. Nurses must communicate effectively, align financial goals with patient care, and promote cost-effective practices. Collaboration and shared accountability are key in optimizing resource utilization and enhancing patient outcomes. By integrating financial considerations into daily practice, Medical Surgical Nurses can drive positive financial outcomes while upholding nursing excellence.

5.5 Disaster Planning and Management

In Disaster Planning and Management, Medical Surgical Nurses must be adept at developing emergency response plans, conducting drills, and coordinating with healthcare teams. Triage and patient prioritization are crucial during crises, ensuring safety and emotional support for all. Effective teamwork and collaboration are vital, requiring clear communication and cooperation among all healthcare professionals. Nurses work alongside physicians, first responders, and community partners to ensure a coordinated response, enhancing patient outcomes and safety. Disaster Planning and Management within Nursing Teamwork is essential for Medical Surgical Nurses to navigate various disasters successfully.

5.5.1 Emergency procedures

In disaster planning, emergency procedures are crucial for a prompt response. Nurses must collaborate effectively, triage patients, prioritize care, and communicate well during crises. Training and preparedness are key to a coordinated effort with healthcare professionals and emergency teams. Having well-defined procedures ensures optimal patient care. Regular drills enhance readiness for various emergencies. Teamwork is essential in implementing these procedures to provide efficient care during disasters. Nurses play a vital role in coordinating efforts and ensuring a swift and effective response.

5.5.2 Hospital incident command structure

In disaster planning, Hospital Incident Command Structure (HICS) is vital. It organizes response efforts efficiently. HICS comprises command staff, general staff, and functional units. Nurses play key roles in patient care coordination, communication, and resource management. Effective teamwork among healthcare professionals, especially nurses, is crucial. Collaboration within HICS enhances disaster response and patient outcomes. Nurses ensure smooth operations, provide quality care, and facilitate communication. Their involvement in HICS is essential for a well-coordinated response during emergencies.

CMSRN

Practice

Questions

[SET 1]

Question 1: Ms. Johnson, a 65-year-old patient, is admitted to the medical-surgical unit with a diagnosis of malnutrition. She has a history of diabetes and hypertension. The healthcare team plans to initiate enteral nutrition to meet her individualized nutritional needs. Which complication is a common concern associated with enteral nutrition in patients like Ms. Johnson?
A) Hyperglycemia
B) Hypertension
C) Aspiration pneumonia
D) Hypokalemia

Question 2: Scenario: Mr. Smith, a 65-year-old patient admitted for a surgical procedure, has a history of Methicillin-resistant Staphylococcus aureus (MRSA) colonization. Which infection control measure is most appropriate to prevent the transmission of MRSA in the healthcare setting?
A) Standard Precautions
B) Droplet Precautions
C) Airborne Precautions
D) Contact Precautions

Question 3: Scenario: Ms. Johnson, a 65-year-old patient, is admitted to the medical-surgical unit with a diagnosis of heart failure. During the assessment, the nurse notes crackles in the lung bases, peripheral edema, and increased shortness of breath. The patient is receiving oxygen therapy via nasal cannula at 2 liters per minute. Vital signs are as follows: blood pressure 148/92 mmHg, heart rate 110 bpm, respiratory rate 24 breaths/min, and oxygen saturation of 92%. The nurse identifies the nursing diagnosis as "Impaired Gas Exchange related to decreased oxygen diffusion across the alveolar-capillary membrane as evidenced by crackles, increased shortness of breath, and oxygen saturation of 92%." Which intervention should the nurse prioritize in the plan of care for Ms. Johnson?
A) Administer a diuretic to reduce fluid volume overload.
B) Increase the oxygen flow rate to 4 liters per minute.
C) Assist the patient with activities of daily living (ADLs).
D) Elevate the head of the bed to a semi-Fowler's position.

Question 4: Which of the following best defines implicit bias in the context of healthcare?
A) Conscious stereotypes influencing decision-making
B) Unintentional and unconscious stereotypes affecting behavior
C) Deliberate prejudice guiding patient care
D) Open and transparent biases shaping treatment plans

Question 5: Scenario: Mr. Smith, a 65-year-old patient, is admitted to the medical-surgical unit with a diagnosis of pneumonia. The nurse notes that the prescribed antibiotic is not in line with the hospital's formulary. What action should the nurse take based on quality standards and policies?
A) Administer the prescribed antibiotic as ordered
B) Consult with the healthcare provider to discuss an alternative from the formulary
C) Substitute the antibiotic with a similar one from the hospital pharmacy
D) Disregard the formulary and administer a different antibiotic

Question 6: Scenario: Mrs. Smith, a 65-year-old patient, has been admitted to the medical-surgical unit for a scheduled surgery. She expresses concerns about the upcoming procedure and mentions feeling anxious about the post-operative pain management. As a CMSRN, what is the most appropriate action to address Mrs. Smith's concerns?
A) Provide Mrs. Smith with a detailed explanation of the surgical procedure and pain management plan.
B) Assure Mrs. Smith that post-operative pain is minimal and does not require any interventions.
C) Dismiss Mrs. Smith's concerns as common pre-surgery anxiety.
D) Refer Mrs. Smith to the hospital's social worker for emotional support.

Question 7: Scenario: Mr. Johnson, a postoperative patient, is scheduled for an urgent surgery. As the nurse, you are preparing for a potential downtime situation in the electronic health record system. Which action should you prioritize during this time?
A) Continue documenting on paper and transfer to the electronic system once it is restored.
B) Delay documentation until the system is back online.
C) Use a colleague's login credentials to document in the system.
D) Inform the healthcare team that documentation is not necessary during downtime.

Question 8: Scenario: Mr. Johnson, a 65-year-old patient, is admitted to the medical-surgical unit for the treatment of pneumonia. He has a history of hypertension and diabetes. The healthcare provider prescribes a new antibiotic for his pneumonia. After receiving the first dose of the antibiotic, Mr. Johnson develops a rash, itching, and shortness of breath. His blood pressure is 90/60 mmHg, heart rate is 110 bpm, and oxygen saturation is 92%. What is the most appropriate action for the nurse to take first?
A) Administer an antihistamine to Mr. Johnson
B) Stop the antibiotic infusion immediately
C) Increase the rate of the IV fluids
D) Notify the healthcare provider about the adverse reaction

Question 9: In the context of 'Holistic Patient Care,' which action by the nurse best demonstrates patient-centered care?
A) Providing medication without explaining its purpose
B) Listening actively to the patient's concerns and preferences
C) Making decisions without involving the patient
D) Following only the physician's orders without question

Question 10: Which action by a Certified Medical Surgical Registered Nurse (CMSRN) best demonstrates effective nursing teamwork and collaboration in the context of professional development?
A) Working independently without seeking input from colleagues.
B) Attending regular team meetings to discuss patient care plans.
C) Ignoring suggestions from other healthcare team members.
D) Refusing to assist colleagues with complex procedures.

Question 11: Scenario: Mrs. Smith, a 65-year-old patient, is scheduled for an elective surgical procedure. The healthcare provider explains the details of the surgery, risks involved, and alternative treatment options to her. Mrs. Smith nods in agreement and signs the consent form. However, postoperatively, she claims she did not fully understand the procedure and its implications. Which of the following best describes the situation regarding consent in this scenario?
A) Mrs. Smith's signature on the consent form indicates valid informed consent.
B) Mrs. Smith's verbal agreement suffices as informed consent.
C) Mrs. Smith's lack of understanding invalidates the consent process.
D) Mrs. Smith's age makes her legally unable to provide consent.

Question 12: In a healthcare setting, which communication technique is most effective for de-escalating a tense situation with a patient?
A) Raising your voice to assert authority
B) Using non-verbal cues to show frustration
C) Active listening and maintaining a calm tone
D) Ignoring the patient's concerns

Question 13: Scenario: Mr. Johnson, a 65-year-old postoperative patient, is receiving care on a medical-surgical unit. While performing a routine assessment, the nurse notes that Mr. Johnson is experiencing shortness of breath, tachycardia, and confusion. The nurse suspects that Mr. Johnson may be developing sepsis. What is the priority action for the nurse to take in this situation?
A) Administer pain medication
B) Notify the healthcare provider immediately
C) Increase the rate of intravenous fluids
D) Reassure the patient and continue routine care

Question 14: In a healthcare organization, the nursing team leader is responsible for coordinating patient care, managing staff, and ensuring quality outcomes. Which organizational structure best supports effective leadership, nursing teamwork, and collaboration?
A) Hierarchical structure
B) Flat structure
C) Matrix structure
D) Functional structure

Question 15: Which approach is essential in ensuring patient satisfaction in the context of Patient-Centered Care and Holistic Patient Care?
A) Focusing solely on physical symptoms
B) Prioritizing efficient treatment over patient preferences
C) Engaging patients in shared decision-making
D) Minimizing communication with patients

Question 16: When conducting a speech consultation for a patient requiring alternate nutrition administration, which of the following considerations is essential?
A) Assessing the patient's swallowing ability
B) Reviewing the patient's medication history
C) Evaluating the patient's mental health status
D) Checking the patient's blood pressure

Question 17: Scenario: Mr. Johnson, a 65-year-old patient, is admitted to the medical-surgical unit with a diagnosis of pneumonia. The healthcare team has initiated a care bundle protocol to improve patient outcomes. As part of the care bundle, which algorithm is most commonly used to prevent ventilator-associated pneumonia (VAP) in hospitalized patients?
A) Early Goal-Directed Therapy (EGDT)
B) Sequential Organ Failure Assessment (SOFA) score
C) Ventilator Bundle
D) Sepsis Bundle

Question 18: Scenario: Mr. Johnson, a 65-year-old patient, is admitted to the medical-surgical unit for post-operative care following a hip replacement surgery. While reviewing his medication orders, the nurse notices that the prescribed dose of pain medication is higher than the recommended safe dosage. Mr. Johnson complains of severe pain but is drowsy and slightly confused. What should the nurse do first to ensure patient safety?
A) Administer the prescribed dose of pain medication to alleviate

Mr. Johnson's pain.
B) Consult with the healthcare provider to clarify the medication order.
C) Wait for the next scheduled dose of pain medication to avoid any potential risks.
D) Inform the patient's family about the situation and seek their advice.

Question 19: In the context of patient grievances, which action by a Certified Medical Surgical Registered Nurse (CMSRN) best demonstrates patient-centered care?
A) Ignoring a patient's complaint about post-operative pain.
B) Listening actively to a patient's concerns and involving them in the care plan.
C) Dismissing a patient's feedback about the cleanliness of their room.
D) Providing medication without explaining the potential side effects.

Question 20: In the context of Change Management, Leadership, Nursing Teamwork, and Collaboration, what is a key ability that a Certified Medical Surgical Registered Nurse (CMSRN) should possess?
A) Technical skills only
B) Communication skills only
C) Critical thinking skills only
D) All of the above

Question 21: Ms. Johnson, a 68-year-old patient with advanced cancer, expresses a desire to explore her spiritual beliefs and find comfort in her faith during her end-of-life care. As her CMSRN, how should you best address her spiritual needs?
A) Encourage her to participate in a support group with individuals of similar beliefs.
B) Provide her with information on local religious services and clergy members for spiritual guidance.
C) Suggest she focuses solely on medical treatments to alleviate physical symptoms.
D) Recommend engaging in activities that distract from spiritual contemplation.

Question 22: During a hand-off report between nurses, which action is most appropriate for ensuring effective communication and patient safety?
A) Using vague language to quickly summarize patient conditions
B) Providing detailed information in an organized manner
C) Skipping over past medical history to save time
D) Omitting any changes in the patient's condition

Question 23: Scenario: Mr. Johnson, a 65-year-old patient, is admitted to the medical-surgical unit with a diagnosis of acute respiratory distress syndrome (ARDS). Despite initial interventions, his condition deteriorates rapidly, and he develops severe hypoxemia. The healthcare team decides to initiate prone positioning to improve oxygenation. As the nurse caring for Mr. Johnson, what is the priority action during the prone positioning of the patient?
A) Ensure proper alignment of the endotracheal tube.
B) Monitor for signs of pressure ulcers on bony prominences.
C) Administer intravenous pain medication for comfort.
D) Check the patency of the nasogastric tube.

Question 24: Ms. Johnson, a 55-year-old patient with chronic lower back pain, is interested in trying acupuncture as a complementary therapy. As a CMSRN, you explain to her that acupuncture involves the insertion of thin needles into specific points on the body to help alleviate pain and promote

healing. **Which of the following statements regarding acupuncture is true?**
A) Acupuncture is based on the principle of restoring the flow of Qi, or vital energy, within the body.
B) Acupuncture primarily works by blocking pain signals in the brain and spinal cord.
C) Acupuncture is only effective for acute pain conditions, not chronic conditions.
D) Acupuncture can cause infections due to the insertion of needles.

Question 25: Scenario: Mr. Smith, a 45-year-old patient, is admitted to the medical-surgical unit following a work-related injury. He is complaining of lower back pain and muscle stiffness after lifting heavy boxes at his workplace. As a CMSRN, what is the most appropriate intervention to promote workplace safety and prevent similar incidents in the future for Mr. Smith?
A) Educate Mr. Smith on proper body mechanics and safe lifting techniques.
B) Provide Mr. Smith with pain medication to alleviate his symptoms.
C) Instruct Mr. Smith to continue lifting heavy objects to strengthen his back muscles.
D) Advise Mr. Smith to ignore the pain and continue working as usual.

Question 26: In multimodal pain management, which intervention combines pharmacological and non-pharmacological approaches to optimize patient outcomes?
A) Administering opioids only
B) Using heat therapy exclusively
C) Employing cognitive-behavioral therapy alone
D) Integrating physical therapy with analgesic medications

Question 27: Scenario: Mrs. Smith, a 65-year-old patient, was admitted to the medical-surgical unit for a total knee replacement surgery. As part of the hospital's commitment to value-based purchasing, the nursing staff ensured that Mrs. Smith received personalized care tailored to her needs. They regularly assessed her pain levels, provided education on post-operative exercises, and encouraged her to actively participate in her recovery process. Mrs. Smith expressed satisfaction with the care she received during her stay. Which aspect of value-based purchasing is exemplified in the scenario involving Mrs. Smith?
A) Patient satisfaction and experience based on personalized care
B) Cost reduction through minimizing nursing interventions
C) Length of hospital stay irrespective of patient needs
D) Standardized care without considering individual preferences

Question 28: Scenario: During the morning rounds, Nurse Sarah notices that Mr. Johnson, a post-operative patient, is displaying signs of increasing confusion and restlessness. She observes that his vital signs are fluctuating, and he appears to be in distress. Despite this, the primary physician on duty seems to overlook these changes and proceeds to discharge orders. What should Nurse Sarah do in this situation?
A) Proceed with the discharge orders as directed by the physician.
B) Document her concerns in the patient's chart and inform the nursing supervisor.
C) Ignore the situation and continue with her routine tasks.
D) Administer sedatives to help calm the patient down.

Question 29: Scenario: Mrs. Smith, a 65-year-old patient, has been diagnosed with a complex medical condition and is seeking a second opinion to explore alternative treatment
options. She expresses concerns about the current treatment plan and wishes to discuss her case with another healthcare provider. **Which action by the Certified Medical Surgical Registered Nurse (CMSRN) best demonstrates patient-centered care in this situation?**
A) Providing Mrs. Smith with information on support groups for patients with similar conditions.
B) Scheduling an appointment with a different specialist for Mrs. Smith to obtain a second opinion.
C) Explaining the risks and benefits of the current treatment plan to Mrs. Smith in detail.
D) Assuring Mrs. Smith that the initial diagnosis and treatment plan are accurate and comprehensive.

Question 30: When applying restraints to a patient, which action is essential for the Certified Medical Surgical Registered Nurse (CMSRN) to take to ensure patient safety?
A) Secure the restraints with a single knot
B) Tie the restraints to the side rails of the bed
C) Ensure that two fingers can be inserted between the restraint and the patient's skin
D) Apply restraints without informing the patient or family members

Question 31: Which of the following best describes a patient's right to informed consent?
A) The patient has the right to refuse treatment.
B) The patient has the right to receive all information about their condition and treatment options.
C) The patient has the right to demand specific medications.
D) The patient has the right to choose their healthcare provider.

Question 32: Scenario: Mr. Johnson, a 65-year-old patient, is admitted to the medical-surgical unit with a history of chronic lower back pain due to degenerative disc disease. The healthcare provider prescribes medication for pain management. Which pharmacological agent is most appropriate for Mr. Johnson's chronic pain?
A) Acetaminophen
B) Ibuprofen
C) Morphine sulfate
D) Gabapentin

Question 33: Scenario: Mrs. Smith, a 65-year-old patient diagnosed with terminal cancer, expresses her wishes to the healthcare team regarding her end-of-life care preferences. She is considering creating an advance directive to ensure her wishes are respected. Which of the following statements best describes an advance directive?
A) A legal document that designates a healthcare proxy to make decisions on behalf of the patient if they become incapacitated.
B) A form that specifies the medical treatments a patient does or does not wish to receive in specific situations.
C) A document that outlines the patient's preferences for spiritual care and rituals at the end of life.
D) A written statement expressing the patient's desire to donate organs after death.

Question 34: Which complementary therapy involves the use of fine needles inserted at specific points on the body to promote healing and pain relief?
A) Aromatherapy
B) Acupuncture
C) Reflexology
D) Reiki

Question 35: Scenario: Mr. Johnson, a 65-year-old patient, was prescribed a new medication for his hypertension. The nurse administered the medication as instructed, but later

discovered that the patient experienced severe allergic reactions. This unintended consequence led to a medical emergency. Which of the following best describes the unintended consequence in this scenario?
A) Adverse drug reaction
B) Therapeutic success
C) Patient satisfaction
D) Routine side effect

Question 36: During a patient assessment, which action by the nurse best demonstrates effective information sharing and communication?
A) Providing vague and ambiguous instructions to the patient.
B) Using medical jargon without explaining terms to the patient.
C) Asking open-ended questions to gather detailed information from the patient.
D) Interrupting the patient frequently during the assessment process.

Question 37: Ms. Johnson, a 65-year-old patient, is admitted to the medical-surgical unit with a diagnosis of Clostridium difficile infection. The healthcare provider prescribes probiotics as part of the treatment plan. Which of the following is the primary rationale for administering probiotics to this patient?
A) To promote the growth of pathogenic bacteria
B) To suppress the immune response
C) To restore the balance of intestinal flora
D) To increase the risk of antibiotic resistance

Question 38: Which of the following is a crucial step in safe medication administration practices for a Certified Medical Surgical Registered Nurse (CMSRN)?
A) Administering medications based on verbal orders
B) Double-checking the medication with another nurse before administration
C) Crushing medications without consulting the pharmacist
D) Using the same syringe to administer multiple medications

Question 39: When considering budgetary considerations in nursing teamwork and collaboration, which approach is most effective for cost-saving measures without compromising patient care?
A) Decreasing the number of nursing staff on each shift
B) Implementing evidence-based practice to reduce unnecessary tests and procedures
C) Cutting down on staff education and training programs
D) Using outdated medical equipment to save on initial costs

Question 40: Which risk assessment method is commonly used to evaluate a patient's risk of developing pressure ulcers in a healthcare setting?
A) Braden Scale
B) Glasgow Coma Scale
C) Morse Fall Scale
D) Wong-Baker FACES Pain Rating Scale

Question 41: In the context of Career Development Relationships, Nursing Teamwork, and Collaboration, which role is exemplified by a Certified Medical Surgical Registered Nurse (CMSRN)?
A) Administrative duties
B) Patient advocacy
C) Facility maintenance
D) Supply chain management

Question 42: Scenario: Mr. Johnson, a 65-year-old patient, has been prescribed a new medication for hypertension. He

expresses concerns about the potential side effects and interactions with his current medications. As a CMSRN providing medication education, what is the most appropriate action to take?
A) Provide Mr. Johnson with a detailed list of potential side effects and interactions.
B) Encourage Mr. Johnson to research the medication online for more information.
C) Offer Mr. Johnson a pamphlet from the pharmaceutical company that manufactures the medication.
D) Schedule a one-on-one session with Mr. Johnson to discuss his concerns and provide personalized education.

Question 43: In the context of 'consent' within Pre- and post-procedural unit standards, Surgical/Procedural Nursing Management, and Patient/Care Management, which statement best describes informed consent?
A) Informed consent is not required for routine procedures.
B) Informed consent is only needed for high-risk procedures.
C) Informed consent is a process where the patient is provided with information about a procedure.
D) Informed consent is solely the responsibility of the healthcare provider.

Question 44: Which practice is essential for ensuring patient-centered care in a medical-surgical setting?
A) Focusing solely on physical symptoms
B) Disregarding patient preferences and values
C) Engaging patients in shared decision-making
D) Providing care without considering emotional well-being

Question 45: Which action by a nurse best demonstrates patient-centered care in a medical-surgical setting?
A) Providing the patient with detailed information about their diagnosis and treatment plan.
B) Making decisions about the patient's care without involving the patient in the process.
C) Following only the physician's orders without considering the patient's preferences.
D) Disregarding the patient's cultural beliefs and practices during care delivery.

Question 46: Which of the following is a modifiable risk factor for patient safety in the context of Patient/Care Management?
A) Age
B) Gender
C) Smoking
D) Genetic predisposition

Question 47: In the context of Elements of Interprofessional Care, which action is essential for effective interprofessional collaboration in a medical-surgical setting?
A) Working in silos without sharing information
B) Avoiding communication with other healthcare team members
C) Respecting the expertise of other team members
D) Ignoring the input from other disciplines

Question 48: Scenario: Sarah, a newly hired nurse, is eager to develop her career in the medical-surgical unit. She is looking for guidance on how to build effective relationships with her nursing team to enhance teamwork and collaboration. Which action by Sarah demonstrates a proactive approach towards career development relationships?
A) Attending mandatory staff meetings only
B) Volunteering to assist colleagues with complex patient cases
C) Keeping interactions with team members to a minimum
D) Avoiding participation in unit-based projects

Question 49: Scenario: Ms. Johnson, a 65-year-old postoperative patient, has been admitted to the medical-surgical unit following a total knee replacement surgery. The nursing team is closely monitoring her progress to ensure optimal recovery and prevent complications. As part of evidence-based practice, which nursing-sensitive indicator should the nurse prioritize to assess Ms. Johnson's postoperative care quality?
A) Pain management
B) Patient falls
C) Pressure ulcers
D) Medication errors

Question 50: Scenario: Mrs. Patel, a 65-year-old Indian American woman, is admitted to the medical-surgical unit with a diagnosis of pneumonia. She speaks limited English and prefers to have her daughter present during medical discussions. Mrs. Patel follows traditional Ayurvedic practices and prefers vegetarian meals. Which action by the nurse best demonstrates cultural and linguistic sensitivity for Mrs. Patel?
A) Providing Mrs. Patel with a menu that includes vegetarian meal options.
B) Using medical jargon when explaining the treatment plan to Mrs. Patel.
C) Excluding Mrs. Patel's daughter from medical discussions to maintain patient confidentiality.
D) Disregarding Mrs. Patel's cultural practices and focusing solely on Western medicine.

Question 51: Which medication is commonly used for the management of chronic neuropathic pain?
A) Ibuprofen
B) Acetaminophen
C) Gabapentin
D) Aspirin

Question 52: In the context of 'Elements of Interprofessional Care,' how does technology impact communication among healthcare teams?
A) Technology enhances communication by providing real-time messaging and video conferencing capabilities.
B) Technology hinders communication by creating barriers and delays in information sharing.
C) Technology has no significant impact on communication within healthcare teams.
D) Technology only allows for basic email communication, limiting effective collaboration.

Question 53: When conducting an educational needs assessment for nursing teamwork and collaboration, which of the following methods is most effective in identifying gaps in knowledge and skills?
A) Sending out a general survey to all nursing staff
B) Observing nursing staff during their daily interactions
C) Reviewing incident reports related to teamwork issues
D) Conducting individual interviews with nursing team members

Question 54: Scenario: Mr. Johnson, a 65-year-old patient with diabetes and hypertension, is admitted to the medical-surgical unit with complaints of chest pain and shortness of breath. The patient is diaphoretic and anxious. Vital signs: BP 160/90 mmHg, HR 110 bpm, RR 24/min, SpO2 92% on room air. The healthcare provider orders stat ECG, oxygen therapy, nitroglycerin sublingual, and labs. The unit is busy, and you are the only nurse available. Which action should the nurse prioritize first for Mr. Johnson?
A) Administer nitroglycerin sublingual
B) Perform a stat ECG

C) Initiate oxygen therapy
D) Draw blood for labs

Question 55: Scenario: Mr. Johnson, a 78-year-old patient with a history of dementia, has been admitted to the medical-surgical unit. Due to his confusion and tendency to pull out medical devices, the healthcare team is considering the use of restraints. As the CMSRN on duty, what is the most appropriate action regarding the use of restraints for Mr. Johnson?
A) Apply wrist restraints to prevent him from pulling out medical devices.
B) Use chemical restraints to keep him sedated and calm.
C) Implement alternative measures such as frequent monitoring and family presence.
D) Apply ankle restraints to limit his movement and ensure safety.

Question 56: Scenario: Mr. Johnson, a 45-year-old patient admitted for exacerbation of COPD, becomes agitated and starts yelling at the nursing staff due to feeling short of breath. He is demanding immediate attention and is refusing to comply with treatment. As a CMSRN, which de-escalation technique would be most appropriate to use in this situation?
A) Ignoring the patient's demands and walking away
B) Speaking calmly and reassuringly, acknowledging his feelings and offering to help
C) Raising your voice to match the patient's intensity to gain control of the situation
D) Threatening the patient with consequences if he does not calm down

Question 57: In the context of 'Interprofessional Collaboration' within 'Elements of Interprofessional Care,' which action best exemplifies effective interprofessional teamwork?
A) Working in isolation without consulting other healthcare team members.
B) Communicating patient updates only within the same discipline.
C) Attending interprofessional team meetings to discuss patient care.
D) Disregarding input from other healthcare professionals during rounds.

Question 58: Which of the following best describes professional empowerment in the context of Career Development Relationships, Nursing Teamwork, and Collaboration for Certified Medical Surgical Registered Nurses (CMSRN)?
A) Seeking approval from superiors before making decisions.
B) Relying solely on individual efforts without seeking input from colleagues.
C) Taking initiative in decision-making and actively participating in team discussions.
D) Following instructions without questioning authority.

Question 59: Scenario: Mr. Johnson, a 65-year-old patient, is admitted to the medical-surgical unit with a diagnosis of congestive heart failure. He appears anxious and expresses concerns about his condition and treatment plan. As a CMSRN providing patient-centered care, which action would be most appropriate to address Mr. Johnson's anxiety and concerns?
A) Provide detailed explanations using medical jargon to educate Mr. Johnson about his condition.
B) Listen actively to Mr. Johnson's concerns, validate his feelings, and involve him in the care planning process.
C) Minimize interactions with Mr. Johnson to avoid escalating his anxiety.
D) Implement the care plan without discussing it with Mr. Johnson to prevent further stress.

Question 60: Which of the following actions by a nurse demonstrates proper use of technology in a medical-surgical setting?
A) Using a smartphone to take pictures of patient records
B) Utilizing a barcode scanner to verify medication administration
C) Sending patient information through unsecured email
D) Storing patient data on a personal USB drive

Question 61: Scenario: Sarah, a Certified Medical Surgical Registered Nurse, is working in a busy hospital. She is assigned to care for Mr. Johnson, a terminally ill patient who has expressed his wish to pass away peacefully at home. However, due to his deteriorating condition, the healthcare team decides to transfer him to the Intensive Care Unit (ICU) against his wishes for better monitoring. Sarah strongly believes in honoring patients' end-of-life preferences. Which action by Sarah best demonstrates advocacy for Mr. Johnson and addresses moral distress?
A) Sarah follows the team's decision and transfers Mr. Johnson to the ICU.
B) Sarah discusses Mr. Johnson's wishes with the healthcare team and advocates for palliative care in a private meeting.
C) Sarah avoids the situation to prevent conflict with the healthcare team.
D) Sarah informs Mr. Johnson about the transfer and leaves the decision to him.

Question 62: Scenario: Nurse Sarah has been working long hours without breaks, feeling emotionally drained and physically exhausted. She notices a decrease in her ability to concentrate and a lack of motivation. Despite feeling overwhelmed, she continues to push herself to meet the demands of her job. Which of the following actions by Nurse Sarah demonstrates a lack of self-care and may contribute to burnout?
A) Taking short breaks to practice deep breathing exercises during shifts.
B) Engaging in regular physical exercise outside of work hours.
C) Seeking support from colleagues and attending stress management workshops.
D) Ignoring her own needs and consistently working overtime without rest.

Question 63: In the context of the 'local governing Scope of Practice' for nurses, which action by a Certified Medical Surgical Registered Nurse (CMSRN) would be considered a violation of the scope of practice?
A) Administering medications without proper training
B) Providing wound care within the established protocols
C) Performing a procedure authorized by the hospital policy
D) Initiating a new treatment without physician approval

Question 64: In dietary consultation for a patient requiring alternate nutrition administration, which factor should be considered most important by the CMSRN?
A) Patient's favorite food
B) Patient's cultural dietary preferences
C) Patient's current medical condition
D) Patient's preferred meal timings

Question 65: Which non-pharmacological intervention is recommended for promoting relaxation and reducing anxiety in medical-surgical patients?
A) Deep breathing exercises
B) Administering sedatives
C) Increasing caffeine intake
D) Encouraging vigorous physical activity

Question 66: Scenario: Mrs. Smith, a 65-year-old female patient, is admitted to the medical-surgical unit with a history of hypertension, diabetes, and obesity. During the assessment, the nurse notes that Mrs. Smith has a body mass index (BMI) of 32, blood pressure of 150/90 mmHg, and a random blood glucose level of 200 mg/dL. Which demographic factor places Mrs. Smith at an increased risk for developing complications during her hospital stay?
A) Age
B) Gender
C) BMI
D) Blood pressure

Question 67: Scenario: Mr. Smith, a 65-year-old male, is admitted to the medical-surgical unit with a diagnosis of pneumonia. The healthcare provider orders antibiotic therapy to treat the infection. As the CMSRN, you understand the importance of antimicrobial stewardship and the need to select the most appropriate antibiotic for Mr. Smith. Which of the following antibiotics is commonly used in the treatment of community-acquired pneumonia and covers typical pathogens such as Streptococcus pneumoniae, Haemophilus influenzae, and atypical pathogens like Mycoplasma pneumoniae?
A) Ciprofloxacin
B) Vancomycin
C) Azithromycin
D) Metronidazole

Question 68: Scenario: Mr. Johnson, a 65-year-old male patient, is admitted to the medical-surgical unit with a history of hypertension, diabetes, and obesity. He is scheduled for a cholecystectomy due to symptomatic gallstones. During the preoperative assessment, the nurse identifies several risk factors that may impact Mr. Johnson's surgical outcome. Which of the following risk factors is most likely to increase the postoperative complications for Mr. Johnson?
A) Controlled diabetes
B) Well-managed hypertension
C) Obesity
D) Non-smoker

Question 69: Which of the following is an example of a career development resource that promotes Nursing Teamwork and Collaboration?
A) Online courses on conflict resolution
B) Solo study guides for personal growth
C) Time management apps for individual use
D) Social media platforms for networking with other nurses

Question 70: Ms. Johnson, a 65-year-old patient, has been admitted for a surgical procedure. During the pre-operative assessment, the nurse realizes that Ms. Johnson has limited health literacy. Which action by the nurse would be most appropriate to ensure effective communication with Ms. Johnson regarding her upcoming surgery?
A) Provide written instructions with medical jargon to encourage learning.
B) Use complex medical terminologies to ensure accuracy in communication.
C) Utilize visual aids and plain language to explain the procedure and post-operative care.
D) Speak quickly to save time and cover all necessary information efficiently.

Question 71: Which teaching method is most effective for educating patients and families in a holistic patient care approach?

A) Lecture-based sessions
B) Hands-on interactive workshops
C) Providing written materials only
D) Group discussions and role-playing activities

Question 72: Scenario: Mr. Johnson, a 68-year-old patient with end-stage heart failure, is admitted to the medical-surgical unit. During the admission process, the nurse asks Mr. Johnson about his preferences regarding resuscitation in case of cardiac arrest. Mr. Johnson expresses his wish to receive full resuscitative measures. What would be the appropriate code status for Mr. Johnson based on his expressed preference?
A) DNR (Do Not Resuscitate)
B) Full Code
C) DNI (Do Not Intubate)
D) Comfort Measures Only

Question 73: Scenario: Mr. Johnson, a 65-year-old patient, has been admitted to the medical-surgical unit with a diagnosis of heart failure. As the CMSRN on duty, you notice a discrepancy in the medication orders for Mr. Johnson. One order specifies a dosage of 20mg of furosemide, while another order indicates 40mg of furosemide. What is the appropriate action for the CMSRN to take in this situation?
A) Administer 20mg of furosemide as per one of the orders.
B) Consult with the healthcare provider to clarify the medication dosage.
C) Administer 40mg of furosemide to ensure adequate diuresis.
D) Hold the medication until the discrepancy is resolved.

Question 74: Ms. Johnson, a 65-year-old patient with diabetes, is admitted to the medical-surgical unit for a foot ulcer. The healthcare team is discussing the implementation of a new wound care protocol based on recent research findings. What is the initial step in the research process that the team should undertake to ensure evidence-based practice?
A) Formulating a research question
B) Conducting a literature review
C) Designing the research study
D) Analyzing the research data

Question 75: Which of the following best defines polypharmacy in the context of medication management for Certified Medical Surgical Registered Nurses (CMSRN)?
A) The use of multiple medications by a patient for the treatment of various conditions.
B) The use of only one medication to treat multiple conditions in a patient.
C) The use of herbal remedies alongside prescribed medications.
D) The use of over-the-counter medications without consulting a healthcare provider.

Question 76: Which communication technique is most effective in ensuring patient understanding and compliance with medical instructions?
A) Using complex medical jargon
B) Speaking quickly to save time
C) Providing clear and simple explanations
D) Avoiding eye contact to respect privacy

Question 77: Scenario: Mr. Smith, a 65-year-old patient, was admitted to the medical-surgical unit for a routine surgical procedure. During his stay, he developed a post-operative infection that required additional treatment. A Root Cause Analysis (RCA) was conducted to investigate the factors contributing to this adverse event. It was identified that the surgical site was not adequately prepped before the procedure, leading to the infection. Which of the following is the most appropriate action to prevent similar incidents in the future?
A) Increase the frequency of staff hand hygiene audits.
B) Implement a checklist to ensure proper surgical site preparation.
C) Conduct more frequent patient education sessions on post-operative care.
D) Review and update the hospital's visitor policy to limit exposure to infections.

Question 78: Ms. Johnson, a 65-year-old patient recovering from a surgical procedure, expresses concerns about managing her medications at home post-discharge. As a CMSRN, which resource would be most appropriate to assist Ms. Johnson in medication management?
A) Providing a list of local pharmacies for her to choose from
B) Scheduling a follow-up appointment with the primary care physician
C) Referring her to a community health nurse for home visits
D) Educating her on medication adherence techniques and providing a pill organizer

Question 79: When utilizing interpreter services for a patient with limited English proficiency, the nurse should:
A) Use family members as interpreters
B) Rely on non-certified bilingual staff
C) Utilize professional medical interpreters
D) Avoid using any form of interpretation services

Question 80: Scenario: Mrs. Smith, a 65-year-old patient, is admitted to the medical-surgical unit for post-operative care following a hip replacement surgery. Her family members are eager to participate in her care and support her during this recovery period. As a CMSRN, what is the most appropriate action regarding family involvement in Mrs. Smith's care?
A) Encourage family members to visit only during designated visiting hours.
B) Allow family members to actively participate in Mrs. Smith's care and decision-making process.
C) Restrict family involvement to prevent interference with the medical team's interventions.
D) Discourage family members from asking questions about Mrs. Smith's condition.

Question 81: Scenario: During a busy shift, a Certified Medical Surgical Registered Nurse (CMSRN) is assigned to a patient who requires wound dressing changes every 4 hours. The nurse notices that the patient's wound appears infected with signs of redness, warmth, and increased pain. The nurse decides to consult the healthcare provider immediately. What action by the nurse is appropriate in this situation regarding delegation and supervision?
A) Delegate the wound dressing change task to a nursing assistant.
B) Collaborate with the wound care nurse specialist for guidance.
C) Ask the patient's family member to assist with the wound dressing.
D) Seek advice from the unit clerk on wound care management.

Question 82: In high accountable organizations focusing on patient safety culture, which of the following is a key component to promote patient safety?
A) Blaming individuals for errors
B) Lack of communication among healthcare team members
C) Encouraging reporting of near-misses and adverse events
D) Ignoring safety protocols and guidelines

Question 83: Scenario: Mr. Johnson, a 65-year-old patient,

was admitted to the medical-surgical unit for a scheduled hip replacement surgery. As part of the care plan, the healthcare team has implemented a care bundle to prevent surgical site infections. Which intervention is NOT typically included in a surgical site infection prevention care bundle?
A) Administering prophylactic antibiotics within one hour before surgery
B) Maintaining normothermia during the perioperative period
C) Encouraging early ambulation post-surgery
D) Using sterile technique during dressing changes

Question 84: In the context of 'Leadership, Nursing Teamwork, and Collaboration,' what is a key role of a Certified Medical Surgical Registered Nurse (CMSRN) in staff advocacy?
A) Advocating for fair compensation and benefits for all staff members
B) Advocating for increased workload without considering staff well-being
C) Advocating for hierarchical structures within the nursing team
D) Advocating for individual recognition over team success

Question 85: In the context of teamwork within the interdisciplinary healthcare team, which role best exemplifies the essence of interprofessional collaboration?
A) The nurse who works independently without consulting other team members.
B) The physician who makes decisions without considering input from other healthcare professionals.
C) The pharmacist who communicates effectively with other team members to ensure medication safety.
D) The technician who performs tasks without interacting with other healthcare team members.

Question 86: Scenario: Ms. Johnson, a 68-year-old patient, was admitted to the medical-surgical unit with a diagnosis of pneumonia. As the CMSRN, you are responsible for documenting the care provided to Ms. Johnson accurately. While reviewing the patient's chart, you notice that the previous nurse did not document the administration of prescribed antibiotics to Ms. Johnson. What should be your immediate action regarding this documentation error?
A) Document the antibiotic administration in your shift notes without mentioning the previous nurse's error.
B) Inform the charge nurse about the documentation error and request assistance in rectifying it.
C) Ignore the error as it was made by the previous nurse and focus on current patient care tasks.
D) Wait until the end of the shift to document the antibiotic administration to avoid any conflict.

Question 87: Scenario: During the morning shift handover, the charge nurse assigns a nursing assistant to assist a patient, Mr. Smith, who is recovering from abdominal surgery. The nurse instructs the nursing assistant to help Mr. Smith with ambulation and to report any signs of pain or discomfort. The nurse emphasizes the importance of monitoring Mr. Smith's incision site for any signs of infection. Which action by the nursing assistant would require immediate intervention by the registered nurse?
A) Assisting Mr. Smith with ambulation as instructed
B) Reporting to the nurse that Mr. Smith's incision site appears red and swollen
C) Notifying the nurse that Mr. Smith is complaining of mild incisional pain
D) Applying a warm compress to Mr. Smith's incision site without informing the nurse

Question 88: Which of the following is an essential component

of effective verbal communication in the healthcare setting?
A) Using complex medical jargon
B) Speaking rapidly to convey urgency
C) Active listening and empathy
D) Interrupting the patient to save time

Question 89: Which of the following is an effective strategy to promote nurse resiliency and well-being in a medical-surgical setting?
A) Encouraging nurses to work overtime regularly
B) Providing access to mental health resources and support groups
C) Assigning heavy workloads without breaks
D) Ignoring signs of burnout and stress in nurses

Question 90: Which of the following statements best describes an advance directive?
A) A legal document that specifies a person's healthcare preferences in case they are unable to communicate
B) A form of emergency medical treatment provided without consent
C) A document that designates financial beneficiaries in case of illness
D) A written record of a patient's daily medication schedule

Question 91: In the context of Nursing Informatics, which element is essential for effective interprofessional care coordination?
A) Electronic Health Records (EHR)
B) Social Media Platforms
C) Online Gaming Platforms
D) Virtual Reality Headsets

Question 92: In the context of "just culture" within Patient Safety, which of the following best defines the concept of "just culture"?
A) Blaming individuals for errors
B) Encouraging open communication about errors
C) Punishing healthcare providers for system failures
D) Ignoring errors to maintain harmony

Question 93: Mr. Johnson, a 55-year-old patient, is admitted to the medical-surgical unit for a scheduled surgery. As a Certified Medical Surgical Registered Nurse (CMSRN), you understand the importance of professional concepts in nursing practice. Which action by the nurse best demonstrates the professional concept of advocacy for the patient?
A) Administering medications as per the physician's orders without discussing potential side effects with the patient.
B) Ensuring the patient receives adequate pain relief post-surgery and advocating for additional pain management if needed.
C) Following the hospital protocol strictly without considering the patient's preferences or concerns.
D) Disregarding the patient's questions about the surgery and recovery process to save time.

Question 94: When interpreting a patient's lab results, which finding would require immediate intervention by the Certified Medical Surgical Registered Nurse (CMSRN)?
A) Hemoglobin level of 12 g/dL
B) Potassium level of 3.5 mEq/L
C) Platelet count of 150,000/mm3
D) Sodium level of 125 mEq/L

Question 95: Scenario: During morning rounds, Nurse Sarah notices that Mr. Johnson, a post-operative patient, is avoiding eye contact, crossing his arms, and turning away when she approaches him. He responds with short, monosyllabic

answers to her questions. What non-verbal cues is Mr. Johnson displaying?
A) Open body language, direct eye contact, and engaged posture
B) Avoiding eye contact, crossed arms, and turning away
C) Smiling, nodding, and maintaining eye contact
D) Fidgeting, looking around the room, and tapping his foot

Question 96: Scenario: Sarah, a newly hired nurse on a medical-surgical unit, is seeking guidance and support to enhance her clinical skills and knowledge. She is interested in finding a mentor who can provide valuable insights and advice to help her navigate her career development in the nursing field. Which of the following resources would be most suitable for Sarah in this situation?
A) Attending a one-time workshop on career development
B) Joining a nursing professional organization
C) Watching online educational videos on nursing skills
D) Participating in a mentorship program offered by the hospital

Question 97: When considering cultural and linguistic needs in healthcare, which written language approach is most appropriate for ensuring holistic patient care?
A) Using only the English language for all written materials
B) Providing written materials in multiple languages spoken by the local community
C) Using complex medical terminology in written materials to maintain professionalism
D) Ignoring written materials as verbal communication is sufficient for patient care

Question 98: Which interdisciplinary collaboration method is most effective in promoting patient mobility in a medical-surgical setting?
A) Conducting regular team meetings to discuss patient progress
B) Implementing individualized care plans for each patient
C) Using technology to track patient movement and activity
D) Administering medications to keep patients sedated

Question 99: In the context of patient safety protocols, what is the primary purpose of hourly rounding by nurses?
A) To check on the patient's pain levels
B) To ensure the patient's room is tidy
C) To provide proactive care and address patient needs promptly
D) To document vital signs every hour

Question 100: In a high accountable organization focused on patient safety culture, which of the following best describes the key aspect of patient/care management?
A) Prioritizing cost-effectiveness over patient outcomes
B) Implementing evidence-based practice guidelines
C) Ignoring staff feedback on safety concerns
D) Minimizing patient education and involvement

Question 101: In the context of Professional Development, Nursing Teamwork, and Collaboration, which action best demonstrates clinical judgment by a Certified Medical Surgical Registered Nurse (CMSRN)?
A) Seeking input from other healthcare team members before making a critical decision.
B) Making decisions independently without consulting other healthcare team members.
C) Following the same routine for patient care without considering individual needs.
D) Avoiding communication with other healthcare team members during patient care.

Question 102: Which of the following is an essential component of infection prevention in patient care

management?
A) Administering antibiotics for all patients
B) Proper hand hygiene practices
C) Reusing disposable gloves
D) Ignoring isolation precautions

Question 103: Scenario: Mr. Smith, a 65-year-old patient, was admitted to the medical-surgical unit for a routine surgical procedure. During his stay, he developed a post-operative infection that required additional treatment. A Root Cause Analysis (RCA) was conducted to investigate the factors contributing to this adverse event. The team identified that the infection might have originated from improper hand hygiene practices among the healthcare staff. Which of the following is the most appropriate action to prevent similar incidents in the future?
A) Conduct a staff training session on the importance of hand hygiene.
B) Increase the use of antibiotics in all post-operative patients.
C) Implement a new electronic medical record system.
D) Change the type of surgical instruments used in procedures.

Question 104: Which action by the nurse best demonstrates a commitment to patient safety in the context of Patient/Care Management?
A) Double-checking the patient's identification before administering medication.
B) Skipping a step in the prescribed wound care procedure to save time.
C) Ignoring a patient's call light while attending to paperwork.
D) Administering a medication without checking the patient's allergies.

Question 105: Scenario: Mr. Johnson, a 65-year-old patient, is admitted to the medical-surgical unit for the treatment of pneumonia. He has a history of hypertension and type 2 diabetes. The physician orders the following medications: 1. Amoxicillin 500mg PO every 8 hours 2. Metformin 1000mg PO twice daily 3. Lisinopril 10mg PO daily Which of the following actions should the nurse take first regarding Mr. Johnson's medication management?
A) Administer all medications as ordered
B) Check Mr. Johnson's blood glucose levels before administering Metformin
C) Administer Lisinopril first, followed by the other medications
D) Consult the pharmacist regarding potential drug interactions

Question 106: Scenario: During a surgical scrub preparation, the nurse notices a colleague not following the correct protocol. The nurse observes the colleague washing hands for only 15 seconds with plain soap before donning sterile gloves. What action should the nurse take next to ensure proper surgical scrub technique?
A) Inform the colleague that the scrub should last for at least 2 minutes with an antimicrobial soap.
B) Proceed with the scrub as usual to avoid confrontation.
C) Ignore the situation as it is the colleague's responsibility to follow correct protocols.
D) Report the incident to the charge nurse after the procedure.

Question 107: Scenario: Mr. Johnson, a 65-year-old male patient, is admitted to the medical-surgical unit with a diagnosis of pneumonia. The healthcare team has initiated a care bundle protocol to ensure optimal patient outcomes. As part of the care bundle, which algorithm is most crucial for preventing ventilator-associated pneumonia (VAP) in Mr. Johnson?
A) Early Ambulation Algorithm

B) Hand Hygiene Algorithm
C) Head-of-Bed Elevation Algorithm
D) Oral Care Algorithm

Question 108: Scenario: Mr. Smith, a 55-year-old patient with a history of recurrent chemotherapy treatments for colon cancer, is scheduled for a new port placement due to complications with his current port. As the CMSRN overseeing his care, you are educating Mr. Smith about the new port. Which statement by Mr. Smith indicates a need for further teaching regarding the port care?
A) "I will avoid lifting heavy objects with the arm on the side of the port."
B) "I will clean the port site daily with alcohol and apply an antibiotic ointment."
C) "I understand that the port should be flushed regularly to prevent clot formation."
D) "I will notify my healthcare provider if I notice any redness, swelling, or drainage around the port site."

Question 109: Which statement best describes a key aspect of verbal intervention in de-escalation techniques for Certified Medical Surgical Registered Nurses (CMSRNs)?
A) Using aggressive language to assert authority
B) Employing active listening and empathy to understand the patient's perspective
C) Ignoring the patient's concerns to maintain control
D) Threatening consequences if the patient does not comply

Question 110: In the context of 'Peer accountability' within the 'Healthy Practice Environment, Professional Concepts,' which statement best describes the concept of peer accountability?
A) Peer accountability involves blaming others for mistakes.
B) Peer accountability is the act of taking responsibility for one's actions and decisions.
C) Peer accountability means avoiding confrontation with colleagues.
D) Peer accountability is solely the responsibility of the team leader.

Question 111: Scenario: Mr. Johnson, a 68-year-old male, is being discharged from the hospital after a surgical procedure. During the medication reconciliation process, the nurse notes that Mr. Johnson has been prescribed multiple medications for his chronic conditions. The nurse ensures that the list of medications is accurate and up-to-date to prevent any adverse events post-discharge. Which of the following best describes the purpose of medication reconciliation in the context of Mr. Johnson's discharge?
A) To increase the cost of healthcare services
B) To expedite the discharge process
C) To identify and resolve discrepancies in medication information
D) To reduce patient satisfaction

Question 112: Scenario: Mrs. Smith, a 65-year-old patient, has been admitted to the medical-surgical unit for a complex surgical procedure. She expresses concerns about the upcoming surgery and feels overwhelmed by the information provided. As a CMSRN, what is the most appropriate action to demonstrate patient advocacy in this situation?
A) Provide Mrs. Smith with additional detailed medical information to address her concerns.
B) Listen actively to Mrs. Smith's fears and provide emotional support.
C) Inform Mrs. Smith that the surgical team is highly experienced and there is no need to worry.
D) Quickly reassure Mrs. Smith that everything will be fine without addressing her specific concerns.

Question 113: Scenario: Mr. Johnson, a 65-year-old patient, is scheduled for discharge after undergoing a surgical procedure. The healthcare team has initiated the discharge planning process to ensure a smooth transition from the hospital to home care. As the CMSRN overseeing Mr. Johnson's case, which action is essential during the discharge planning process to promote effective care coordination and transition management?
A) Providing the patient with a list of community resources without assessing his understanding.
B) Engaging only the patient in the discharge planning process, excluding family members.
C) Discharging the patient without a comprehensive medication reconciliation.
D) Collaborating with the interdisciplinary team to develop a personalized care plan for Mr. Johnson.

Question 114: Scenario: Mr. Johnson, a postoperative patient recovering from abdominal surgery, is under the care of Nurse Smith. The physician verbally orders a change in Mr. Johnson's pain medication from oral to intravenous due to inadequate pain control. Nurse Smith receives the verbal order from the physician. What is the appropriate action for Nurse Smith to take regarding the verbal order for changing Mr. Johnson's pain medication?
A) Implement the change immediately and document the verbal order in the patient's chart.
B) Ask the physician to provide the order in writing before making any changes.
C) Consult with another nurse to confirm the physician's verbal order.
D) Disregard the verbal order and continue with the current pain medication regimen.

Question 115: Scenario: Mr. Smith, a 65-year-old patient, is admitted to the medical-surgical unit with a diagnosis of heart failure. The healthcare team includes the medical doctor, nurse, physical therapist, and dietitian. The team meets to discuss Mr. Smith's care plan, which involves medication management, dietary modifications, and physical therapy exercises. The nurse ensures that all team members are informed about the plan and collaborates to provide comprehensive care. Which action by the nurse best demonstrates effective care coordination in this scenario?
A) Providing medication education to the patient
B) Scheduling a follow-up appointment with the cardiologist
C) Communicating Mr. Smith's progress to his family members
D) Facilitating a team meeting to discuss the care plan

Question 116: Which of the following equipment is essential for ensuring patient safety during a surgical procedure?
A) Blood pressure cuff
B) Stethoscope
C) Pulse oximeter
D) Intravenous (IV) pole

Question 117: When analyzing a patient's condition, which action demonstrates critical thinking skills by a Certified Medical Surgical Registered Nurse (CMSRN)?
A) Making assumptions based on personal beliefs
B) Consulting evidence-based practice guidelines
C) Relying solely on past experiences
D) Disregarding patient preferences

Question 118: Scenario: Mr. Smith, a 65-year-old patient admitted for a surgical procedure, is diagnosed with a healthcare-associated infection. The healthcare team is

implementing infection control measures to prevent the spread of infection to other patients and healthcare workers. Which precaution should be followed specifically for Mr. Smith to prevent transmission of the infection?
A) Droplet precautions
B) Contact precautions
C) Airborne precautions
D) Standard precautions

Question 119: Which demographic factor is considered a significant risk factor in patient safety and care management?
A) Age
B) Hair color
C) Shoe size
D) Favorite food

Question 120: Scenario: Mr. Smith, a 65-year-old postoperative patient, has a surgical wound that is healing well. During your assessment, you notice that the wound dressing is intact, dry, and without any signs of infection. Mr. Smith mentions feeling a bit warm but denies any chills or other symptoms. What is the most appropriate action for the nurse to take regarding infection control practices?
A) Notify the healthcare provider immediately.
B) Document the findings and continue to monitor the patient.
C) Remove the dressing to inspect the wound closely.
D) Initiate contact precautions for the patient.

Question 121: Scenario: Mrs. Smith, a 65-year-old patient, is admitted to the medical-surgical unit for post-operative care following a hip replacement surgery. She expresses concerns about managing her pain and being able to walk independently after discharge. Mrs. Smith's daughter, who lives in another state, calls the nurse frequently to inquire about her mother's progress and care plan. The nurse recognizes the importance of involving the patient and family in the care process to ensure a smooth transition from hospital to home. Which action by the nurse best demonstrates patient/family-centered care in this scenario?
A) Providing Mrs. Smith with pain medication without discussing potential side effects.
B) Updating Mrs. Smith's daughter on her mother's condition without seeking Mrs. Smith's permission.
C) Collaborating with Mrs. Smith and her daughter to develop a personalized pain management and mobility plan.
D) Discharging Mrs. Smith without any education on post-operative care instructions.

Question 122: Which of the following best defines a positive patient safety culture in a healthcare setting?
A) Blaming individuals for errors
B) Prioritizing speed over accuracy in patient care
C) Open communication about errors and near misses
D) Ignoring staff concerns about patient safety

Question 123: Scenario: Mrs. Smith, a 65-year-old patient, has been admitted to the medical-surgical unit for post-operative care following a knee replacement surgery. She is experiencing severe pain in her surgical site despite receiving prescribed pain medication. Mrs. Smith expresses her concerns about the pain not being adequately controlled and requests a different pain management approach. Which action by the nurse best demonstrates patient advocacy in this situation?
A) Explaining to Mrs. Smith that she needs to endure the pain as it is expected after surgery.
B) Consulting with the healthcare team to discuss alternative pain management options for Mrs. Smith.

C) Dismissing Mrs. Smith's concerns and reassuring her that the current pain medication is sufficient.
D) Delaying Mrs. Smith's pain medication administration to see if the current regimen eventually provides relief.

Question 124: In the context of patient safety culture, which action best exemplifies the concept of "speaking up" for a Certified Medical Surgical Registered Nurse (CMSRN)?
A) Ignoring a medication error made by a colleague
B) Reporting a near-miss incident to the supervisor
C) Keeping quiet about a safety concern to avoid conflict
D) Disregarding a patient's request for additional information

Question 125: Which resource is commonly utilized for providing emotional support and guidance to patients and caregivers facing end-of-life situations?
A) Hospice care services
B) Chemotherapy treatments
C) Surgical interventions
D) Physical therapy sessions

Question 126: Scenario: Sarah, a Certified Medical Surgical Registered Nurse, is conducting a coaching session with a colleague on documentation performance improvement. During the session, the colleague mentions that they find it challenging to accurately document wound care procedures. Sarah advises her colleague to focus on using precise and descriptive language while documenting wound assessments and treatments to ensure clarity and accuracy. Which of the following best describes the key aspect of coaching for documentation performance improvement highlighted in the scenario?
A) Using vague language to allow for interpretation
B) Including unnecessary details to enhance documentation
C) Prioritizing speed over accuracy in documentation
D) Using precise and descriptive language for clarity and accuracy

Question 127: Which of the following is considered a social determinant of health?
A) Access to healthcare facilities
B) Genetic predisposition to certain diseases
C) Level of education
D) Blood pressure measurement

Question 128: During downtime procedures in a medical-surgical unit, which action by the nurse is essential for ensuring accurate documentation?
A) Delaying documentation until the system is back online
B) Using paper-based documentation as a temporary measure
C) Documenting on a random piece of paper to transfer later
D) Not documenting until the system is restored

Question 129: Scenario: Mr. Smith, a 65-year-old patient, is admitted to the medical-surgical unit with a diagnosis of heart failure. The healthcare team notices a trend of medication errors related to incorrect dosages being administered to patients on the unit. As part of the continuous quality and process improvement initiative, what action should the CMSRN take first?
A) Conduct an in-depth analysis of the medication administration process.
B) Implement a new electronic health record system for medication orders.
C) Provide additional training to the nursing staff on medication administration.
D) Report the issue to the hospital administration for immediate action.

Question 130: Which cultural factor should a Certified Medical Surgical Registered Nurse (CMSRN) consider when addressing individualized nutritional needs for patients?
A) Religious dietary restrictions
B) Preferred meal times based on cultural practices
C) Traditional healing practices
D) Social media influence on dietary choices

Question 131: Scenario: Mrs. Smith, a 65-year-old patient, is admitted to the medical-surgical unit with a history of heart failure. She appears anxious and expresses concerns about her upcoming cardiac procedure. As a CMSRN providing patient-centered care, what action should you prioritize to address Mrs. Smith's anxiety?
A) Provide detailed information about the procedure and potential complications.
B) Administer a sedative medication to help Mrs. Smith relax before the procedure.
C) Encourage Mrs. Smith to focus on positive thinking and distract herself from worries.
D) Listen actively to Mrs. Smith's concerns, validate her feelings, and offer emotional support.

Question 132: Scenario: Mrs. Smith, a 65-year-old patient admitted for postoperative care following abdominal surgery, is experiencing anxiety and difficulty sleeping. As a CMSRN, which nonpharmacological intervention would be most appropriate to address Mrs. Smith's symptoms?
A) Administering a sedative medication
B) Encouraging relaxation techniques such as deep breathing exercises
C) Providing a high dose of pain medication to induce sleep
D) Allowing unrestricted visitation hours for family and friends

Question 133: In physical therapy for postoperative care, which intervention is essential to prevent deep vein thrombosis (DVT) in surgical patients?
A) Passive range of motion exercises
B) Ambulation and early mobilization
C) Application of heat packs
D) Isometric strengthening exercises

Question 134: Scenario: Mr. Johnson, a 65-year-old postoperative patient, has a central venous catheter in place. The nurse notes redness, warmth, and tenderness at the catheter site. Upon assessment, there is purulent drainage present. Mr. Johnson also has a low-grade fever. Which of the following actions is the priority for the nurse to take in this situation?
A) Administering an antipyretic medication
B) Notifying the healthcare provider immediately
C) Documenting the findings in the patient's chart
D) Applying a warm compress to the catheter site

Question 135: Ms. Johnson, a 68-year-old postoperative patient, has been admitted to the medical-surgical unit. She underwent abdominal surgery yesterday and is currently on bed rest. The nurse understands the importance of repositioning Ms. Johnson to prevent complications. Which action is most appropriate for the nurse to take regarding repositioning?
A) Reposition Ms. Johnson every 4 hours.
B) Reposition Ms. Johnson every 2 hours.
C) Reposition Ms. Johnson every 6 hours.
D) Reposition Ms. Johnson every 8 hours.

Question 136: Scenario: During a shift hand-off report, the nurse is discussing a patient, Mr. Smith, who is scheduled for surgery in the morning. The outgoing nurse mentions that Mr. Smith has a known allergy to penicillin and requires preoperative antibiotics. The nurse also informs that Mr. Smith's daughter will be arriving early in the morning to provide support during the surgery. Which action by the incoming nurse demonstrates effective hand-off communication?
A) Asking the outgoing nurse about Mr. Smith's preferred pain management methods.
B) Documenting the allergy to penicillin in Mr. Smith's medical record.
C) Contacting the pharmacy to inquire about the availability of the preoperative antibiotics.
D) Informing the surgical team about Mr. Smith's daughter coming in the morning.

Question 137: Which spiritual intervention is most appropriate for a patient receiving palliative care at the end of life?
A) Encouraging the patient to engage in prayer and meditation
B) Suggesting the patient to avoid discussing spiritual matters
C) Discouraging the patient from participating in religious rituals
D) Ignoring the patient's spiritual needs

Question 138: Which environmental factor poses the highest risk to patient safety in a healthcare setting?
A) Noise pollution
B) Improper lighting
C) Airborne pathogens
D) Improper waste disposal

Question 139: Ms. Johnson, a 68-year-old patient, expresses dissatisfaction with the care provided by the nursing staff. She feels her concerns are not being addressed promptly. As a CMSRN, what is the most appropriate initial action to take in this situation?
A) Apologize to Ms. Johnson and assure her that her concerns will be looked into.
B) Inform Ms. Johnson that the nursing staff is doing their best and she should be patient.
C) Document Ms. Johnson's grievances in detail and escalate them to the appropriate channels.
D) Disregard Ms. Johnson's complaints as part of her emotional state due to her medical condition.

Question 140: According to Standard V of the AMSN Scope and Standards, what is a key aspect of a Certified Medical Surgical Registered Nurse's scope of practice?
A) Performing complex surgical procedures
B) Providing direct care to patients with medical-surgical conditions
C) Conducting advanced diagnostic tests
D) Administering anesthesia during surgeries

Question 141: Which step is essential in the process of implementing evidence-based practice principles?
A) Ignoring current research findings
B) Relying solely on personal experience
C) Consulting the latest clinical practice guidelines
D) Disregarding patient preferences

Question 142: Which type of port is implanted completely beneath the skin and requires no external components?
A) Tunneled catheter
B) Implanted port
C) External catheter
D) Peripherally inserted central catheter (PICC)

Question 143: In the context of discharge planning for a patient being prepared for transition to home, which action by

the Certified Medical Surgical Registered Nurse (CMSRN) best demonstrates effective interdisciplinary collaboration?
A) Providing the patient with a list of community resources for follow-up care.
B) Holding a team meeting involving the patient, family, social worker, and physical therapist to discuss the discharge plan.
C) Discharging the patient without involving other healthcare team members.
D) Instructing the patient to follow up with their primary care physician without further guidance.

Question 144: Ms. Johnson, a 55-year-old patient diagnosed with chronic lower back pain, expresses interest in trying complementary and alternative therapies to manage her discomfort. As a CMSRN, you educate her about various non-pharmacological interventions. Which therapy involves the use of fine needles inserted at specific points on the body to alleviate pain and improve overall well-being?
A) Aromatherapy
B) Acupuncture
C) Reflexology
D) Reiki

Question 145: In value-based purchasing, what is the primary focus when evaluating patient customer experience based on data results?
A) Cost-effectiveness
B) Timeliness of care
C) Patient satisfaction
D) Healthcare provider convenience

Question 146: Which demographic factor is considered a significant risk factor in patient safety and care management?
A) Gender
B) Marital status
C) Age
D) Blood type

Question 147: Which of the following best describes the concept of nursing teamwork and collaboration in professional nursing practice?
A) Working independently without seeking input from other healthcare team members.
B) Engaging in interdisciplinary communication and cooperation to provide optimal patient care.
C) Ignoring the contributions of other healthcare professionals in patient management.
D) Refusing to participate in team meetings and care planning sessions.

Question 148: Scenario: Sarah, a 45-year-old patient with end-stage liver disease, has been deemed a candidate for organ donation. As her CMSRN, you are discussing the organ donation process with Sarah and her family. Sarah expresses concerns about the impact of organ donation on her religious beliefs and wishes to explore options that align with her faith. Which of the following statements best reflects a holistic approach to addressing Sarah's concerns regarding organ donation?
A) "Organ donation is a medical procedure that can save multiple lives, and it is important to prioritize the needs of those awaiting transplants."
B) "Sarah, your religious beliefs are important, but saving lives through organ donation should be the primary focus at this time."
C) "Let's explore how we can respect your religious beliefs while also considering the possibility of organ donation to help others in need."
D) "Sarah, organ donation is a routine process, and your concerns

about religious beliefs should not interfere with the decision to donate."

Question 149: Which physical symptom is commonly associated with patients receiving palliative or end-of-life care?
A) Increased appetite
B) Improved mobility
C) Decreased pain
D) Fatigue

Question 150: What is the primary purpose of safety huddles in a medical-surgical setting?
A) To discuss staff scheduling issues
B) To review patient satisfaction surveys
C) To identify and address potential safety concerns
D) To plan social events for the healthcare team

ANSWER WITH DETAILED EXPLANATION SET [1]

Question 1: Correct Answer: C) Aspiration pneumonia
Rationale: In patients receiving enteral nutrition, such as Ms. Johnson, the risk of aspiration pneumonia is a significant concern. Aspiration pneumonia can occur when food, liquid, or gastric contents enter the lungs, leading to inflammation and infection. This risk is higher in patients with conditions like diabetes and hypertension due to impaired swallowing reflexes or altered sensorium. Hyperglycemia (Option A) and hypertension (Option B) are common comorbidities in such patients but are not direct complications of enteral nutrition. Hypokalemia (Option D) may occur due to various reasons but is not a primary complication associated with enteral nutrition in this scenario.

Question 2: Correct Answer: D) Contact Precautions
Rationale: Contact Precautions are essential for preventing the transmission of MRSA, as it is primarily spread through direct or indirect contact. Standard Precautions involve basic infection prevention practices for all patient care, while Droplet Precautions are used for diseases transmitted by respiratory droplets larger than 5 microns. Airborne Precautions are for diseases transmitted by smaller droplets or particles that remain infectious over long distances. In this scenario, the most appropriate measure to prevent MRSA transmission is Contact Precautions due to the nature of MRSA spread through direct contact with the patient or contaminated surfaces.

Question 3: Correct Answer: D) Elevate the head of the bed to a semi-Fowler's position.
Rationale: Elevating the head of the bed to a semi-Fowler's position helps improve ventilation and oxygenation by reducing pressure on the diaphragm and promoting lung expansion. This position facilitates better gas exchange and can alleviate dyspnea in patients with heart failure. Administering a diuretic (Option A) may be necessary to address fluid volume overload but is not the priority in this scenario. Increasing the oxygen flow rate (Option B) without addressing the positioning first may not be as effective in improving oxygenation. Assisting with ADLs (Option C) is important for overall patient care but does not directly address the impaired gas exchange in this case.

Question 4: Correct Answer: B) Unintentional and unconscious stereotypes affecting behavior
Rationale: Implicit bias refers to the unconscious attitudes or stereotypes that can influence our actions, decisions, and understanding in an unconscious manner. Option A is incorrect as implicit bias is not conscious. Option C is incorrect as implicit bias is not deliberate. Option D is incorrect as implicit bias is not open or transparent. Understanding implicit bias is crucial in providing holistic patient care as it can impact patient outcomes, treatment decisions, and overall healthcare experiences. Healthcare providers must actively work to recognize and address their implicit biases to ensure equitable and inclusive patient care.

Question 5: Correct Answer: B) Consult with the healthcare provider to discuss an alternative from the formulary
Rationale: In this scenario, the correct action based on quality standards and policies is to consult with the healthcare provider to discuss an alternative antibiotic from the hospital's formulary. It is essential to adhere to the formulary to ensure patient safety, cost-effectiveness, and compliance with institutional guidelines. Option A is incorrect as administering a non-formulary medication without consultation can lead to adverse effects and non-compliance. Option C is incorrect as substituting without proper authorization can violate policies. Option D is incorrect as disregarding the formulary compromises quality standards and policies. Consulting with the healthcare provider promotes collaborative decision-making and upholds quality care practices.

Question 6: Correct Answer: A) Provide Mrs. Smith with a detailed explanation of the surgical procedure and pain management plan.
Rationale: It is essential for CMSRNs to address patient concerns regarding procedures and pain management effectively. Option A is the correct choice as it demonstrates patient-centered care by providing Mrs. Smith with the necessary information to alleviate her anxiety. Options B and C are incorrect as they disregard Mrs. Smith's feelings and may lead to inadequate pain management. Option D is not the best initial action as the CMSRN should first attempt to address Mrs. Smith's concerns directly before involving additional support services.

Question 7: Correct Answer: A) Continue documenting on paper and transfer to the electronic system once it is restored.
Rationale: During downtime procedures, the priority is to ensure accurate and timely documentation to maintain continuity of care. Option A is the correct choice as it allows for immediate documentation on paper, ensuring essential information is recorded and can be later transferred to the electronic system. Options B and D are incorrect as delaying documentation or neglecting it altogether can compromise patient safety and continuity of care. Option C is also incorrect as using another colleague's login credentials violates patient privacy and is against healthcare regulations.

Question 8: Correct Answer: B) Stop the antibiotic infusion immediately
Rationale: Stopping the antibiotic infusion is the priority in this situation as Mr. Johnson is displaying signs of a severe allergic reaction, which could progress to anaphylaxis. Administering an antihistamine (Option A) can be considered after stopping the infusion, but the immediate action should be to halt the administration of the offending medication. Increasing IV fluids (Option C) may be necessary later, but it is not the initial priority. Notifying the healthcare provider (Option D) is important, but stopping the infusion takes precedence to prevent further harm to the patient.

Question 9: Correct Answer: B) Listening actively to the patient's concerns and preferences
Rationale: Patient-centered care emphasizes the importance of involving patients in their care. Actively listening to the patient's concerns and preferences is a fundamental aspect of patient-centered care as it shows respect for the patient's autonomy, promotes shared decision-making, and enhances the overall quality of care. Options A, C, and D do not align with patient-centered care principles as they disregard the patient's voice and preferences, highlighting the significance of active listening in fostering a holistic approach to patient care.

Question 10: Correct Answer: B) Attending regular team meetings to discuss patient care plans.
Rationale: Attending regular team meetings to discuss patient care plans is a key aspect of nursing teamwork and collaboration. It allows nurses to share knowledge, coordinate care, and make informed decisions collectively. This fosters a collaborative environment where input from all team members is valued, leading to improved patient outcomes. Options A, C, and D promote individualism and hinder teamwork, which is contrary to the principles of effective collaboration in professional development within the nursing context.

Question 11: Correct Answer: C) Mrs. Smith's lack of understanding invalidates the consent process.

Rationale: Informed consent requires the patient to fully comprehend the procedure, risks, benefits, and alternatives before providing consent. Mrs. Smith's lack of understanding indicates that true informed consent was not obtained, making the consent process invalid. While her signature is important, it is not sufficient if she did not grasp the information provided. Verbal agreement alone is not considered valid informed consent. Age alone does not determine a patient's ability to provide consent; understanding is key in the consent process.

Question 12: Correct Answer: C) Active listening and maintaining a calm tone

Rationale: Active listening and maintaining a calm tone are crucial components of effective communication in de-escalating tense situations with patients. By actively listening, nurses show empathy and understanding, which can help diffuse the situation. Maintaining a calm tone conveys professionalism and reassurance, helping to prevent further escalation. Options A and B can exacerbate the situation by escalating tension and displaying unprofessional behavior. Option D, ignoring the patient's concerns, is not a recommended approach as it can lead to increased frustration and lack of trust.

Question 13: Correct Answer: B) Notify the healthcare provider immediately

Rationale: In this scenario, the nurse should prioritize notifying the healthcare provider immediately because Mr. Johnson is displaying signs and symptoms of sepsis, a life-threatening condition that requires prompt medical intervention. Administering pain medication (Option A) is not the priority as addressing the underlying cause of Mr. Johnson's symptoms is crucial. Increasing intravenous fluids (Option C) may be necessary but should not delay contacting the healthcare provider. Reassuring the patient and continuing routine care (Option D) is not appropriate when sepsis is suspected, as urgent medical attention is required to prevent further deterioration.

Question 14: Correct Answer: C) Matrix structure

Rationale: In a matrix organizational structure, nurses report both to their nursing team leader and to the department head or clinical manager. This dual reporting system fosters collaboration, communication, and shared decision-making among nursing staff and other healthcare professionals. Unlike a hierarchical structure where communication flows strictly from top to bottom, or a functional structure where departments work in silos, a matrix structure encourages interdisciplinary teamwork and a patient-centered approach to care. This structure enhances leadership effectiveness, promotes nursing teamwork, and facilitates collaboration across departments, ultimately leading to improved patient outcomes.

Question 15: Correct Answer: C) Engaging patients in shared decision-making

Rationale: In patient satisfaction management, engaging patients in shared decision-making is crucial for providing Patient-Centered Care and Holistic Patient Care. This approach involves actively involving patients in their treatment plans, considering their preferences, values, and beliefs. By fostering open communication and collaboration between healthcare providers and patients, shared decision-making enhances patient autonomy, trust, and satisfaction. Options A, B, and D are incorrect as they contradict the principles of patient-centered care by neglecting the importance of involving patients in decision-making, focusing solely on physical aspects, and minimizing communication, which can lead to decreased patient satisfaction and outcomes.

Question 16: Correct Answer: A) Assessing the patient's swallowing ability

Rationale: When conducting a speech consultation for a patient requiring alternate nutrition administration, assessing the patient's swallowing ability is crucial. This evaluation helps determine the patient's ability to safely swallow food and liquids, which is essential for determining the appropriate method of nutrition administration. Reviewing the patient's medication history (option B) is important but not directly related to speech consultation. Evaluating the patient's mental health status (option C) is important for overall patient care but not specific to speech consultation. Checking the patient's blood pressure (option D) is important for general health assessment but not a primary consideration in speech consultation for nutrition administration.

Question 17: Correct Answer: C) Ventilator Bundle

Rationale: The correct answer is C) Ventilator Bundle. The Ventilator Bundle is a set of evidence-based practices aimed at preventing VAP in patients on mechanical ventilation. It includes interventions such as elevating the head of the bed, daily sedation vacations, peptic ulcer disease prophylaxis, and deep vein thrombosis prophylaxis. Options A, B, and D are not specific to preventing VAP but rather focus on other aspects of patient care such as sepsis management (Sepsis Bundle), hemodynamic optimization (EGDT), and organ dysfunction assessment (SOFA score). Therefore, the Ventilator Bundle is the most appropriate algorithm in this scenario to prevent VAP and improve patient safety.

Question 18: Correct Answer: B) Consult with the healthcare provider to clarify the medication order.

Rationale: In this scenario, the nurse's priority should be patient safety. Administering a dose higher than the recommended safe dosage can lead to adverse effects, especially in an elderly patient who is drowsy and confused. Consulting with the healthcare provider to clarify the medication order ensures that the patient receives the appropriate and safe dose of pain medication. Waiting for the next scheduled dose or informing the family without taking immediate action can compromise patient safety. By consulting with the healthcare provider, the nurse upholds the principles of patient safety and effective communication in care management.

Question 19: Correct Answer: B) Listening actively to a patient's concerns and involving them in the care plan.

Rationale: Patient-centered care is a fundamental aspect of nursing practice that focuses on involving patients in their care decisions and respecting their preferences. By actively listening to a patient's concerns and involving them in the care plan, the nurse demonstrates empathy, respect, and a commitment to addressing the patient's needs. Ignoring complaints, dismissing feedback, or providing medication without explanation are not aligned with patient-centered care principles and may lead to increased grievances and decreased patient satisfaction. Active listening and collaboration with patients promote trust, communication, and better outcomes in healthcare delivery.

Question 20: Correct Answer: D) All of the above

Rationale: A Certified Medical Surgical Registered Nurse (CMSRN) needs to possess a combination of technical, communication, and critical thinking skills to excel in their role. While technical skills are essential for providing quality patient care, communication skills are crucial for effective interaction with patients, families, and the healthcare team. Additionally, critical thinking skills enable nurses to make sound clinical judgments and decisions. Therefore, having all these abilities collectively (option D) is vital for a CMSRN to navigate the complexities of healthcare delivery, promote positive patient outcomes, and contribute to a collaborative healthcare environment.

Question 21: Correct Answer: B) Provide her with information on local religious services and clergy members for spiritual guidance.

Rationale: Addressing the spiritual needs of a patient like Ms. Johnson is crucial in providing holistic care. Option A may be beneficial, but it does not directly address Ms. Johnson's individual spiritual beliefs. Option C overlooks the importance of spiritual comfort in end-of-life care. Option D may hinder Ms. Johnson's coping mechanisms. Providing information on local religious services and clergy members allows Ms. Johnson to seek spiritual guidance aligned with her beliefs, promoting emotional well-being and comfort during this challenging time.

Question 22: Correct Answer: B) Providing detailed information in an organized manner

Rationale: Providing detailed information in an organized manner during a hand-off report is crucial for effective communication and patient safety. This approach ensures that essential patient data, including current status, medications, treatments, and any recent changes, are accurately conveyed. Using vague language (Option A) can lead to misunderstandings and errors. Skipping over past medical history (Option C) can result in overlooking important details. Omitting changes in the patient's condition (Option D) can jeopardize patient safety by failing to communicate critical updates. Therefore, option B is the most appropriate choice for a successful hand-off report.

Question 23: Correct Answer: A) Ensure proper alignment of the endotracheal tube.

Rationale: During prone positioning, ensuring the proper alignment of the endotracheal tube is crucial to maintain adequate oxygenation and prevent complications such as accidental extubation or endobronchial intubation. Monitoring for pressure ulcers is important but not the priority during the prone positioning procedure. Administering pain medication and checking the nasogastric tube are essential aspects of care but do not take precedence over ensuring the airway patency and oxygenation of the patient in this critical situation.

Question 24: Correct Answer: A) Acupuncture is based on the principle of restoring the flow of Qi, or vital energy, within the body.

Rationale: Acupuncture is rooted in traditional Chinese medicine, where it is believed that the body's vital energy, Qi, flows along meridians. By inserting needles at specific points, acupuncturists aim to restore the balance and flow of Qi to promote healing and alleviate pain. Option B is incorrect as acupuncture also stimulates the release of endorphins and other neurotransmitters to reduce pain perception. Option C is incorrect as acupuncture has been shown to be effective for both acute and chronic pain conditions. Option D is incorrect as long as proper sterile techniques are followed during acupuncture sessions, the risk of infection is minimal.

Question 25: Correct Answer: A) Educate Mr. Smith on proper body mechanics and safe lifting techniques.

Rationale: Option A is the correct answer as educating Mr. Smith on proper body mechanics and safe lifting techniques is crucial in preventing work-related injuries. By teaching him the correct way to lift heavy objects, such as bending at the knees and keeping the back straight, the risk of further injury can be minimized. Option B is incorrect as solely providing pain medication does not address the root cause of the issue. Option C is incorrect as continuing to lift heavy objects without proper technique can exacerbate the injury. Option D is incorrect as ignoring the pain and continuing to work can lead to further harm and complications.

Question 26: Correct Answer: D) Integrating physical therapy with analgesic medications

Rationale: Multimodal pain management involves utilizing a combination of interventions to address pain effectively. Option A is incorrect as relying solely on opioids does not constitute a multimodal approach. Option B is incorrect because using heat therapy alone is not considered multimodal. Option C is incorrect as cognitive-behavioral therapy alone is not a multimodal strategy. The correct answer, Option D, is supported by evidence showing that integrating physical therapy with analgesic medications can lead to better pain control, functional improvement, and reduced reliance on medications, making it a comprehensive multimodal approach.

Question 27: Correct Answer: A) Patient satisfaction and experience based on personalized care

Rationale: In the given scenario, the correct answer is A) Patient satisfaction and experience based on personalized care. This aligns with the core principle of value-based purchasing, which emphasizes providing high-quality, individualized care to enhance patient outcomes and satisfaction. Option B is incorrect as cost reduction should not compromise the quality of care provided. Option C is incorrect as value-based purchasing focuses on meeting patient needs effectively, which may impact the length of hospital stay. Option D is incorrect as standardized care may not always address individual patient preferences, which is essential in value-based purchasing to improve outcomes and experiences.

Question 28: Correct Answer: B) Document her concerns in the patient's chart and inform the nursing supervisor.

Rationale: In this scenario, the correct course of action for Nurse Sarah is to document her observations and concerns in the patient's chart and then escalate the issue by informing the nursing supervisor. This aligns with the concept of "speaking up" in patient care management, where healthcare professionals are encouraged to voice their concerns regarding patient safety. Option A is incorrect as it disregards the patient's deteriorating condition. Option C is incorrect as ignoring the situation compromises patient safety. Option D is incorrect as administering sedatives without addressing the underlying issue can be harmful to the patient. By documenting and escalating her concerns, Nurse Sarah ensures that appropriate actions are taken promptly to address Mr. Johnson's changing health status, promoting patient safety and effective care management.

Question 29: Correct Answer: B) Scheduling an appointment with a different specialist for Mrs. Smith to obtain a second opinion.

Rationale: Providing patient-centered care involves respecting the patient's autonomy and preferences. In this scenario, scheduling an appointment with a different specialist aligns with patient-centered care by empowering Mrs. Smith to seek a second opinion and explore other treatment options. Option A focuses on emotional support, Option C emphasizes education, and Option D disregards Mrs. Smith's request for a second opinion, making them less suitable choices in this context.

Question 30: Correct Answer: C) Ensure that two fingers can be inserted between the restraint and the patient's skin

Rationale: It is crucial for the CMSRN to maintain proper restraint application by ensuring that there is enough slack to insert two fingers between the restraint and the patient's skin. This practice prevents skin breakdown, nerve damage, and circulation impairment. Options A and B are incorrect as they can lead to skin injuries and compromise patient safety. Option D is inappropriate as it violates ethical principles and patient rights by not involving them in the decision-making process. Therefore, option C is the correct choice for ensuring patient safety and quality care.

Question 31: Correct Answer: B) The patient has the right to receive all information about their condition and treatment options.

Rationale: Informed consent is a crucial aspect of a patient's rights, ensuring they receive all necessary information regarding their condition, treatment options, risks, and benefits before making a decision. Option A is incorrect as it only addresses the right to refuse treatment, which is part of informed consent but not the complete definition. Option C is incorrect as patients do not have the right to demand specific medications without medical justification. Option D is incorrect as patients can choose their healthcare provider but this is not directly related to informed consent.

Question 32: Correct Answer: D) Gabapentin

Rationale: Gabapentin is a medication commonly used in the management of chronic neuropathic pain, such as that experienced by patients with degenerative disc disease. It works by stabilizing electrical activity in the brain and nervous system. Acetaminophen (Option A) is more suitable for mild pain relief and is not as effective for chronic neuropathic pain. Ibuprofen (Option B) is a nonsteroidal anti-inflammatory drug (NSAID) that is more appropriate for acute pain and inflammation. Morphine sulfate (Option C) is an opioid analgesic typically reserved for severe acute pain or end-of-life care, not for chronic pain management like in Mr. Johnson's case. Therefore, Gabapentin is the most suitable option for managing Mr. Johnson's chronic lower back pain.

Question 33: Correct Answer: B) A form that specifies the medical treatments a patient does or does not wish to receive in specific situations.

Rationale: Option A is incorrect as it describes a healthcare proxy or durable power of attorney, which is a separate legal document from an advance directive. Option C is incorrect as it refers to a spiritual care plan, which is not the primary focus of an advance directive. Option D is incorrect as it pertains to organ donation preferences, which although important, are not directly related to advance directives. The correct answer, Option B, accurately defines an advance directive as a document that allows individuals to outline their preferences for medical treatments in advance, ensuring their wishes are known and respected during end-of-life care.

Question 34: Correct Answer: B) Acupuncture

Rationale: Acupuncture is a traditional Chinese medicine practice that involves inserting thin needles into specific points on the body to stimulate energy flow and promote healing. Aromatherapy (Option A) uses essential oils for therapeutic purposes, Reflexology (Option C) involves applying pressure to specific points on the feet, hands, or ears, and Reiki (Option D) is a form of energy healing. Acupuncture has been widely studied and shown to be effective in managing various conditions such as chronic pain, nausea, and anxiety, making it a popular choice among patients seeking complementary therapies.

Question 35: Correct Answer: A) Adverse drug reaction

Rationale: In this scenario, the unintended consequence is an adverse drug reaction, as the patient experienced severe allergic reactions after taking the prescribed medication. This outcome was not the intended therapeutic effect of the medication but rather a harmful reaction. Option B, therapeutic success, is incorrect as the patient did not experience the desired therapeutic outcome. Option C, patient satisfaction, is incorrect as the patient faced a medical emergency due to the adverse reaction. Option D, routine side effect, is also incorrect as the allergic reaction was severe and unexpected, not a common or anticipated side effect.

Question 36: Correct Answer: C) Asking open-ended questions to gather detailed information from the patient.

Rationale: Asking open-ended questions during a patient assessment encourages the patient to provide detailed information, enabling the nurse to gather comprehensive data for accurate evaluation and care planning. Options A and B hinder effective communication by creating confusion and barriers to understanding. Option D disrupts the flow of information exchange and may lead to incomplete assessment data. Effective communication in assessment involves active listening, clear explanations, and open-ended questions to promote patient-centered care and holistic understanding of the patient's health status.

Question 37: Correct Answer: C) To restore the balance of intestinal flora

Rationale: Probiotics are beneficial bacteria that help restore the natural balance of gut flora, which can be disrupted during antibiotic therapy or infections like Clostridium difficile. Option A is incorrect as probiotics actually help inhibit the growth of pathogenic bacteria by competing for nutrients and adhesion sites. Option B is incorrect as probiotics support the immune system. Option D is incorrect as probiotics do not increase the risk of antibiotic resistance; in fact, they may help reduce it by restoring healthy gut flora.

Question 38: Correct Answer: B) Double-checking the medication with another nurse before administration

Rationale: Double-checking the medication with another nurse before administration is a vital step in ensuring medication safety. This practice helps in verifying the right patient, medication, dose, route, and time, reducing the risk of medication errors. Administering medications based on verbal orders (Option A) can

lead to miscommunication errors. Crushing medications without consulting the pharmacist (Option C) can alter the drug's effectiveness or cause harm. Using the same syringe to administer multiple medications (Option D) can result in cross-contamination and adverse reactions. Double-checking with another nurse enhances patient safety and minimizes medication errors.

Question 39: Correct Answer: B) Implementing evidence-based practice to reduce unnecessary tests and procedures

Rationale: Implementing evidence-based practice to reduce unnecessary tests and procedures is the most effective approach for cost-saving measures without compromising patient care. This strategy ensures that resources are utilized efficiently, avoiding unnecessary expenses while maintaining high-quality care standards. Decreasing the number of nursing staff on each shift (Option A) can lead to increased workload, compromising patient safety. Cutting down on staff education and training programs (Option C) can hinder professional development and quality of care. Using outdated medical equipment (Option D) may result in higher maintenance costs and compromise patient outcomes. Therefore, Option B is the most appropriate choice for optimizing budgetary considerations in nursing teamwork and collaboration.

Question 40: Correct Answer: A) Braden Scale

Rationale: The Braden Scale is a widely recognized risk assessment tool used to evaluate a patient's risk of developing pressure ulcers. It assesses six criteria: sensory perception, moisture, activity, mobility, nutrition, and friction/shear. The other options, Glasgow Coma Scale, Morse Fall Scale, and Wong-Baker FACES Pain Rating Scale, are used for assessing different aspects of patient care such as neurological status, fall risk, and pain assessment, respectively. However, when specifically focusing on assessing the risk of pressure ulcers, the Braden Scale is the most appropriate tool due to its comprehensive evaluation criteria.

Question 41: Correct Answer: B) Patient advocacy

Rationale: Patient advocacy is a crucial role for a CMSRN as it involves ensuring that patients' rights and preferences are respected, promoting their well-being, and acting as a liaison between patients and the healthcare team. This role focuses on empowering patients to make informed decisions about their care and advocating for their best interests. While administrative duties, facility maintenance, and supply chain management are important aspects of healthcare delivery, they do not directly align with the core responsibilities of a CMSRN in terms of patient-centered care and advocacy.

Question 42: Correct Answer: D) Schedule a one-on-one session with Mr. Johnson to discuss his concerns and provide personalized education.

Rationale: Option A is incorrect because simply providing a list of potential side effects and interactions may overwhelm the patient and not address his specific concerns. Option B is incorrect as relying on online research may lead to misinformation and confusion for the patient. Option C is incorrect as pharmaceutical pamphlets may not address Mr. Johnson's individual questions and may contain complex medical jargon. The correct answer is D as scheduling a personalized session allows for tailored education, addressing Mr. Johnson's concerns directly and ensuring clear understanding of his new medication.

Question 43: Correct Answer: C) Informed consent is a process where the patient is provided with information about a procedure.

Rationale: Informed consent is a crucial aspect of patient care, ensuring that patients have a clear understanding of the risks, benefits, and alternatives to a procedure before providing their consent. Option A is incorrect as informed consent is necessary for all procedures, not just routine ones. Option B is incorrect as informed consent is required for all procedures, regardless of risk level. Option D is incorrect as informed consent involves shared decision-making between the healthcare provider and the patient, with both parties actively participating in the process.

Question 44: Correct Answer: C) Engaging patients in shared decision-making

Rationale: Patient-centered care emphasizes the importance of involving patients in their care decisions, considering their preferences, values, and beliefs. By engaging patients in shared decision-making, healthcare providers can tailor treatment plans to individual needs, leading to improved patient satisfaction and outcomes. Options A, B, and D are incorrect as they go against the principles of patient-centered care, which requires a holistic approach that addresses not only physical symptoms but also emotional, social, and spiritual aspects of care.

Question 45: Correct Answer: A) Providing the patient with detailed information about their diagnosis and treatment plan.

Rationale: Patient-centered care emphasizes the importance of involving patients in their care decisions and providing them with comprehensive information about their health status, treatment options, and care plans. Option A reflects the core principle of patient-centered care by empowering the patient with knowledge and involving them in the decision-making process. Options B, C, and D are not aligned with patient-centered care as they disregard the patient's autonomy, preferences, and cultural considerations, which are essential aspects of holistic patient care.

Question 46: Correct Answer: C) Smoking

Rationale: Smoking is a modifiable risk factor that directly impacts patient safety and care management. By quitting smoking, patients can reduce the risk of various health complications such as respiratory issues, cardiovascular diseases, and surgical complications. Age and gender are non-modifiable risk factors that may influence patient outcomes but cannot be altered. Genetic predisposition, while significant, is also non-modifiable. Therefore, smoking stands out as a crucial risk factor that healthcare providers can actively address to improve patient safety and care management.

Question 47: Correct Answer: C) Respecting the expertise of other team members

Rationale: In interprofessional care, respecting the expertise of other team members is crucial for effective collaboration. This fosters a culture of mutual respect, trust, and understanding among healthcare professionals, leading to improved patient outcomes. Options A and B hinder collaboration by promoting isolation and lack of communication, which can result in fragmented care. Option D dismisses the value of input from different disciplines, which is counterproductive to achieving comprehensive patient care. Therefore, option C stands out as the correct choice for promoting successful interprofessional teamwork.

Question 48: Correct Answer: B) Volunteering to assist colleagues with complex patient cases

Rationale: Option B is the correct answer as it showcases Sarah's proactive attitude towards career development relationships. By offering help to colleagues with complex cases, Sarah not only demonstrates teamwork and collaboration but also shows her willingness to learn and grow within the nursing team. Options A, C, and D are incorrect as they reflect passive or negative behaviors that do not contribute to building strong relationships or fostering career development. It is essential for nurses to actively engage with their team, seek learning opportunities, and support each other to promote a positive work environment and professional growth.

Question 49: Correct Answer: A) Pain management

Rationale: Pain management is a crucial nursing-sensitive indicator in postoperative care as effective pain control is essential for patient comfort, early mobilization, and overall recovery. Monitoring and addressing pain promptly align with evidence-based guidelines to enhance patient outcomes. Patient falls, pressure ulcers, and medication errors are also important indicators; however, in the immediate postoperative period, pain management takes precedence to ensure patient comfort and facilitate early ambulation, which are key factors in preventing complications and promoting recovery.

Question 50: Correct Answer: A) Providing Mrs. Patel with a menu that includes vegetarian meal options.

Rationale: Option A is the correct answer as it demonstrates cultural sensitivity by respecting Mrs. Patel's dietary preferences based on her cultural background. Traditional Ayurvedic practices often include vegetarianism, and offering suitable meal options aligns with holistic patient care. Options B, C, and D are incorrect as they do not address Mrs. Patel's cultural and linguistic needs. Using medical jargon may confuse her due to limited English proficiency, excluding her daughter can hinder effective communication, and disregarding her cultural practices goes against providing patient-centered care.

Question 51: Correct Answer: C) Gabapentin

Rationale: Gabapentin is a medication frequently prescribed for chronic neuropathic pain due to its mechanism of action in modulating calcium channels and reducing excitatory neurotransmitter release. Ibuprofen and acetaminophen are more commonly used for acute pain and have different mechanisms of action. Aspirin, although effective for certain types of pain, is not typically the first-line choice for chronic neuropathic pain. Therefore, the correct answer is Gabapentin as it specifically targets the neuropathic pain pathways, making it a suitable option for chronic pain management.

Question 52: Correct Answer: A) Technology enhances communication by providing real-time messaging and video conferencing capabilities.

Rationale: Technology plays a crucial role in improving communication among healthcare teams by offering tools such as real-time messaging platforms and video conferencing, which facilitate quick information exchange and seamless collaboration. These technological advancements enable healthcare professionals to communicate efficiently, share updates on patient care, and consult with team members regardless of physical location. In contrast, options B, C, and D are incorrect as they do not acknowledge the positive impact that technology has on enhancing communication within interprofessional healthcare teams.

Question 53: Correct Answer: B) Observing nursing staff during their daily interactions

Rationale: Observing nursing staff during their daily interactions is the most effective method for identifying gaps in knowledge and skills related to teamwork and collaboration. This approach provides direct insight into how team members communicate, coordinate care, and work together in real-time situations. Unlike sending out a general survey (Option A), which may not capture the nuances of actual teamwork dynamics, or reviewing incident reports (Option C), which only highlight specific issues after they have occurred, observation allows for a comprehensive understanding of the team's strengths and areas needing improvement. Conducting individual interviews (Option D) may provide valuable insights but may not offer a holistic view of teamwork practices within the nursing team.

Question 54: Correct Answer: C) Initiate oxygen therapy

Rationale: In this scenario, the nurse should prioritize initiating oxygen therapy (Option C) for Mr. Johnson. Oxygen therapy is crucial in the management of a patient with chest pain and shortness of breath to improve oxygenation and reduce the workload on the heart. Administering nitroglycerin (Option A) and performing a stat ECG (Option B) are important interventions but should follow the initiation of oxygen therapy. Drawing blood for labs (Option D) can be delegated to a support staff member once the patient's respiratory status is stabilized. Prioritizing oxygen therapy ensures the patient's immediate safety and addresses the most critical need in this situation.

Question 55: Correct Answer: C) Implement alternative measures such as frequent monitoring and family presence.

Rationale: Option A is incorrect as using wrist restraints solely to prevent Mr. Johnson from pulling out medical devices may compromise his circulation and mobility, leading to potential complications. Option B is not the best choice as chemical restraints should be avoided unless absolutely necessary due to the associated risks and ethical considerations. Option D is not recommended as ankle restraints can increase the risk of falls and skin breakdown. Option C is the most appropriate answer as it promotes patient safety through non-restraint interventions such as frequent monitoring and involving family members in the care process, aligning with patient-centered and evidence-based care practices.

Question 56: Correct Answer: B) Speaking calmly and reassuringly, acknowledging his feelings and offering to help

Rationale: In this scenario, the most appropriate de-escalation technique is to choose option B, which involves speaking calmly and reassuringly to the patient, acknowledging his feelings, and offering assistance. This approach aims to validate the patient's emotions, show empathy, and establish a connection to address his needs effectively. Options A, C, and D are incorrect as they do not promote a therapeutic nurse-patient relationship and may further escalate the situation by disregarding the patient's feelings, matching aggression, or using threats, which can be counterproductive in managing agitation and promoting patient cooperation.

Question 57: Correct Answer: C) Attending interprofessional team meetings to discuss patient care.

Rationale: Effective interprofessional collaboration involves active participation in team meetings where healthcare professionals from various disciplines come together to discuss and plan patient care. Option A is incorrect as working in isolation hinders collaboration. Option B is inadequate as communication should extend beyond the same discipline for comprehensive care. Option D is counterproductive as disregarding input undermines the value of diverse perspectives in improving patient outcomes. Therefore, attending interprofessional team meetings promotes shared decision-making, enhances communication, and fosters holistic patient care.

Question 58: Correct Answer: C) Taking initiative in decision-making and actively participating in team discussions.

Rationale: Professional empowerment in nursing involves nurses taking charge of their practice, making autonomous decisions, and actively engaging in collaborative teamwork. Option A is incorrect as seeking approval hinders empowerment. Option B is incorrect as teamwork and collaboration are essential in nursing practice. Option D is incorrect as empowerment encourages questioning and critical thinking, not blind obedience. Therefore, the correct choice is C, where nurses demonstrate empowerment by actively participating in decision-making and teamwork, fostering a culture of professional growth and development.

Question 59: Correct Answer: B) Listen actively to Mr. Johnson's concerns, validate his feelings, and involve him in the care planning process.

Rationale: Option B is the correct answer as it aligns with the principles of patient-centered care, emphasizing active listening, empathy, and involving the patient in decision-making. By listening to Mr. Johnson's concerns, validating his feelings, and involving him in the care planning process, the CMSRN can address his anxiety, build trust, and promote a collaborative approach to his care. Options A, C, and D are incorrect as they do not prioritize patient-centered care. Providing detailed explanations using medical jargon (Option A) may further confuse and overwhelm the patient. Minimizing interactions (Option C) and implementing care plans without discussion (Option D) disregard the patient's emotional needs and preferences, contradicting the holistic approach of patient-centered care.

Question 60: Correct Answer: B) Utilizing a barcode scanner to verify medication administration

Rationale: Utilizing a barcode scanner to verify medication administration is a standard practice in medical-surgical settings to ensure patient safety and accuracy in medication administration. This technology helps in matching the right medication with the right patient, dosage, and time, reducing medication errors. Options A, C, and D pose serious risks to patient confidentiality and data security, violating HIPAA regulations and compromising patient privacy. It is crucial for nurses to adhere to best practices and use technology appropriately to provide safe and effective patient care.

Question 61: Correct Answer: B) Sarah discusses Mr. Johnson's wishes with the healthcare team and advocates for palliative care in a private meeting.

Rationale: Option B is the correct answer as it showcases Sarah's advocacy for the patient's autonomy and end-of-life wishes, aligning with ethical principles and professional concepts. By initiating a discussion with the healthcare team and advocating for palliative care, Sarah addresses moral distress by promoting patient-centered care and ethical decision-making. Options A, C, and D do not effectively address the moral distress experienced by Sarah, as they either neglect the patient's wishes or fail to actively advocate for patient-centered care, highlighting the importance of effective communication and advocacy in nursing practice.

Question 62: Correct Answer: D) Ignoring her own needs and consistently working overtime without rest.

Rationale: Option D is the correct answer as it highlights a behavior that contributes to burnout. Ignoring personal needs, such as rest and work-life balance, can lead to physical and emotional exhaustion, impacting overall well-being. Options A, B, and C promote self-care practices and seeking support, which are essential for nurse resiliency and well-being. Taking breaks, engaging in physical exercise, and seeking support from colleagues are positive strategies to prevent burnout and promote a healthy practice environment.

Question 63: Correct Answer: A) Administering medications without proper training

Rationale: Administering medications without proper training is a clear violation of the nurse's scope of practice as it poses serious risks to patient safety. Nurses must adhere to the local governing regulations and only perform tasks within their scope of practice to ensure the highest quality of care. Options B, C, and D are within the nurse's scope of practice as long as they align with established protocols, policies, and physician approval, respectively. It is crucial for nurses to always practice within the boundaries of their training and expertise to maintain patient safety and uphold professional standards.

Question 64: Correct Answer: C) Patient's current medical condition

Rationale: When providing dietary consultation for a patient requiring alternate nutrition administration, the most crucial factor to consider is the patient's current medical condition. This includes assessing the patient's nutritional needs based on their diagnosis, medical history, and any ongoing treatments. While considering the patient's favorite food and cultural dietary preferences is important for enhancing compliance and satisfaction, the primary focus should always be on meeting the patient's specific nutritional requirements to support their health and recovery. Preferred meal timings, although relevant, are secondary to ensuring that the patient's medical condition is appropriately addressed through the dietary plan.

Question 65: Correct Answer: A) Deep breathing exercises

Rationale: Deep breathing exercises are a widely recognized non-pharmacological intervention for promoting relaxation and reducing anxiety in medical-surgical patients. These exercises help patients focus on their breathing patterns, leading to decreased stress levels and improved oxygenation. Administering sedatives (option B) may have adverse effects and is not the first-line approach for anxiety management. Increasing caffeine intake (option C) can exacerbate anxiety symptoms due to its stimulant properties. Encouraging vigorous physical activity (option D) may not always be suitable for all patients, especially those with physical limitations or acute conditions. Therefore, deep breathing exercises are the most appropriate and effective intervention in this scenario.

Question 66: Correct Answer: C) BMI

Rationale: The correct answer is C) BMI. Mrs. Smith's BMI of 32 indicates obesity, which is a significant risk factor for developing complications such as pressure ulcers, deep vein thrombosis, and surgical site infections during her hospital stay. While age (option A) is a consideration in overall health assessment, it is not the primary factor in this scenario. Gender (option B) does not directly impact the risk of complications related to obesity. Blood pressure (option D) is important but not as directly linked to the increased risk of complications as BMI in this case. Therefore, the most relevant demographic factor in this scenario is Mrs. Smith's BMI.

Question 67: Correct Answer: C) Azithromycin

Rationale: Azithromycin is a macrolide antibiotic commonly used in the treatment of community-acquired pneumonia due to its coverage of typical and atypical pathogens involved in such infections. Ciprofloxacin (Option A) is a fluoroquinolone antibiotic more commonly used for urinary tract infections. Vancomycin (Option B) is a glycopeptide antibiotic reserved for serious gram-positive infections like MRSA. Metronidazole (Option D) is an antibiotic primarily used for anaerobic infections. Therefore, the correct choice for Mr. Smith's pneumonia treatment would be Azithromycin due to its spectrum of coverage for the likely pathogens involved in community-acquired pneumonia.

Question 68: Correct Answer: C) Obesity

Rationale: Obesity is a significant risk factor for surgical complications due to its association with impaired wound healing, increased risk of infection, and respiratory issues. While controlled diabetes (option A) and well-managed hypertension (option B) are important considerations, obesity poses a higher risk in surgical patients. Being a non-smoker (option D) is beneficial for postoperative recovery but does not outweigh the impact of obesity on surgical outcomes. In Mr. Johnson's case, addressing his obesity preoperatively and providing appropriate perioperative care will be crucial in reducing the risk of complications.

Question 69: Correct Answer: A) Online courses on conflict resolution

Rationale: Online courses on conflict resolution are a valuable career development resource that enhances Nursing Teamwork and Collaboration skills. These courses provide nurses with the necessary knowledge and techniques to effectively manage conflicts within the healthcare team, leading to improved teamwork and collaboration. Options B and C focus on individual development rather than teamwork, while option D, social media platforms, although useful for networking, may not directly contribute to enhancing teamwork and collaboration skills within the nursing team. Therefore, option A is the most relevant choice for career development in Nursing Teamwork and Collaboration.

Question 70: Correct Answer: C) Utilize visual aids and plain language to explain the procedure and post-operative care.

Rationale: Health literacy is crucial in ensuring patients understand their conditions, treatments, and instructions. In this scenario, the most appropriate action for the nurse is to utilize visual aids and plain language to effectively communicate with Ms. Johnson. Providing written instructions with medical jargon (Option A) would not be helpful for a patient with limited health literacy. Using complex medical terminologies (Option B) can further confuse the patient. Speaking quickly to save time (Option D) may lead to misunderstandings and hinder effective communication. Therefore, utilizing visual aids and plain language (Option C) is the best approach to promote understanding and ensure Ms. Johnson's active participation in her care.

Question 71: Correct Answer: B) Hands-on interactive workshops

Rationale: Hands-on interactive workshops are the most effective teaching method for educating patients and families in a holistic patient care approach. This method allows for active participation, engagement, and practical application of knowledge, leading to better retention and understanding of the information provided. In contrast, lecture-based sessions (option A) may be passive and less engaging, written materials only (option C) may not cater to different learning styles, and group discussions and role-playing activities (option D) may not provide the hands-on experience necessary for effective learning in this context.

Question 72: Correct Answer: B) Full Code

Rationale: In this scenario, Mr. Johnson has clearly stated his preference to receive full resuscitative measures in case of cardiac arrest. Therefore, the appropriate code status for him would be "Full Code." Option A, DNR (Do Not Resuscitate), is incorrect as it contradicts Mr. Johnson's expressed preference. Option C, DNI (Do Not Intubate), is also incorrect as it specifically refers to intubation and not overall resuscitative measures. Option D, Comfort Measures Only, is not applicable in this case as Mr. Johnson has opted for full resuscitation. It is crucial for healthcare providers to respect and honor patients' end-of-life preferences to provide patient-centered care.

Question 73: Correct Answer: B) Consult with the healthcare provider to clarify the medication dosage.

Rationale: In this scenario, the correct action for the CMSRN is to consult with the healthcare provider to clarify the medication dosage discrepancy. It is essential to ensure patient safety and accuracy in medication administration by seeking clarification from the prescriber when encountering conflicting orders. Administering the incorrect dosage could lead to adverse effects on the patient's condition. Holding the medication until clarification is obtained is the appropriate course of action to prevent errors and prioritize patient well-being. Administering either of the conflicting dosages without clarification poses a risk to the patient's health, highlighting the importance of effective communication and professional reporting in healthcare settings.

Question 74: Correct Answer: A) Formulating a research question

Rationale: Formulating a research question is the initial step in the research process. It involves identifying a specific area of interest or concern that needs to be addressed through research. In this scenario, before conducting a literature review, designing a research study, or analyzing research data, the healthcare team must first formulate a clear and focused research question related to wound care protocols for diabetic foot ulcers. This question will guide the subsequent steps in the research process, ensuring that the team's efforts are directed towards addressing the specific needs of the patient population. Conducting a literature review, designing a research study, and analyzing research data are important subsequent steps in the research process but come after formulating a research question.

Question 75: Correct Answer: A) The use of multiple medications by a patient for the treatment of various conditions.

Rationale: Polypharmacy refers to the concurrent use of multiple medications by a patient, often involving several healthcare providers. It is a common concern in healthcare as it can lead to adverse drug interactions, non-adherence to treatment plans, and increased risk of medication errors. Option A is the correct definition as it accurately describes the practice of using multiple medications to manage various health conditions. Options B, C, and D are incorrect as they do not capture the essence of polypharmacy and may lead to misconceptions about this important concept in medication management.

Question 76: Correct Answer: C) Providing clear and simple explanations

Rationale: Clear and simple explanations enhance patient understanding and compliance with medical instructions. Using complex medical jargon (Option A) can confuse patients and hinder effective communication. Speaking quickly (Option B) may lead to misunderstandings and errors. Avoiding eye contact (Option D) can make patients feel disconnected and impact trust. Therefore, the most effective technique is to provide information in a clear and simple manner, ensuring patients comprehend and follow medical guidance effectively.

Question 77: Correct Answer: B) Implement a checklist to ensure proper surgical site preparation.

Rationale: The correct answer is to implement a checklist to ensure proper surgical site preparation. This action directly addresses the root cause identified in the scenario and provides a systematic approach to prevent similar incidents. Option A focuses on hand hygiene, which is important but not directly related to the specific issue of surgical site preparation. Option C addresses patient education, which is valuable but does not address the system-level error identified in the RCA. Option D, reviewing the visitor policy, is important for infection control but does not directly address the root cause of the post-operative infection.

Question 78: Correct Answer: D) Educating her on medication adherence techniques and providing a pill organizer

Rationale: Option A is not the most appropriate resource as simply providing a list of pharmacies does not directly address Ms. Johnson's concerns regarding medication management. Option B, scheduling a follow-up appointment with the primary care physician, is important but may not specifically address her immediate need for medication management support. Option C, referring her to a community health nurse for home visits, could be beneficial but may not be readily available post-discharge. Option D is the correct answer as it directly addresses Ms. Johnson's concerns by providing education on medication adherence techniques and offering a practical solution with a pill organizer, promoting holistic patient care and empowering the patient to manage their medications effectively at home.

Question 79: Correct Answer: C) Utilize professional medical interpreters

Rationale: Utilizing professional medical interpreters is crucial to ensure accurate communication between healthcare providers and patients with limited English proficiency. Using family members as interpreters can lead to breaches in patient confidentiality and misinterpretation of medical information. Relying on non-certified bilingual staff may result in inaccuracies and misunderstandings. Avoiding interpretation services altogether can compromise patient safety and quality of care. Professional medical interpreters are trained to accurately convey medical information, maintain confidentiality, and bridge the communication gap effectively, promoting holistic patient care and upholding diversity and inclusion principles in healthcare settings.

Question 80: Correct Answer: B) Allow family members to actively participate in Mrs. Smith's care and decision-making process.

Rationale: In patient-centered care, involving the patient's family in the care process is crucial for better outcomes. Option A is incorrect as it limits family involvement, which is not aligned with patient-centered care principles. Option C is incorrect as family involvement should be encouraged unless it hinders medical interventions. Option D is incorrect as family members should be encouraged to ask questions to stay informed and involved in the patient's care. Option B is the correct answer as it promotes holistic patient care by recognizing the importance of family support and involvement in the patient's recovery journey.

Question 81: Correct Answer: B) Collaborate with the wound care nurse specialist for guidance.

Rationale: In this scenario, the appropriate action for the CMSRN is to collaborate with the wound care nurse specialist for guidance. Delegating the task to a nursing assistant (Option A) may not be suitable as the wound appears infected, requiring specialized knowledge. Asking the patient's family member to assist (Option C) or seeking advice from the unit clerk (Option D) does not align with the scope of practice for wound care management. Collaborating with the wound care nurse specialist ensures that the patient receives the necessary expertise and care for the infected wound, emphasizing the importance of teamwork and collaboration in nursing practice.

Question 82: Correct Answer: C) Encouraging reporting of near-misses and adverse events

Rationale: Encouraging reporting of near-misses and adverse events is crucial in high accountable organizations to promote patient safety culture. This practice fosters a culture of transparency, continuous improvement, and learning from mistakes. Options A, B, and D are incorrect as they represent practices that are counterproductive to patient safety culture. Blaming individuals for errors creates a culture of fear and hinders reporting, lack of communication leads to errors, and ignoring safety protocols jeopardizes patient safety. Therefore, option C is the most appropriate choice in promoting patient safety within high accountable organizations.

Question 83: Correct Answer: C) Encouraging early ambulation post-surgery

Rationale: In the context of preventing surgical site infections, care bundles are designed to improve patient outcomes by implementing a set of evidence-based practices. Options A, B, and D are commonly included in surgical site infection prevention care bundles. Administering prophylactic antibiotics before surgery helps reduce the risk of infection, maintaining normothermia supports optimal healing, and using sterile technique during dressing changes minimizes the introduction of pathogens. However, encouraging early ambulation post-surgery is more related to preventing complications such as deep vein thrombosis rather than directly preventing surgical site infections.

Question 84: Correct Answer: A) Advocating for fair compensation and benefits for all staff members

Rationale: Staff advocacy is an essential aspect of nursing leadership, emphasizing the importance of supporting and speaking up for the well-being and rights of all staff members. Option A is the correct choice as advocating for fair compensation and benefits ensures that the nursing team feels valued, motivated, and supported, leading to improved job satisfaction and retention rates. Options B, C, and D are incorrect as they do not align with the principles of staff advocacy, which should focus on promoting a positive work environment, fostering teamwork, and prioritizing the collective welfare of the staff over individual interests.

Question 85: Correct Answer: C) The pharmacist who communicates effectively with other team members to ensure medication safety.

Rationale: Effective teamwork in healthcare relies on interprofessional collaboration, where team members work together, communicate, and share responsibilities to provide optimal patient care. The pharmacist plays a crucial role in medication management, requiring constant communication with other team members such as nurses, physicians, and technicians to ensure safe and effective medication administration. Unlike options A, B, and D, which depict isolated or non-collaborative roles, option C highlights the importance of teamwork and communication in achieving positive patient outcomes through interprofessional collaboration.

Question 86: Correct Answer: B) Inform the charge nurse about the documentation error and request assistance in rectifying it.

Rationale: Option A is incorrect because documenting false information is unethical and can lead to serious consequences. Option C is incorrect as ignoring the error does not align with the principles of accurate documentation and patient safety. Option D is incorrect as delaying documentation can compromise the continuity of care and patient outcomes. The correct action, as per best practice, is to promptly report any documentation errors to the charge nurse to ensure accurate and complete patient records, promoting safe and effective interprofessional care.

Question 87: Correct Answer: D) Applying a warm compress to Mr. Smith's incision site without informing the nurse

Rationale: In this scenario, the correct action that would require immediate intervention by the registered nurse is option D. Applying a warm compress to the incision site without informing the nurse can potentially introduce infection or disrupt the healing process. It is crucial for the nursing assistant to communicate any changes or interventions related to the patient's condition to the registered nurse for proper assessment and management. Options A, B, and C are all appropriate actions that align with the nursing assistant's scope of practice and delegation instructions, emphasizing the importance of teamwork and collaboration in patient care.

Question 88: Correct Answer: C) Active listening and empathy

Rationale: Active listening and empathy are crucial elements of effective verbal communication in healthcare. By actively listening to patients, nurses can better understand their concerns, provide appropriate support, and build trust. Empathy allows nurses to connect with patients on a deeper level, showing understanding and compassion. In contrast, using complex medical jargon may confuse patients, speaking rapidly can increase anxiety, and interrupting patients can hinder the therapeutic relationship. Therefore, active listening and empathy are the most important aspects of verbal communication in healthcare.

Question 89: Correct Answer: B) Providing access to mental health resources and support groups

Rationale: Providing access to mental health resources and support groups is crucial in promoting nurse resiliency and well-being. It allows nurses to seek help, share experiences, and learn coping strategies. Options A, C, and D are detrimental to nurse well-being as they contribute to burnout, fatigue, and decreased job satisfaction. Working overtime regularly, heavy workloads without breaks, and ignoring signs of burnout can lead to increased stress levels, decreased productivity, and overall negative impact on nurses' mental and physical health. Therefore, option B is the most appropriate choice to support nurse resiliency and well-being in a medical-surgical setting.

Question 90: Correct Answer: A) A legal document that specifies a person's healthcare preferences in case they are unable to communicate

Rationale: An advance directive is a legal document that allows individuals to express their healthcare preferences in advance, particularly regarding end-of-life care, in case they become unable to communicate their wishes. Option B is incorrect as it refers to emergency medical treatment without consent, which is not related to advance directives. Option C is incorrect as advance directives focus on healthcare decisions, not financial matters. Option D is incorrect as it pertains to medication records, not advance directives. Therefore, the correct answer is A, as it accurately defines the purpose of an advance directive in healthcare settings.

Question 91: Correct Answer: A) Electronic Health Records (EHR)

Rationale: Electronic Health Records (EHR) play a crucial role in facilitating communication and information sharing among healthcare team members, enabling seamless coordination of care. EHRs provide a centralized platform for healthcare professionals to access and update patient information, track interventions, and collaborate on patient care plans. In contrast, social media platforms, online gaming platforms, and virtual reality headsets are not designed for secure healthcare communication or interprofessional collaboration, making them unsuitable for effective care coordination in the healthcare setting.

Question 92: Correct Answer: B) Encouraging open communication about errors

Rationale: "Just culture" in Patient Safety emphasizes creating an environment where healthcare professionals feel safe to report errors without fear of retribution. Option A is incorrect as blaming individuals discourages reporting and learning from mistakes. Option C is incorrect because the focus should be on addressing system failures rather than punishing individuals. Option D is incorrect as ignoring errors hinders improvement in patient safety. Encouraging open communication about errors fosters a culture of transparency, accountability, and continuous improvement in healthcare practices.

Question 93: Correct Answer: B) Ensuring the patient receives adequate pain relief post-surgery and advocating for additional pain management if needed.

Rationale: Advocacy is a crucial professional concept in nursing that involves standing up for the patient's rights and needs. In this scenario, ensuring the patient receives adequate pain relief post-surgery and advocating for additional pain management if needed demonstrates advocacy. Option A is incorrect as it neglects the patient's right to information and informed consent. Option C is incorrect as it overlooks individualized patient care. Option D is incorrect as it goes against effective communication and patient education, essential components of advocacy in nursing practice.

Question 94: Correct Answer: D) Sodium level of 125 mEq/L

Rationale: A sodium level of 125 mEq/L indicates hyponatremia, which is a critical condition requiring immediate intervention to prevent neurological complications such as seizures, confusion, and coma. Hemoglobin level of 12 g/dL, potassium level of 3.5 mEq/L, and platelet count of 150,000/mm3 are within normal ranges and do not pose immediate life-threatening risks. Therefore, the CMSRN must prioritize addressing the low sodium level to ensure patient safety and prevent adverse outcomes.

Question 95: Correct Answer: B) Avoiding eye contact, crossed arms, and turning away

Rationale: Mr. Johnson's non-verbal cues of avoiding eye contact, crossing his arms, and turning away indicate discomfort, defensiveness, and a desire to create physical distance. These behaviors suggest that he may be feeling anxious, in pain, or unwilling to engage in conversation. Option A is incorrect as it describes open and engaged body language, which is not displayed by Mr. Johnson. Option C describes positive non-verbal cues that are not present in this scenario. Option D portrays signs of restlessness and distraction, which are not exhibited by Mr. Johnson.

Question 96: Correct Answer: D) Participating in a mentorship program offered by the hospital

Rationale: Participating in a mentorship program offered by the hospital is the most appropriate option for Sarah as it provides her with a structured and ongoing relationship with an experienced nurse who can offer guidance, support, and advice tailored to her needs. This resource allows for personalized mentorship, fostering a nurturing environment for professional growth and development. Option A, attending a one-time workshop, may offer general information but lacks the personalized guidance and support that a mentorship program provides. Option B, joining a nursing professional organization, is beneficial for networking but may not offer the individualized support that a mentor can offer. Option C, watching online educational videos, is valuable for self-learning but does not provide the interactive guidance and support that a mentorship relationship entails.

Question 97: Correct Answer: B) Providing written materials in multiple languages spoken by the local community

Rationale: Providing written materials in multiple languages spoken by the local community is crucial for addressing cultural and linguistic needs in healthcare. This approach promotes diversity and inclusion, enhances patient understanding, and fosters effective communication between healthcare providers and patients from different linguistic backgrounds. Using only the English language (Option A) may create barriers for non-English speakers, leading to misunderstandings and potential risks to patient safety. Using complex medical terminology (Option C) can further alienate patients who may not be familiar with such terms. Ignoring written materials (Option D) disregards the importance of written communication in reinforcing verbal instructions and patient education, which are essential components of holistic patient care.

Question 98: Correct Answer: B) Implementing individualized care plans for each patient

Rationale: Implementing individualized care plans for each patient is crucial in promoting mobility as it tailors interventions to the specific needs and abilities of the patient. Regular team meetings (Option A) are important but may not directly address individual patient needs. While technology (Option C) can aid in monitoring, it does not replace personalized care plans. Administering sedating medications (Option D) can hinder mobility and should be avoided unless medically necessary. By focusing on individualized care plans, healthcare teams can optimize patient mobility outcomes through tailored interventions and support.

Question 99: Correct Answer: C) To provide proactive care and address patient needs promptly

Rationale: Hourly rounding plays a crucial role in patient safety by allowing nurses to anticipate and address patient needs before they escalate. Option A is incorrect as pain assessment is just one aspect of rounding, not the sole purpose. Option B focuses on the environment rather than the patient's well-being. Option D is incorrect as vital signs are typically not required to be documented every hour unless specified by the healthcare provider. Therefore, the correct answer is C as it aligns with the core objective of hourly rounding, which is to provide proactive care and promptly address patient needs to enhance safety and satisfaction.

Question 100: Correct Answer: B) Implementing evidence-based practice guidelines

Rationale: In high accountable organizations, patient/care management revolves around implementing evidence-based practice guidelines to ensure the best possible patient outcomes. This approach emphasizes using proven methods and protocols to deliver safe and effective care. Prioritizing cost-effectiveness over patient outcomes (Option A) goes against the core principles of patient safety culture. Ignoring staff feedback on safety concerns (Option C) can lead to missed opportunities for improvement. Minimizing patient education and involvement (Option D) hinders the collaborative nature of care delivery, which is essential in high accountable organizations.

Question 101: Correct Answer: A) Seeking input from other healthcare team members before making a critical decision.

Rationale: Clinical judgment in nursing involves the ability to make sound decisions based on critical thinking, evidence-based practice, and collaboration with the healthcare team. Seeking input from other team members before making a critical decision demonstrates the nurse's commitment to teamwork and collaboration, which are essential components of providing safe and effective patient care. Options B, C, and D are incorrect as they do not align with the principles of clinical judgment, which emphasize the importance of teamwork, communication, and individualized patient care.

Question 102: Correct Answer: B) Proper hand hygiene practices

Rationale: Proper hand hygiene is a fundamental aspect of infection prevention in patient care management. It is crucial for healthcare workers to wash their hands regularly and correctly to prevent the spread of infections between patients and healthcare personnel. Administering antibiotics for all patients is not a preventive measure and can lead to antibiotic resistance. Reusing disposable gloves increases the risk of cross-contamination. Ignoring isolation precautions can result in the transmission of infectious agents among patients and healthcare workers. Therefore, the correct answer is B) Proper hand hygiene practices, as it is a simple yet effective way to reduce the spread of infections in healthcare settings.

Question 103: Correct Answer: A) Conduct a staff training session on the importance of hand hygiene.

Rationale: The correct answer is to conduct a staff training session on the importance of hand hygiene. This action directly addresses the root cause identified in the RCA, which was improper hand hygiene practices among the healthcare staff. By educating and reinforcing proper hand hygiene protocols, the risk of similar infections can be significantly reduced. Increasing antibiotic use (option B) without addressing the root cause can lead to antibiotic resistance and other complications. Implementing a new electronic

medical record system (option C) or changing surgical instruments (option D) does not directly address the issue of hand hygiene compliance, making them less effective in preventing similar incidents in the future.

Question 104: Correct Answer: A) Double-checking the patient's identification before administering medication.

Rationale: Patient safety is a critical aspect of nursing care. Double-checking the patient's identification before medication administration is a key step to prevent medication errors and ensure the right patient receives the right medication. Skipping steps in wound care, ignoring patient calls, or administering medication without checking for allergies can all compromise patient safety. By prioritizing patient identification verification, the nurse demonstrates a proactive approach to preventing errors and promoting a safe care environment, ultimately enhancing patient outcomes and reducing risks associated with medication administration errors.

Question 105: Correct Answer: B) Check Mr. Johnson's blood glucose levels before administering Metformin

Rationale: The correct answer is to check Mr. Johnson's blood glucose levels before administering Metformin. This is crucial as Metformin is an oral antidiabetic medication used to treat type 2 diabetes. It is essential to ensure that the patient's blood glucose levels are within the target range before administering Metformin to prevent hypoglycemia or hyperglycemia. Option A is incorrect as blindly administering all medications without considering specific patient factors can lead to adverse effects. Option C is incorrect as there is no specific order in which the medications need to be administered. Option D is incorrect as consulting the pharmacist should be done after assessing the patient's specific needs and conditions.

Question 106: Correct Answer: A) Inform the colleague that the scrub should last for at least 2 minutes with an antimicrobial soap.

Rationale: Option A is the correct answer as it addresses the incorrect practice observed by the nurse's colleague. A proper surgical scrub should last for at least 2 minutes using an antimicrobial soap to effectively reduce microorganisms on the hands. This action ensures patient safety by minimizing the risk of surgical site infections. Options B and C are incorrect as they do not prioritize patient safety and adherence to proper protocols. Option D, while important, should not be the first step; addressing the issue directly with the colleague is crucial in real-time to prevent potential harm to the patient.

Question 107: Correct Answer: C) Head-of-Bed Elevation Algorithm

Rationale: The correct answer is C) Head-of-Bed Elevation Algorithm. Elevating the head of the bed between 30-45 degrees is a key component in preventing VAP by reducing the risk of aspiration. Option A, Early Ambulation Algorithm, while important for overall patient mobility, is not specifically targeted at preventing VAP. Option B, Hand Hygiene Algorithm, is crucial for infection control but not directly related to VAP prevention. Option D, Oral Care Algorithm, is essential for preventing ventilator-associated pneumonia, but head-of-bed elevation takes precedence in the care bundle for this specific purpose.

Question 108: Correct Answer: B) "I will clean the port site daily with alcohol and apply an antibiotic ointment."

Rationale: Option B is the correct answer as cleaning the port site with alcohol and applying an antibiotic ointment is not recommended for port care. Using alcohol can cause skin irritation and dryness, while applying antibiotic ointment can lead to the development of resistant strains of bacteria. The appropriate method for cleaning a port site involves using sterile saline or chlorhexidine solution as per evidence-based practice guidelines to prevent infection. Options A, C, and D are all correct statements regarding port care, emphasizing the importance of proper arm movement, regular flushing, and monitoring for signs of infection.

Question 109: Correct Answer: B) Employing active listening and empathy to understand the patient's perspective

Rationale: In de-escalation techniques, it is crucial for CMSRNs to utilize active listening and empathy to establish rapport with the patient, understand their emotions, and address their concerns effectively. This approach helps in building trust, reducing anxiety, and fostering a collaborative environment for resolving conflicts peacefully. Options A, C, and D are incorrect as they promote negative and counterproductive behaviors that can escalate the situation further, leading to potential harm to both the patient and the healthcare provider.

Question 110: Correct Answer: B) Peer accountability is the act of taking responsibility for one's actions and decisions.

Rationale: Peer accountability is a crucial aspect of a healthy practice environment where each team member takes ownership of their actions and decisions. Option A is incorrect as peer accountability does not involve blaming others but rather holding oneself responsible. Option C is incorrect as peer accountability encourages open communication and addressing issues directly. Option D is incorrect as peer accountability is a shared responsibility among all team members, not just the team leader. By choosing option B, individuals contribute to a culture of trust, respect, and professionalism within the healthcare team.

Question 111: Correct Answer: C) To identify and resolve discrepancies in medication information

Rationale: Medication reconciliation is a crucial process during transitions of care, such as discharge, to ensure that accurate and complete medication information is communicated between healthcare providers. Option A is incorrect as the purpose of medication reconciliation is not to increase costs but to enhance patient safety. Option B is incorrect as the focus is on accuracy, not speed, to prevent medication errors. Option D is incorrect as the primary goal is patient safety, not patient satisfaction. Therefore, the correct answer is C, as it highlights the key objective of medication reconciliation in preventing medication discrepancies and ensuring patient safety.

Question 112: Correct Answer: B) Listen actively to Mrs. Smith's fears and provide emotional support.

Rationale: Patient advocacy involves actively listening to patients, understanding their concerns, and providing support tailored to their emotional and psychological needs. Option A may overwhelm the patient with more medical information. Option C dismisses the patient's feelings without addressing them directly. Option D provides reassurance without acknowledging Mrs. Smith's specific worries, which may not effectively address her emotional needs. Option B is the most appropriate as it demonstrates empathy, support, and patient-centered care, essential components of patient advocacy in holistic patient care.

Question 113: Correct Answer: D) Collaborating with the interdisciplinary team to develop a personalized care plan for Mr. Johnson.

Rationale: In discharge planning, collaborating with the interdisciplinary team is crucial to ensure comprehensive care coordination and transition management. Option A is incorrect as providing a list of community resources without assessing the patient's understanding may lead to ineffective utilization. Option B is incorrect as family involvement is vital for successful discharge planning. Option C is incorrect as medication reconciliation is essential to prevent medication errors and ensure patient safety. Collaborating with the interdisciplinary team enhances communication, promotes holistic care, and tailors the care plan to meet Mr. Johnson's specific needs, making option D the correct choice.

Question 114: Correct Answer: B) Ask the physician to provide the order in writing before making any changes.

Rationale: The correct action for Nurse Smith in this scenario is to ask the physician to provide the verbal order in writing before implementing any changes to the patient's medication regimen. Verbal orders are prone to miscommunication and errors;

therefore, it is essential to have written documentation to ensure clarity, accuracy, and accountability in patient care. Option A is incorrect as implementing a verbal order without written confirmation can lead to medication errors. Option C is not necessary as the responsibility lies with the receiving nurse to clarify and confirm the verbal order. Option D is unsafe and goes against the standard practice of following proper protocols for medication administration.

Question 115: Correct Answer: D) Facilitating a team meeting to discuss the care plan

Rationale: In this scenario, the nurse's action of facilitating a team meeting to discuss the care plan best demonstrates effective care coordination. This approach ensures that all healthcare team members are on the same page regarding Mr. Smith's treatment plan, promoting collaboration and communication among the interdisciplinary team. Option A is important but does not encompass the entire team's involvement. Option B focuses on a specific specialist rather than the entire team. Option C involves family communication, which is essential but not directly related to interprofessional collaboration within the healthcare team.

Question 116: Correct Answer: C) Pulse oximeter

Rationale: A pulse oximeter is crucial during surgical procedures to continuously monitor a patient's oxygen saturation levels, providing real-time feedback on respiratory status. While a blood pressure cuff and stethoscope are important for monitoring vital signs, they do not provide direct information on oxygen levels. An IV pole is necessary for administering fluids but does not directly contribute to monitoring patient safety during surgery. Therefore, the pulse oximeter is the most essential equipment for ensuring patient safety by promptly detecting any oxygenation issues.

Question 117: Correct Answer: B) Consulting evidence-based practice guidelines

Rationale: Critical thinking in nursing involves using evidence-based practice guidelines to make informed decisions about patient care. Option A is incorrect as making assumptions based on personal beliefs can lead to biased judgments. Option C is incorrect because solely relying on past experiences may not consider current best practices. Option D is incorrect as disregarding patient preferences goes against patient-centered care. By choosing option B, the nurse demonstrates the ability to analyze information critically, leading to better patient outcomes.

Question 118: Correct Answer: B) Contact precautions

Rationale: Contact precautions are essential for patients with known or suspected infections that are spread by direct or indirect contact. In Mr. Smith's case, where he has a healthcare-associated infection, contact precautions are crucial to prevent transmission through contact with the patient or contaminated surfaces. Droplet precautions are for infections spread through respiratory droplets, airborne precautions are for infections transmitted through small droplets that remain in the air, and standard precautions are used for all patients to prevent the spread of infections from blood, body fluids, or contaminated items. In this scenario, contact precautions are the most appropriate measure to prevent transmission of the healthcare-associated infection.

Question 119: Correct Answer: A) Age

Rationale: Age is a crucial demographic factor in patient safety and care management. As individuals age, they are more prone to various health conditions, decreased mobility, and slower healing processes. This impacts their overall safety and care needs, requiring healthcare providers to adapt interventions accordingly. In contrast, hair color, shoe size, and favorite food are not directly linked to increased risk factors in patient safety or care management. Understanding the impact of age on patient outcomes is essential for providing effective and tailored care to different age groups, making it the correct choice among the options provided.

Question 120: Correct Answer: B) Document the findings and continue to monitor the patient.

Rationale: In this scenario, the correct action for the nurse is to document the findings and continue to monitor the patient. The wound appears to be healing well without signs of infection, and the patient only reports feeling warm without other concerning symptoms. It is essential to maintain a record of the assessment findings and observe the patient for any changes in condition. Notifying the healthcare provider immediately or removing the dressing without indication can disrupt the healing process. Initiating contact precautions is unnecessary as there are no indications of an infectious process. Monitoring and documentation are key components of infection control practices to ensure patient safety and appropriate care.

Question 121: Correct Answer: C) Collaborating with Mrs. Smith and her daughter to develop a personalized pain management and mobility plan.

Rationale: In this scenario, the nurse exemplifies patient/family-centered care by involving both Mrs. Smith and her daughter in the care planning process. Collaborating with the patient and family members ensures that their preferences, concerns, and needs are considered when creating a personalized care plan. Option A is incorrect as providing medication without discussing side effects does not involve the patient in decision-making. Option B is incorrect as updating the daughter without Mrs. Smith's permission disregards patient confidentiality. Option D is incorrect as discharging the patient without proper education on post-operative care violates the principles of patient-centered care.

Question 122: Correct Answer: C) Open communication about errors and near misses

Rationale: A positive patient safety culture is characterized by open communication among healthcare team members regarding errors and near misses. Option A is incorrect as blaming individuals for errors fosters a culture of fear and hinders reporting. Option B is incorrect as prioritizing speed over accuracy can compromise patient safety. Option D is incorrect as ignoring staff concerns undermines the importance of addressing potential safety issues. In contrast, open communication promotes transparency, learning from mistakes, and continuous improvement in patient care, making it essential for a positive patient safety culture.

Question 123: Correct Answer: B) Consulting with the healthcare team to discuss alternative pain management options for Mrs. Smith.

Rationale: Patient advocacy involves actively supporting and promoting the patient's best interests, including ensuring their voice is heard and respected in decision-making processes. In this scenario, the nurse advocating for Mrs. Smith's well-being would involve collaborating with the healthcare team to explore alternative pain management strategies that could better address her needs. Options A, C, and D do not align with patient advocacy principles as they either dismiss the patient's concerns, ignore her requests, or compromise her comfort and safety. Option B is the most appropriate as it involves proactive communication and collaboration to address the patient's unmet needs effectively.

Question 124: Correct Answer: B) Reporting a near-miss incident to the supervisor

Rationale: Speaking up in healthcare settings is crucial for patient safety. Option B is the correct choice as it demonstrates the nurse's commitment to reporting potential risks, promoting a culture of transparency and continuous improvement. Options A, C, and D are incorrect as they involve behaviors that compromise patient safety by either overlooking errors, avoiding confrontation, or neglecting patient needs. By choosing option B, the nurse fulfills their ethical duty to prioritize patient well-being and contribute to a culture of open communication and accountability in healthcare settings.

Question 125: Correct Answer: A) Hospice care services

Rationale: Hospice care services are specialized in providing comprehensive support, including emotional, spiritual, and physical care, to patients and their families during the end-of-life phase.

These services focus on enhancing quality of life, managing symptoms, and offering comfort. In contrast, options B, C, and D are not primarily aimed at addressing the holistic needs of patients and caregivers in end-of-life situations. Chemotherapy treatments and surgical interventions are more focused on disease management rather than palliative care, while physical therapy sessions may not provide the emotional support and guidance crucial during this sensitive time.

Question 126: Correct Answer: D) Using precise and descriptive language for clarity and accuracy

Rationale: In the scenario, Sarah emphasizes the importance of using precise and descriptive language in documentation to ensure clarity and accuracy. This approach helps in conveying information effectively, promoting patient safety, and facilitating continuity of care. Options A, B, and C are incorrect as they do not align with best practices in documentation, which require clear, specific, and accurate language to support quality patient care and communication among healthcare team members.

Question 127: Correct Answer: C) Level of education

Rationale: Social determinants of health are non-medical factors that can greatly impact an individual's health outcomes. Level of education is a key social determinant as it influences access to job opportunities, income, living conditions, and overall health literacy. While access to healthcare facilities is important, it falls under the category of healthcare services rather than social determinants. Genetic predisposition relates to biological factors, not social determinants. Blood pressure measurement is a healthcare intervention, not a social determinant of health. Therefore, the correct option is C) Level of education.

Question 128: Correct Answer: B) Using paper-based documentation as a temporary measure

Rationale: During downtime, using paper-based documentation is crucial to ensure continuity of care and accurate recording of patient information. Delaying documentation (option A) can lead to missed details, documenting on random paper (option C) may result in lost information, and not documenting at all (option D) is a violation of patient safety protocols. Paper-based documentation allows for immediate recording of essential data, which can later be transferred into the electronic system, maintaining the integrity of patient records and ensuring seamless care delivery.

Question 129: Correct Answer: A) Conduct an in-depth analysis of the medication administration process.

Rationale: Conducting an in-depth analysis of the medication administration process is the initial step in continuous quality and process improvement. This action involves identifying the root causes of the medication errors, evaluating current practices, and implementing necessary changes to prevent future errors. Implementing a new electronic health record system (Option B) may be a solution but should come after the analysis. Providing additional training (Option C) is beneficial but not the first step. Reporting the issue to hospital administration (Option D) should be done after the analysis to propose informed solutions.

Question 130: Correct Answer: A) Religious dietary restrictions

Rationale: When addressing individualized nutritional needs, a CMSRN must consider religious dietary restrictions as they significantly impact food choices and meal planning for patients. Religious beliefs often dictate what foods are allowed or prohibited, influencing the patient's dietary requirements. Option B, preferred meal times, while important, may vary among individuals regardless of culture. Option C, traditional healing practices, focuses more on medical interventions rather than dietary considerations. Option D, social media influence, is not a direct cultural factor affecting individualized nutritional needs in the healthcare setting.

Question 131: Correct Answer: D) Listen actively to Mrs. Smith's concerns, validate her feelings, and offer emotional support.

Rationale: In patient-centered care, it is essential to prioritize active listening, validation of feelings, and emotional support to address patient anxiety effectively. Option A focuses more on providing information rather than emotional support. Option B may not align with Mrs. Smith's preferences or holistic care approach. Option C, while promoting positivity, may not address the root cause of Mrs. Smith's anxiety. Therefore, actively listening, validating feelings, and offering emotional support are crucial components of patient-centered care in this scenario.

Question 132: Correct Answer: B) Encouraging relaxation techniques such as deep breathing exercises

Rationale: Nonpharmacological interventions play a crucial role in managing anxiety and sleep disturbances in postoperative patients. Option A is incorrect as administering sedative medication should be avoided unless absolutely necessary due to potential side effects and interactions. Option C is incorrect as using pain medication solely for inducing sleep may not address the underlying anxiety. Option D is incorrect as unrestricted visitation hours may not directly address Mrs. Smith's anxiety and sleep issues. Encouraging relaxation techniques like deep breathing exercises promotes natural relaxation and can help Mrs. Smith manage her symptoms effectively without the risks associated with medications.

Question 133: Correct Answer: B) Ambulation and early mobilization

Rationale: Ambulation and early mobilization play a crucial role in preventing deep vein thrombosis (DVT) in surgical patients by enhancing blood circulation, reducing stasis, and preventing clot formation. Passive range of motion exercises (Option A) may help with joint flexibility but do not directly address DVT prevention. Application of heat packs (Option C) is more suitable for muscle relaxation and pain relief rather than DVT prevention. Isometric strengthening exercises (Option D) focus on muscle strength and may not directly impact DVT prevention as ambulation does. Early mobilization is key to preventing complications such as DVT in postoperative patients.

Question 134: Correct Answer: B) Notifying the healthcare provider immediately

Rationale: In this scenario, the priority action for the nurse is to notify the healthcare provider immediately. The presence of redness, warmth, tenderness, purulent drainage, and fever at the central venous catheter site indicates a potential catheter-related bloodstream infection. Prompt notification of the healthcare provider is crucial to initiate appropriate interventions such as possible removal of the catheter, initiation of antibiotic therapy, and further evaluation to prevent complications. Administering an antipyretic medication (Option A) may help reduce the fever but does not address the underlying infection. Documenting the findings (Option C) is important but not the priority over immediate notification. Applying a warm compress (Option D) can exacerbate the infection and is contraindicated in this situation.

Question 135: Correct Answer: B) Reposition Ms. Johnson every 2 hours.

Rationale: Repositioning postoperative patients, like Ms. Johnson, every 2 hours is crucial to prevent pressure ulcers, improve circulation, and maintain skin integrity. Repositioning every 4, 6, or 8 hours increases the risk of pressure ulcers due to prolonged pressure on specific areas. Frequent repositioning ensures adequate blood flow to tissues, reducing the likelihood of skin breakdown and other complications. Therefore, the most appropriate action for the nurse in this scenario is to reposition Ms. Johnson every 2 hours to promote optimal patient outcomes.

Question 136: Correct Answer: B) Documenting the allergy to penicillin in Mr. Smith's medical record.

Rationale: Documenting the allergy to penicillin in Mr. Smith's medical record is crucial for patient safety and ensures that all healthcare providers involved in Mr. Smith's care are aware of this important information. Option A is incorrect as pain management methods, while important, are not directly related to the immediate preoperative care. Option C is incorrect as the availability of

preoperative antibiotics should have been addressed during the outgoing nurse's report. Option D is incorrect as informing the surgical team about Mr. Smith's daughter, while thoughtful, is not as critical as documenting the allergy for immediate patient care.

Question 137: Correct Answer: A) Encouraging the patient to engage in prayer and meditation

Rationale: In palliative or end-of-life care, addressing the spiritual needs of patients is crucial for holistic patient care. Encouraging the patient to engage in prayer and meditation can provide comfort, solace, and a sense of peace during this challenging time. It allows the patient to connect with their beliefs, find meaning, and cope with the emotional and existential aspects of their illness. Suggesting avoidance of spiritual matters (option B), discouraging religious rituals (option C), or ignoring spiritual needs (option D) can neglect an essential aspect of the patient's well-being and may hinder their coping mechanisms and quality of life.

Question 138: Correct Answer: C) Airborne pathogens

Rationale: Airborne pathogens, such as bacteria and viruses, present a significant risk to patient safety in healthcare settings due to their potential to cause infections and spread diseases. Noise pollution and improper lighting can affect patient comfort but are not as directly linked to infection control. Improper waste disposal, while important for infection prevention, is not as immediate a threat as airborne pathogens, which can quickly lead to outbreaks and compromise patient health. Therefore, identifying and mitigating risks associated with airborne pathogens is crucial in maintaining a safe healthcare environment.

Question 139: Correct Answer: C) Document Ms. Johnson's grievances in detail and escalate them to the appropriate channels.

Rationale: It is crucial for a CMSRN to take patient grievances seriously and ensure they are documented accurately. By documenting Ms. Johnson's concerns, the nurse can initiate the appropriate steps to address and resolve the issues effectively. Option A is not sufficient as just apologizing may not address the underlying problems. Option B dismisses the patient's concerns and lacks empathy. Option D is inappropriate as ignoring patient grievances can lead to further dissatisfaction and compromise patient-centered care.

Question 140: Correct Answer: B) Providing direct care to patients with medical-surgical conditions

Rationale: Certified Medical Surgical Registered Nurses are responsible for providing direct care to patients with medical-surgical conditions, which includes assessing, diagnosing, planning, implementing, and evaluating patient care. This role does not involve performing complex surgical procedures (Option A), conducting advanced diagnostic tests (Option C), or administering anesthesia during surgeries (Option D). The focus is on holistic patient care within the medical-surgical specialty, emphasizing the importance of comprehensive nursing interventions and patient education.

Question 141: Correct Answer: C) Consulting the latest clinical practice guidelines

Rationale: Consulting the latest clinical practice guidelines is crucial in evidence-based practice as it integrates the best available research evidence with clinical expertise and patient values. Ignoring current research findings (Option A) goes against evidence-based practice principles. Relying solely on personal experience (Option B) may not align with the most current evidence. Disregarding patient preferences (Option D) overlooks the patient-centered aspect of evidence-based care, which is essential for successful implementation. Therefore, the correct answer is C) Consulting the latest clinical practice guidelines.

Question 142: Correct Answer: B) Implanted port

Rationale: An implanted port is a type of port that is completely implanted beneath the skin, requiring no external components. It consists of a reservoir attached to a catheter. This design reduces the risk of infection and allows for easy access to administer medications or draw blood. In contrast, tunneled catheters have an external portion that exits the skin, external catheters are entirely external, and PICCs are inserted into a peripheral vein and threaded towards the heart, all of which pose higher infection risks and are more prone to dislodgement compared to implanted ports.

Question 143: Correct Answer: B) Holding a team meeting involving the patient, family, social worker, and physical therapist to discuss the discharge plan.

Rationale: Effective discharge planning involves interdisciplinary collaboration to ensure comprehensive care continuity. Option B is the correct choice as it demonstrates the involvement of key team members in the decision-making process, promoting a holistic approach to the patient's transition. Options A, C, and D lack the essential aspect of teamwork and coordination among healthcare professionals, which are crucial in achieving successful patient outcomes during the discharge process.

Question 144: Correct Answer: B) Acupuncture

Rationale: Acupuncture is a traditional Chinese medicine practice that involves the insertion of thin needles at specific points on the body to stimulate energy flow and promote healing. In contrast, aromatherapy (Option A) uses essential oils for therapeutic purposes, reflexology (Option C) involves applying pressure to specific points on the feet/hands, and Reiki (Option D) is a form of energy healing. By comparing these options, acupuncture stands out as the correct choice for Ms. Johnson's chronic lower back pain, as it targets pain relief through precise needle placement based on traditional Chinese medicine principles.

Question 145: Correct Answer: C) Patient satisfaction

Rationale: Patient satisfaction is a crucial aspect of value-based purchasing as it directly reflects the quality of care provided. While cost-effectiveness and timeliness of care are important factors, patient satisfaction encompasses the overall experience, including communication, empathy, and patient-centered care. Healthcare provider convenience, although relevant, is not the primary focus when evaluating patient customer experience in value-based purchasing. By prioritizing patient satisfaction, healthcare facilities can improve outcomes, enhance patient loyalty, and ultimately drive better results in value-based care models.

Question 146: Correct Answer: C) Age

Rationale: Age is a crucial demographic factor in patient care as it influences various aspects of health and well-being. Older age is associated with a higher risk of developing chronic conditions, decreased physiological reserves, and increased susceptibility to infections. These factors can impact patient safety by affecting medication metabolism, surgical outcomes, and overall care management. Gender and marital status, while important in certain contexts, do not have as direct an impact on patient safety and care management as age. Blood type, although relevant for transfusions, is not a primary demographic factor influencing patient outcomes in the same way age does.

Question 147: Correct Answer: B) Engaging in interdisciplinary communication and cooperation to provide optimal patient care.

Rationale: Nursing teamwork and collaboration are essential components of professional nursing practice. Option A is incorrect as nursing practice involves collaboration with other healthcare team members to ensure comprehensive care. Option C is incorrect as recognizing and valuing the contributions of all team members is crucial for effective patient outcomes. Option D is incorrect as active participation in team meetings and care planning sessions enhances patient care through shared decision-making and coordinated efforts. Option B is the correct answer as it highlights the importance of interdisciplinary communication and cooperation in providing the best possible care for patients.

Question 148: Correct Answer: C) "Let's explore how we can respect your religious beliefs while also considering the possibility of organ donation to help others in need."

Rationale: Option C demonstrates a holistic approach by acknowledging Sarah's religious beliefs and involving her in the decision-making process regarding organ donation. It shows respect for her values while also considering the potential benefits of organ donation. Options A, B, and D do not prioritize Sarah's holistic care needs and fail to address her concerns about the impact of organ donation on her religious beliefs. By choosing option C, the CMSRN can support Sarah in making a well-informed decision that aligns with her values and promotes holistic patient care.

Question 149: Correct Answer: D) Fatigue

Rationale: Fatigue is a prevalent physical symptom experienced by patients in palliative or end-of-life care. It is often a result of the underlying illness, treatments, or the emotional burden of the situation. Increased appetite (Option A) is less common due to various factors affecting appetite in such patients. Improved mobility (Option B) may not be typical as the patient's condition may limit physical abilities. While decreasing pain (Option C) is a crucial goal, it may not always be achievable in these care settings where comfort and quality of life are prioritized over complete pain relief. Therefore, fatigue (Option D) stands out as the most common physical symptom in this context.

Question 150: Correct Answer: C) To identify and address potential safety concerns

Rationale: Safety huddles in a medical-surgical setting are structured brief meetings where healthcare team members come together to proactively identify and address potential safety concerns related to patient care. Option A is incorrect as safety huddles focus on patient safety, not staff scheduling. Option B is incorrect as patient satisfaction surveys are not the primary focus of safety huddles. Option D is incorrect as the purpose of safety huddles is not to plan social events but to enhance patient safety and quality of care through open communication and problem-solving.

CMSRN Exam Practice Questions [SET 2]

Question 1: During bedside report, the nurse is discussing the care plan for a patient named Mr. Johnson who is scheduled for discharge the next day. The nurse should prioritize which information to include in the report?
A) The patient's preferred meal choices
B) The patient's family contact information
C) The patient's mobility status and any assistance needed
D) The patient's favorite TV shows

Question 2: Which of the following is a key component of effective written communication in the healthcare setting?
A) Using complex medical jargon
B) Providing vague and ambiguous information
C) Ensuring clarity and simplicity
D) Including personal opinions and biases

Question 3: Ms. Johnson, a 65-year-old patient, is being discharged from the hospital after a surgical procedure. She lives alone and requires assistance with wound care and medication management. Which community resource would be most appropriate for ensuring Ms. Johnson receives the necessary support at home?
A) Local pharmacy for medication delivery service
B) Senior center for social activities
C) Grocery store for meal delivery service
D) Fitness center for exercise classes

Question 4: Ms. Johnson, a 68-year-old postoperative patient, is being cared for on a medical-surgical unit. The nurse documents the patient's vital signs every 4 hours, wound appearance, and intake and output. Which of the following statements regarding documentation is accurate in this scenario?
A) The nurse should document vital signs every 6 hours.
B) The nurse should document wound appearance once a day.
C) The nurse should document intake and output every shift.
D) The nurse should document vital signs every 4 hours.

Question 5: Scenario: Ms. Johnson, a postoperative patient, requires a dressing change on her surgical wound. As a Certified Medical Surgical Registered Nurse (CMSRN), you gather the necessary supplies for the procedure. Which of the following supplies is essential for maintaining a sterile environment during the dressing change?
A) Sterile gloves
B) Non-sterile gloves
C) Regular gauze pads
D) Alcohol wipes

Question 6: Scenario: Mr. Smith, a 65-year-old patient, is admitted to the medical-surgical unit with a history of heart failure and diabetes. He requires frequent monitoring of vital signs, strict intake and output measurements, and administration of intravenous medications. As a Certified Medical Surgical Registered Nurse (CMSRN), what is within your scope of practice regarding Mr. Smith's care?
A) Adjusting the dosage of intravenous medications based on the patient's response.
B) Collaborating with the dietitian to modify Mr. Smith's meal plan.
C) Providing education to the patient on managing his diabetes.
D) Monitoring and documenting Mr. Smith's vital signs and intake and output.

Question 7: In the context of 'Continuum of care' within 'Care Coordination and Transition Management, Elements of Interprofessional Care,' which action best exemplifies effective care coordination for a patient transitioning from hospital to home?
A) Providing the patient with a list of community resources before discharge.
B) Discharging the patient without a follow-up appointment.
C) Instructing the patient to manage medications without any guidance.
D) Failing to communicate the discharge plan with the primary care provider.

Question 8: Scenario: Mr. Johnson, a 65-year-old patient, is admitted to the medical-surgical unit with a history of hypertension, diabetes, and recent myocardial infarction. During the initial assessment, the nurse notes that Mr. Johnson is at risk for developing pressure ulcers due to his limited mobility and poor nutritional status. Which risk assessment method would be most appropriate for evaluating Mr. Johnson's risk of developing pressure ulcers?
A) Braden Scale
B) Glasgow Coma Scale
C) Morse Fall Scale
D) Katz Index of Independence in Activities of Daily Living

Question 9: Scenario: Ms. Smith, a 65-year-old patient, is admitted to the medical-surgical unit for postoperative care following a hip replacement surgery. The healthcare team is implementing a checklist to ensure comprehensive care and patient safety. Which item is most likely to be included in the checklist for Ms. Smith's care?
A) Ensuring the patient receives adequate pain management
B) Monitoring the patient's blood pressure every 4 hours
C) Administering antibiotics as prescribed
D) Providing a foot massage for comfort

Question 10: Which pharmacological intervention is commonly used to reduce the risk of blood clots in postoperative patients?
A) Antibiotics
B) Antihypertensives
C) Anticoagulants
D) Antidepressants

Question 11: Which of the following best describes the scope of practice for a Certified Medical Surgical Registered Nurse (CMSRN)?
A) Performing surgical procedures independently
B) Prescribing medications without physician oversight
C) Collaborating with the healthcare team to provide comprehensive care to surgical patients
D) Making unilateral decisions regarding patient care without consulting other healthcare professionals

Question 12: Scenario: Mr. Johnson, a 65-year-old postoperative patient, has a central venous catheter in place. The nurse notes redness, warmth, and tenderness at the catheter site. Upon assessment, there is purulent drainage present. Mr. Johnson has a low-grade fever. Which infection prevention measure is the nurse most likely to implement

first?
A) Administering broad-spectrum antibiotics
B) Notifying the healthcare provider
C) Removing the central venous catheter
D) Applying a warm compress to the site

Question 13: Scenario: Mr. Johnson, a 65-year-old patient, is admitted to the medical-surgical unit with complaints of chest pain and shortness of breath. His vital signs are as follows: blood pressure 160/90 mmHg, heart rate 110 bpm, respiratory rate 24/min, and oxygen saturation 92% on room air. He has a history of hypertension and hyperlipidemia. The nurse notes crackles in his lung bases and bilateral pedal edema. Mr. Johnson is diaphoretic and anxious. Which action should the nurse prioritize?
A) Administer oxygen therapy at 2 L/min via nasal cannula.
B) Obtain a 12-lead electrocardiogram (ECG) immediately.
C) Start an intravenous line and draw labs for cardiac enzymes.
D) Assist Mr. Johnson with deep breathing and coughing exercises.

Question 14: In the context of change management, which element of the ADKAR model focuses on ensuring that the change is sustained and reinforced over time?
A) Awareness
B) Desire
C) Knowledge
D) Reinforcement

Question 15: In the context of 'Care bundles' for Patient Safety and Patient/Care Management, which algorithm is commonly used to reduce the risk of central line-associated bloodstream infections (CLABSIs)?
A) Random Forest algorithm
B) Support Vector Machine algorithm
C) Apriori algorithm
D) Central Line Bundle algorithm

Question 16: Scenario: Mr. Johnson, a 65-year-old patient, is admitted to the medical-surgical unit for a complex surgical procedure. As the nurse in charge of his care, you are discussing the financial aspects of his treatment with him. Mr. Johnson expresses concerns about the cost of the procedure and post-operative care. He asks about potential financial assistance programs available to him. Which of the following options best demonstrates the nurse's role in financial stewardship for Mr. Johnson?
A) Providing Mr. Johnson with a detailed breakdown of hospital charges.
B) Explaining the billing process and insurance coverage to Mr. Johnson.
C) Suggesting alternative treatment options to reduce costs.
D) Referring Mr. Johnson to the hospital's financial counselor for assistance.

Question 17: In the context of mediation in healthcare settings, which of the following statements best describes the role of a mediator?
A) The mediator acts as a judge, making final decisions for the parties involved.
B) The mediator provides legal advice to one party to help them gain an advantage.
C) The mediator facilitates communication and negotiation between conflicting parties.
D) The mediator imposes solutions on the parties without their input.

Question 18: Ms. Johnson, a 65-year-old patient, is admitted to the medical-surgical unit with dysphagia and is unable to consume oral intake. The healthcare provider has prescribed enteral nutrition for her. Which of the following resources is most appropriate for alternate nutrition administration for Ms. Johnson?
A) Percutaneous endoscopic gastrostomy (PEG) tube
B) Nasogastric (NG) tube
C) Dobhoff tube
D) Jejunostomy tube

Question 19: Scenario: Mrs. Patel, a 65-year-old female patient of Indian descent, is admitted to the medical-surgical unit with a diagnosis of pneumonia. She speaks limited English and prefers to communicate in her native language, Gujarati. As a CMSRN, what action should you take to ensure effective communication and holistic care for Mrs. Patel?
A) Use a language translation app to communicate with Mrs. Patel in English.
B) Request an interpreter who speaks Gujarati to assist with communication.
C) Ask Mrs. Patel's family members to translate important information.
D) Speak loudly and slowly in English to ensure Mrs. Patel understands.

Question 20: Scenario: Mr. Smith, a 65-year-old patient admitted for a surgical procedure, has a history of Methicillin-resistant Staphylococcus aureus (MRSA) colonization. The nurse is preparing to provide care for Mr. Smith. Which precaution should the nurse implement to prevent the transmission of MRSA to other patients and healthcare workers?
A) Droplet precautions
B) Contact precautions
C) Airborne precautions
D) Standard precautions

Question 21: In the context of 'code status' for patients, what does the code status DNR stand for?
A) Do Not Treat
B) Do Not Resuscitate
C) Do Not Recover
D) Do Not Respond

Question 22: Scenario: Mr. Smith, a 55-year-old patient, is scheduled for a complex surgical procedure. As part of the project development for his care, the healthcare team decides to implement a new quality management initiative to enhance patient outcomes. Which of the following steps is essential in the project development process for quality management in this scenario?
A) Conducting a risk assessment to identify potential issues
B) Skipping the pilot phase to expedite implementation
C) Ignoring feedback from frontline staff
D) Implementing changes without evaluating outcomes

Question 23: Scenario: Mr. Johnson, a 65-year-old patient, is admitted to the medical-surgical unit with a diagnosis of congestive heart failure. The healthcare team consists of a medical doctor, a registered nurse, a physical therapist, and a social worker. The team meets to discuss Mr. Johnson's care plan, including medication management, dietary restrictions, mobility goals, and discharge planning. Which action by the registered nurse best demonstrates effective teamwork in this scenario?
A) Providing medication education to the patient and family.
B) Setting mobility goals for Mr. Johnson without consulting the physical therapist.

C) Making dietary decisions for the patient without involving the healthcare team.
D) Discharging the patient without coordinating with the social worker.

Question 24: In providing holistic patient care, a CMSRN should prioritize which action related to diversity and inclusion?
A) Ignoring cultural differences
B) Providing individualized care based on patient's beliefs and values
C) Excluding family members from the care process
D) Implementing a one-size-fits-all approach to patient care

Question 25: When reporting adverse events, which action should the Certified Medical Surgical Registered Nurse (CMSRN) prioritize to ensure accurate documentation and quality improvement?
A) Delay reporting until all facts are confirmed
B) Report only severe adverse events
C) Document all details promptly and accurately
D) Rely on memory for reporting at a later time

Question 26: Scenario: Mr. Johnson, a 78-year-old patient admitted for postoperative care following hip replacement surgery, has been prescribed the use of restraints due to his tendency to pull out his IV line and attempt to get out of bed unassisted. As the CMSRN on duty, you assess Mr. Johnson's need for restraints. Which action is most appropriate regarding the use of restraints for Mr. Johnson?
A) Apply wrist restraints as ordered to prevent him from pulling out the IV line.
B) Educate Mr. Johnson about the importance of keeping the IV line intact and encourage him to call for assistance.
C) Implement alternative measures such as frequent checks and diversional activities to prevent Mr. Johnson from attempting to get out of bed.
D) Apply ankle restraints in addition to wrist restraints to ensure maximum safety for Mr. Johnson.

Question 27: In the context of patient safety culture, which action best exemplifies the concept of "speaking up" for the benefit of patient care?
A) Ignoring a medication error made by a colleague
B) Reporting a safety concern to the charge nurse
C) Keeping quiet about a mislabeled specimen
D) Concealing a near-miss incident to avoid conflict

Question 28: When providing oral care to a diverse patient population, which approach is most appropriate for a Certified Medical Surgical Registered Nurse (CMSRN) to ensure cultural and linguistic needs are met?
A) Using standardized oral care products for all patients
B) Asking the patient about their preferences and any cultural considerations
C) Avoiding oral care discussions to prevent discomfort
D) Providing care without considering the patient's background

Question 29: When utilizing de-escalation techniques in a medical-surgical setting, which action by the nurse is most appropriate?
A) Raising voice to match the patient's tone
B) Maintaining a safe distance and personal space
C) Making direct threats to assert authority
D) Ignoring the patient's concerns and complaints

Question 30: During a crisis situation in a medical-surgical unit, which resource should the Certified Medical Surgical

Registered Nurse (CMSRN) prioritize for patient care?
A) Administrative paperwork
B) Staffing assignments
C) Patient safety and immediate needs
D) Personal breaks for the nursing team

Question 31: In a healthcare setting, the need for an interpreter or translator arises primarily to overcome which barrier?
A) Physical barrier
B) Emotional barrier
C) Language barrier
D) Cultural barrier

Question 32: Which of the following best describes the term 'cultural competence' in the context of providing holistic patient care?
A) Understanding and respecting the beliefs, values, and practices of individuals from diverse cultural backgrounds.
B) Ignoring cultural differences to focus solely on medical treatment.
C) Assuming that all patients have the same cultural beliefs and practices.
D) Excluding patients from certain treatments based on their cultural background.

Question 33: Scenario: Mr. Johnson, a 65-year-old patient, is admitted to the medical-surgical unit with a diagnosis of pneumonia. The nurse receives an order to administer intravenous antibiotics. Before administering the medication, the nurse double-checks the patient's identification, allergies, and the medication prescribed. The nurse then proceeds to administer the medication. Which action by the nurse best describes the concept of 'check-back' in this scenario?
A) Confirming the patient's identification and allergies before administering the medication.
B) Administering the medication without verifying the patient's identification.
C) Asking the patient if they have any allergies after administering the medication.
D) Checking the patient's identification after administering the medication.

Question 34: Scenario: Mrs. Smith, a 65-year-old patient, is admitted to the medical-surgical unit with a history of COPD exacerbation. While assessing the patient's environment, the nurse identifies the need to prevent falls. Which intervention is most appropriate to ensure patient safety in this situation?
A) Keep the call bell within the patient's reach
B) Place the patient's water pitcher on the bedside table
C) Ensure the room temperature is comfortable for the patient
D) Provide a variety of reading materials for the patient's entertainment

Question 35: In the context of near miss reporting in patient safety culture, which of the following best defines a near miss event?
A) An adverse event that resulted in patient harm
B) A medical error that was successfully intercepted before reaching the patient
C) A routine procedure performed without any complications
D) A delay in administering prescribed medication

Question 36: Which professional behavior is essential for promoting effective nursing teamwork and collaboration in the healthcare setting?
A) Competence and accountability
B) Autonomy and independence

C) Conflict avoidance
D) Hierarchical communication

Question 37: Which of the following best describes the concept of accountability in nursing practice?
A) Taking responsibility for one's actions and decisions
B) Following orders without questioning superiors
C) Blaming others for errors
D) Ignoring patient needs

Question 38: Which healthcare professionals are typically involved in interprofessional rounding?
A) Only physicians
B) Only nurses
C) Physicians, nurses, pharmacists, and social workers
D) Only pharmacists

Question 39: Which of the following is a key component of patient safety assessments and reporting in the context of Patient Safety and Patient/Care Management?
A) Ensuring timely administration of medications
B) Implementing proper hand hygiene protocols
C) Conducting regular patient fall risk assessments
D) Documenting and reporting incidents of medication errors

Question 40: Which nutrient is essential for wound healing in patients with surgical incisions?
A) Vitamin C
B) Sodium
C) Iron
D) Vitamin K

Question 41: Scenario: Mr. Johnson, a 65-year-old patient recovering from abdominal surgery, is on strict bed rest. The nurse is preparing to assist him with ambulation using a walker. Which equipment is essential for the nurse to ensure Mr. Johnson's safety during ambulation?
A) Wheelchair
B) Crutches
C) Cane
D) Walker

Question 42: Ms. Johnson, a 65-year-old patient, is admitted to the medical-surgical unit for a hip replacement surgery. As part of providing patient-centered care, which resource would be most beneficial for promoting holistic patient care in her post-operative recovery?
A) Physical therapy services
B) Social media platforms for patient support groups
C) Hospital cafeteria menu for meal choices
D) Hospital policy handbook for visitors' guidelines

Question 43: In the context of patient safety and care management, which algorithm is commonly used to reduce the risk of central line-associated bloodstream infections (CLABSIs)?
A) Morse Fall Scale
B) RACE Algorithm
C) SBAR Technique
D) Central Line Bundle

Question 44: Which method is most effective for providing health information to meet the holistic needs of patients?
A) Using only written materials
B) Conducting group education sessions
C) Utilizing multimedia resources
D) Engaging in one-on-one counseling sessions

Question 45: As a Certified Medical Surgical Registered Nurse (CMSRN), participating in professional organizations is essential for professional development and networking opportunities. Which of the following is a primary benefit of engaging in professional organizations?
A) Access to discounted healthcare products
B) Opportunities for continuing education and professional growth
C) Free meals at networking events
D) Exclusive access to non-healthcare related events

Question 46: Scenario: During a busy shift at the medical-surgical unit, a Certified Medical Surgical Registered Nurse (CMSRN) notices a colleague struggling to keep up with the workload. The colleague appears overwhelmed and stressed. The nurse observes that the colleague is making frequent errors in medication administration and documentation. What should the CMSRN do in this situation?
A) Offer to help the colleague with some of the tasks.
B) Ignore the situation and focus on completing personal tasks.
C) Report the colleague to the nurse manager immediately.
D) Confront the colleague in front of other staff members.

Question 47: Which action by the nurse best demonstrates holistic patient care in the context of 'Holistic Patient Care'?
A) Administering prescribed medications on time
B) Providing emotional support and actively listening to the patient's concerns
C) Ensuring accurate documentation of vital signs
D) Following strict adherence to hand hygiene protocols

Question 48: Ms. Johnson, a 55-year-old patient, is admitted to the medical-surgical unit for exacerbation of chronic obstructive pulmonary disease (COPD). The nurse is discussing health promotion goals with Ms. Johnson to improve her respiratory status. Which of the following goals is most appropriate for Ms. Johnson at this time?
A) Increase daily intake of caffeinated beverages
B) Engage in regular aerobic exercise
C) Limit fluid intake to 1 liter per day
D) Avoid using prescribed inhalers

Question 49: Scenario: Mrs. Smith, a 65-year-old patient with multiple chronic conditions, is being discharged home with a new medication regimen. She has a history of medication non-adherence. Which intervention by the nurse is most appropriate to promote safe medication management at home?
A) Provide Mrs. Smith with pill organizers labeled for each day of the week.
B) Instruct Mrs. Smith to keep all her medications in one large container for convenience.
C) Advise Mrs. Smith to store her medications in the bathroom to ensure easy access.
D) Recommend Mrs. Smith to share her medications with her neighbor who has similar health conditions.

Question 50: Scenario: Mr. Johnson, a 65-year-old patient, is admitted to the medical-surgical unit with a history of chronic obstructive pulmonary disease (COPD) exacerbation. While assessing the patient's room environment, the nurse identifies potential risk factors that could compromise patient safety. Which intervention by the nurse is most appropriate to address these risk factors related to the environment?
A) Ensuring the room temperature is kept warm to prevent hypothermia.
B) Placing the patient's water pitcher out of reach to prevent overhydration.
C) Keeping the oxygen equipment away from potential ignition

sources.
D) Providing extra blankets to increase the room's humidity level.

Question 51: In the hospital incident command structure, who is responsible for managing the overall incident response and ensuring coordination among all involved parties?
A) Chief Nursing Officer (CNO)
B) Charge Nurse on duty
C) Incident Commander
D) Head of Security

Question 52: Ms. Johnson, a 65-year-old patient, is admitted to the medical-surgical unit with a diagnosis of heart failure. As the CMSRN caring for Ms. Johnson, which action demonstrates adherence to Standard V of the AMSN Scope and Standards?
A) Administering medications without verifying the patient's identity
B) Documenting vital signs only at the beginning of the shift
C) Providing education on dietary sodium restrictions
D) Ignoring the patient's call light for assistance

Question 53: Scenario: Sarah, a registered nurse, has been working in a medical-surgical unit for several years. She is known for her exceptional patient care and dedication to her work. Recently, Sarah has been feeling overwhelmed and stressed due to the increased patient load and administrative tasks. Despite this, she continues to provide quality care to her patients. Which of the following actions by the nurse manager would best demonstrate employee engagement in this scenario?
A) Providing Sarah with additional training on time management.
B) Acknowledging Sarah's hard work and dedication in a team meeting.
C) Assigning Sarah to mentor a new nurse on the unit.
D) Increasing Sarah's workload to challenge her skills.

Question 54: Scenario: Mr. Johnson, a 65-year-old patient, has been admitted to the medical-surgical unit for post-operative care following a hip replacement surgery. During your assessment, you notice that Mr. Johnson appears anxious and is having difficulty expressing his concerns about the pain management plan. He seems hesitant to ask questions or seek clarification. As a CMSRN, what is the most appropriate action to take in this situation?
A) Provide Mr. Johnson with written instructions to read on his own.
B) Ask closed-ended questions to quickly address his concerns.
C) Use open-ended questions to encourage Mr. Johnson to share his thoughts and feelings.
D) Assume Mr. Johnson understands the plan and proceed with the care.

Question 55: Which emotional response is most appropriate for a Certified Medical Surgical Registered Nurse (CMSRN) when faced with a challenging situation in the workplace?
A) Panic and anxiety
B) Anger and frustration
C) Empathy and compassion
D) Indifference and apathy

Question 56: Which of the following is an example of non-verbal communication?
A) Speaking clearly and concisely
B) Making eye contact while listening
C) Using appropriate medical terminology
D) Writing detailed progress notes

Question 57: In the context of training for Certified Medical Surgical Registered Nurses (CMSRN), which method is most effective for promoting Nursing Teamwork and Collaboration?
A) Online modules with individual assessments
B) In-person group workshops with role-playing exercises
C) Self-directed study with periodic progress check-ins
D) Lecture-style presentations with Q&A sessions

Question 58: When coaching for documentation performance improvement, which of the following strategies is most effective in ensuring accurate and comprehensive documentation?
A) Providing generic feedback
B) Conducting regular chart audits
C) Offering rewards for quantity over quality
D) Encouraging interdisciplinary collaboration

Question 59: Scenario: Sarah, a 25-year-old female, presents to the emergency department with multiple unexplained injuries and appears fearful when questioned about how she sustained them. She avoids making eye contact and seems hesitant to provide personal information. The nurse notices that Sarah's companion is overly controlling and answers most of the questions on her behalf. Sarah's behavior raises concerns about potential human trafficking. Which action should the nurse prioritize in this situation?
A) Discharge Sarah with instructions to follow up with a primary care provider.
B) Conduct a thorough physical assessment and document the findings.
C) Ask Sarah's companion to step out of the room for further questioning.
D) Contact the hospital social worker to discuss the situation and seek guidance.

Question 60: Which of the following actions by a patient indicates safe home medication management?
A) Storing medications in a bathroom medicine cabinet
B) Sharing prescription medications with a family member
C) Keeping medications in their original labeled containers
D) Mixing different medications into a single container for convenience

Question 61: Scenario: Mr. Smith, a 65-year-old patient, was admitted to the medical-surgical unit with a diagnosis of congestive heart failure. The healthcare team consists of nurses, physicians, physical therapists, and dietitians working collaboratively to provide comprehensive care. During the interdisciplinary team meeting, the nurse shares vital information about Mr. Smith's deteriorating condition and the need for immediate intervention. Which action best exemplifies effective interdisciplinary communication in this scenario?
A) The nurse updates the patient's family about the treatment plan without consulting other team members.
B) The nurse documents the patient's vital signs in the electronic health record but does not communicate changes to the team.
C) The nurse collaborates with the physical therapist to develop a mobility plan for Mr. Smith.
D) The nurse prescribes new medications for the patient without consulting the physician.

Question 62: When providing translated materials to patients with limited English proficiency, which approach is most appropriate for ensuring effective communication and understanding?
A) Using free online translation tools
B) Asking family members to interpret
C) Utilizing professional medical interpreters
D) Providing written materials in English only

Question 63: When utilizing the SBAR (Situation, Background, Assessment, Recommendation) communication technique, what does the 'R' stand for?
A) Response
B) Reflection
C) Request
D) Review

Question 64: Scenario: During a busy shift, a Certified Medical Surgical Registered Nurse (CMSRN) notices a sudden change in a postoperative patient's condition. The patient, Mr. Smith, who underwent abdominal surgery earlier in the day, is now experiencing increasing abdominal pain, distention, and tachycardia. The nurse suspects a possible complication and needs to escalate the situation promptly. What should be the nurse's immediate action following the chain of command principles?
A) Notify the charge nurse on the unit.
B) Contact the surgeon who performed the procedure.
C) Inform the nursing supervisor of the unit.
D) Call the patient's family to update them on the situation.

Question 65: Scenario: Mrs. Smith, a 65-year-old patient, has been admitted to the medical-surgical unit for post-operative care following a knee replacement surgery. She appears anxious and is having difficulty expressing her concerns about the pain management plan. As a CMSRN, how should you best address Mrs. Smith's communication preferences in this situation?
A) Provide detailed written instructions about the pain medications.
B) Use open-ended questions to encourage Mrs. Smith to share her concerns.
C) Quickly reassure Mrs. Smith that everything will be fine.
D) Discuss pain management options with Mrs. Smith's family instead.

Question 66: In a closed-loop communication system, which of the following best describes the process?
A) One-way communication where feedback is not required
B) Two-way communication where feedback is encouraged and essential
C) Communication only between healthcare providers excluding patients
D) Communication that is open to interpretation without clarification

Question 67: Scenario: Sarah, a newly graduated nurse, is eager to advance her career in medical-surgical nursing. She is seeking guidance on the best educational resources to enhance her knowledge and skills. Which of the following options would be most beneficial for Sarah in her career development journey?
A) Attending a one-time seminar on general nursing topics
B) Enrolling in an accredited online medical-surgical nursing course
C) Participating in a workshop focused on basic nursing skills
D) Reading general healthcare magazines regularly

Question 68: In the context of 'Quality Management' under 'Professional Concepts', which of the following is a key principle of Total Quality Management (TQM)?
A) Focus on individual performance
B) Emphasis on blame culture
C) Continuous improvement
D) Hierarchical decision-making

Question 69: Scenario: Sarah, a CMSRN, is participating in a peer review process at her healthcare facility. During the review, she notices that a fellow nurse consistently fails to document patient assessments accurately, leading to potential patient safety concerns. What is the most appropriate action for Sarah to take in this situation?
A) Confront the nurse publicly during a team meeting about the documentation errors.
B) Report the nurse's actions to the nursing manager or supervisor in a confidential manner.
C) Ignore the situation as it is not Sarah's responsibility to address the peer's documentation errors.
D) Discuss the issue with other colleagues to gather their opinions before taking any action.

Question 70: Scenario: Mr. Johnson, a 65-year-old patient, is admitted to the medical-surgical unit with a complex medical history including diabetes, hypertension, and recent myocardial infarction. The healthcare team consists of nurses, physicians, physical therapists, and dietitians working together to provide comprehensive care. As the CMSRN, you recognize the importance of interdisciplinary collaboration in managing Mr. Johnson's care. Which of the following best exemplifies an effective method of interdisciplinary collaboration in this scenario?
A) The nurse independently develops a care plan without consulting other team members.
B) The physician makes all decisions regarding the patient's treatment without input from other team members.
C) The physical therapist and dietitian work together to create a customized exercise and nutrition plan for the patient.
D) The nurse restricts communication with other team members to written notes in the patient's chart.

Question 71: During safety rounds, which action by the nurse is most appropriate to ensure patient safety?
A) Documenting medication administration
B) Checking the patient's identification band
C) Updating the care plan
D) Reviewing the patient's dietary preferences

Question 72: Which advanced access device is specifically designed for long-term venous access and can remain in place for months to years?
A) Peripheral IV catheter
B) Midline catheter
C) Peripherally inserted central catheter (PICC)
D) Tunneled central venous catheter

Question 73: Which of the following is a crucial step to ensure safe intravenous therapy administration?
A) Using an IV catheter that is larger than necessary
B) Administering medications rapidly to save time
C) Checking the compatibility of medications before mixing in the same IV line
D) Skipping the verification of patient identification before starting IV therapy

Question 74: Which instrument is commonly used to grasp and hold tissues during surgical procedures?
A) Hemostat
B) Ophthalmoscope
C) Stethoscope
D) Sphygmomanometer

Question 75: Scenario: Ms. Smith, a 65-year-old patient, is admitted to the medical-surgical unit with a history of diabetes and hypertension. The nurse is utilizing a new electronic health record system to document Ms. Smith's vital signs. Which action by the nurse demonstrates effective use of nursing informatics?

A) The nurse manually records vital signs on a paper chart and then enters them into the electronic system at the end of the shift.
B) The nurse asks a colleague to document the vital signs in the electronic system to save time.
C) The nurse uses the electronic system to directly input and save Ms. Smith's vital signs during the assessment.
D) The nurse decides not to document the vital signs in the electronic system as it is time-consuming.

Question 76: When utilizing critical thinking skills in problem-solving as a Certified Medical Surgical Registered Nurse (CMSRN), which action is most appropriate?
A) Jumping to conclusions without assessing all available information.
B) Relying solely on past experiences without considering new evidence.
C) Collaborating with the healthcare team to gather diverse perspectives.
D) Making decisions hastily without evaluating potential outcomes.

Question 77: Which risk assessment method is commonly used in healthcare settings to evaluate patient safety and care management?
A) SWOT analysis
B) Failure Mode and Effects Analysis (FMEA)
C) Pareto analysis
D) Delphi technique

Question 78: Scenario: During a safety huddle on a medical-surgical unit, the team discusses a patient, Mr. Johnson, who is at risk for falls due to recent weakness. The team decides to implement fall prevention strategies for Mr. Johnson. Which action by the nurse best demonstrates a proactive approach to prevent falls?
A) Placing a "Fall Risk" sign on Mr. Johnson's door.
B) Ensuring Mr. Johnson's call bell is within reach at all times.
C) Checking on Mr. Johnson every hour.
D) Applying physical restraints to Mr. Johnson's bed.

Question 79: Scenario: Sarah, a Certified Medical Surgical Registered Nurse, is known for her exceptional leadership skills and ability to empower her colleagues. She actively engages in promoting a positive work environment and encourages her team members to voice their opinions and contribute to decision-making processes. Sarah believes in fostering a culture of collaboration and professional growth among her peers. Which action by Sarah best demonstrates professional empowerment in the context of nursing teamwork and collaboration?
A) Assigning tasks without seeking input from team members
B) Encouraging open communication and idea-sharing among colleagues
C) Making unilateral decisions without considering team feedback
D) Micromanaging every aspect of her team's work

Question 80: Scenario: Mrs. Smith, a 55-year-old patient, is admitted to the medical-surgical unit for exacerbation of chronic obstructive pulmonary disease (COPD). During the assessment, the nurse notes that Mrs. Smith has a history of smoking for the past 30 years. She expresses her willingness to quit smoking and asks for guidance on smoking cessation programs. Which intervention by the nurse would be most appropriate to assist Mrs. Smith in smoking cessation?
A) Providing information on the harmful effects of smoking
B) Recommending nicotine replacement therapy
C) Suggesting joining a support group for smokers
D) Encouraging gradual reduction of smoking

Question 81: In the context of near miss reporting in patient safety culture, which of the following best defines a near miss event?
A) An adverse event that resulted in patient harm
B) An event that had the potential to cause harm but did not reach the patient
C) A routine procedure without any complications
D) A medical error that was successfully intercepted before reaching the patient

Question 82: In the context of mentoring and coaching resources for career development in nursing teamwork and collaboration, which of the following is a key characteristic of an effective mentor?
A) Providing all the answers and solutions
B) Being overly critical and discouraging
C) Offering guidance, support, and constructive feedback
D) Ignoring the mentee's progress and challenges

Question 83: Scenario: Ms. Rodriguez, a 45-year-old Hispanic female, presents to the medical-surgical unit with complaints of severe abdominal pain. She appears distressed and is having difficulty communicating in English. The nurse on duty notices that Ms. Rodriguez seems hesitant to provide information about her symptoms. Which of the following actions by the nurse best demonstrates an understanding of implicit bias in this situation?
A) Assuming Ms. Rodriguez is exaggerating her symptoms due to language barriers.
B) Asking a colleague to communicate with Ms. Rodriguez instead.
C) Providing a professional interpreter to facilitate communication.
D) Dismissing Ms. Rodriguez's concerns as cultural differences.

Question 84: Which intervention is a priority in providing holistic end-of-life care to a terminally ill patient?
A) Administering high-dose pain medication
B) Initiating aggressive life-sustaining treatments
C) Encouraging the patient to discuss their fears and concerns
D) Placing the patient in isolation to prevent infections

Question 85: Ms. Rodriguez, a 68-year-old Hispanic patient, was admitted to the medical-surgical unit with a diagnosis of pneumonia. She speaks limited English and prefers to communicate in Spanish. The healthcare team needs to provide her with educational materials about her condition. Which of the following resources would be most appropriate to ensure effective communication and understanding for Ms. Rodriguez?
A) Using an online translation tool to convert the materials into Spanish.
B) Providing written materials in English with a list of local translation services.
C) Utilizing a professional medical interpreter to verbally translate the materials into Spanish.
D) Asking a bilingual staff member who speaks some Spanish to explain the materials to Ms. Rodriguez.

Question 86: Ms. Johnson, a 65-year-old patient, is admitted to the medical-surgical unit with a history of heart failure. The healthcare team plans to utilize telemonitoring technology to remotely track her vital signs and symptoms. This technology allows real-time data transmission to the healthcare provider for prompt intervention. Which benefit of telemonitoring technology is most significant for Ms. Johnson's care?
A) Improved patient satisfaction
B) Enhanced communication among healthcare team members
C) Early detection of clinical deterioration
D) Cost savings for the healthcare facility

Question 87: In the context of 'timeout' procedures in surgical settings, what is the primary purpose of implementing a timeout before a procedure?
A) To delay the procedure
B) To verify patient identity, surgical site, and procedure
C) To rush through the pre-procedural checklist
D) To skip unnecessary safety steps

Question 88: Scenario: Mr. Johnson, a 65-year-old male patient, is admitted to the medical-surgical unit with complaints of severe abdominal pain and distention. Upon assessment, the nurse notes absent bowel sounds, guarding, and rebound tenderness in the lower right quadrant. The patient has a history of hypertension and diabetes. Vital signs are stable except for a slightly elevated temperature. The healthcare provider suspects appendicitis and orders further diagnostic tests. Which action should the nurse prioritize in the care of Mr. Johnson?
A) Administer pain medication as ordered.
B) Prepare the patient for an emergency appendectomy.
C) Insert a nasogastric tube for decompression.
D) Initiate intravenous (IV) fluid therapy.

Question 89: In the context of patient safety and care management, which statement regarding the use of checklists is accurate?
A) Checklists are only beneficial for routine tasks.
B) Checklists are not effective in reducing medical errors.
C) Checklists help standardize care processes and improve patient outcomes.
D) Checklists are time-consuming and should be avoided in healthcare settings.

Question 90: Scenario: During a busy shift on a medical-surgical unit, a patient with a history of heart failure starts experiencing shortness of breath and chest pain. The patient's vital signs are unstable, and the nurse suspects a potential cardiac event. As the charge nurse, what is your primary responsibility in this situation?
A) Delegate the patient's care to another nurse and continue with administrative tasks.
B) Immediately assess the patient, initiate appropriate interventions, and notify the healthcare provider.
C) Wait for the primary nurse to return and handle the situation.
D) Document the patient's condition and wait for the next shift to address the issue.

Question 91: Which statement best describes reflective practice in the context of Career Development Relationships, Nursing Teamwork, and Collaboration?
A) Reflective practice involves solely focusing on personal achievements and goals.
B) Reflective practice is a structured process that involves looking back on experiences to learn and improve.
C) Reflective practice is a passive activity that does not require action or change.
D) Reflective practice is a one-time activity and does not contribute to professional growth.

Question 92: During safety rounds, which action by the nurse is most appropriate to ensure patient safety?
A) Checking the patient's identification band before administering medication.
B) Skipping hand hygiene if the nurse is wearing gloves.
C) Ignoring a patient's call light if the nurse is busy with another task.
D) Administering medication without verifying the patient's allergies.

Question 93: Which of the following is a common consequence of burnout among medical surgical nurses?
A) Increased job satisfaction
B) Improved patient outcomes
C) Decreased empathy towards patients
D) Enhanced teamwork skills

Question 94: Which of the following actions by a nurse best demonstrates adherence to patient safety protocols in a medical-surgical setting?
A) Administering medication without checking the patient's identification band
B) Double-checking the patient's allergies before administering a new medication
C) Disregarding hand hygiene before and after patient contact
D) Ignoring a patient's call light for assistance

Question 95: Scenario: Ms. Smith, a 55-year-old patient, is scheduled for a laparoscopic cholecystectomy in the morning. As the Certified Medical Surgical Registered Nurse (CMSRN) responsible for her care, which of the following pre-procedural actions is essential to ensure compliance with unit standards?
A) Administering a dose of aspirin for pain relief
B) Verifying the patient's identity and surgical site with another nurse
C) Allowing the patient to eat a heavy meal the night before surgery
D) Skipping the pre-operative checklist to expedite the process

Question 96: Ms. Johnson, a 65-year-old patient, has been admitted for a surgical procedure. As part of her pre-operative education, the nurse should prioritize teaching Ms. Johnson about:
A) The importance of deep breathing exercises post-surgery
B) The history of surgical procedures
C) The hospital's financial policies
D) The nurse's personal experiences with surgery

Question 97: Scenario: Ms. Smith, a 45-year-old postoperative patient, is exhibiting signs of emotional distress following her surgery. She appears tearful, anxious, and expresses concerns about her recovery process. As a CMSRN, what is the most appropriate initial action to address Ms. Smith's emotional needs?
A) Provide her with a list of community support groups for postoperative patients.
B) Encourage her to practice relaxation techniques such as deep breathing exercises.
C) Administer a sedative medication to help alleviate her anxiety.
D) Refer her to a mental health professional for counseling services.

Question 98: When prioritizing care for multiple patients, which patient should the Certified Medical Surgical Registered Nurse (CMSRN) attend to first?
A) A patient with stable vital signs who requires routine medication administration.
B) A patient who is experiencing chest pain and shortness of breath.
C) A patient requesting assistance with personal hygiene tasks.
D) A patient awaiting discharge instructions.

Question 99: Scenario: Mr. Johnson, a 65-year-old patient, has been admitted to the medical-surgical unit for post-operative care following a hip replacement surgery. As the CMSRN on duty, you notice that Mr. Johnson is experiencing increased

pain and restlessness. Upon assessment, you find that his surgical wound is warm, red, and swollen, with purulent drainage. His temperature is 101.5 蚌, heart rate 110 bpm, and blood pressure 150/90 mmHg. Mr. Johnson is also complaining of chills and feeling unwell. What is the most appropriate initial action by the CMSRN?
A) Administer acetaminophen for pain relief.
B) Notify the healthcare provider immediately.
C) Apply a warm compress to the surgical wound.
D) Increase the intravenous fluid rate.

Question 100: Scenario: Mr. Johnson, a 68-year-old patient, was admitted to the medical-surgical unit following a hip replacement surgery. He has a history of hearing impairment and relies on lip-reading to aid in communication. During the morning rounds, the nurse notices that Mr. Johnson is having difficulty understanding the instructions given by the healthcare team due to his hearing impairment. Which action by the nurse would be most appropriate to facilitate effective communication with Mr. Johnson?
A) Speaking loudly to ensure Mr. Johnson can hear clearly.
B) Using written notes or gestures to supplement verbal communication.
C) Asking Mr. Johnson's family to interpret the instructions for him.
D) Limiting communication with Mr. Johnson to essential information only.

Question 101: Scenario: Mrs. Smith, a 65-year-old patient, has been admitted to the medical-surgical unit for post-operative care following a hip replacement surgery. The hospital has implemented a new electronic health record system to enhance patient care and streamline documentation processes. As a CMSRN, how can you best support the nursing team during this change management process?
A) Attend training sessions on how to use the new electronic health record system.
B) Ignore the change and continue using the previous documentation methods.
C) Provide feedback to the nursing leadership about the challenges faced with the new system.
D) Encourage other nurses to resist the change and voice their concerns collectively.

Question 102: In the context of self-regulation, a Certified Medical Surgical Registered Nurse (CMSRN) demonstrates the ability to:
A) Recognize personal biases and work to minimize their impact on patient care.
B) Ignore feedback from colleagues to maintain autonomy in decision-making.
C) Rely solely on intuition without considering evidence-based practice.
D) Disregard ethical principles when faced with challenging situations.

Question 103: Scenario: Mrs. Smith, a 65-year-old patient, is admitted to the medical-surgical unit following a fall at home. During the assessment, the nurse discovers that Mrs. Smith lives alone, has limited mobility due to arthritis, and struggles with managing her medications independently. She expresses concerns about feeling isolated and unable to attend follow-up appointments due to transportation issues. Which social determinant of health is most likely impacting Mrs. Smith's current situation?
A) Socioeconomic status
B) Health literacy
C) Transportation access
D) Social support

Question 104: Scenario: Sarah, a Certified Medical Surgical Registered Nurse (CMSRN), is considering joining a professional organization related to medical-surgical nursing. She believes that being part of such an organization will enhance her professional development and provide opportunities for networking and continuing education. Which of the following is the most appropriate benefit of Sarah's decision to participate in a professional organization?
A) Access to discounted medical supplies and equipment
B) Opportunities for interprofessional collaboration
C) Increased administrative responsibilities
D) Mandatory overtime shifts

Question 105: Which resource is essential for promoting patient-centered care in a medical-surgical setting?
A) Advanced medical equipment
B) Comprehensive patient education materials
C) Increased nurse-to-patient ratio
D) Updated hospital policies and procedures

Question 106: Scenario: Mr. Johnson, a 65-year-old postoperative patient, is admitted to the medical-surgical unit following a hip replacement surgery. The unit is short-staffed due to unexpected call-outs, and the nurse is struggling to provide adequate care to all patients. Mr. Johnson requires frequent monitoring of vital signs and assistance with mobility. Despite the challenges, the nurse ensures that Mr. Johnson receives his medications on time and is comfortable. Which action by the nurse best demonstrates effective resource allocation in this staffing situation?
A) Prioritizing medication administration over vital sign monitoring
B) Delaying assistance with mobility to focus on other patients
C) Seeking assistance from other healthcare team members when needed
D) Decreasing communication with Mr. Johnson to save time

Question 107: Scenario: Mr. Smith, a 65-year-old patient, was admitted to the medical-surgical unit with a diagnosis of malnutrition. The nurse is assessing Mr. Smith's nutritional status. Which finding would be most indicative of malnutrition in this patient?
A) BMI of 28
B) Albumin level of 4.2 g/dL
C) Hemoglobin level of 12 g/dL
D) Serum transferrin level of 150 mg/dL

Question 108: During the assessment phase of the nursing process, the nurse should prioritize which action?
A) Administering medications
B) Developing a care plan
C) Collecting patient data
D) Implementing interventions

Question 109: Scenario: Mrs. Smith, a 72-year-old female patient with a history of hypertension, diabetes, and osteoarthritis, presents to the clinic with complaints of dizziness, confusion, and falls. Upon reviewing her medication list, it is noted that she is taking multiple medications prescribed by different specialists. Which of the following is the most appropriate intervention for Mrs. Smith's condition related to polypharmacy?
A) Discontinue all medications and start fresh.
B) Conduct a comprehensive medication review and deprescribe unnecessary medications.
C) Increase the dosage of all current medications.
D) Add more medications to address the symptoms.

Question 110: When sharing patient information with other healthcare team members, which method ensures confidentiality and privacy?
A) Sending patient details via unsecured email
B) Discussing patient information in a crowded hallway
C) Using a secure hospital communication system
D) Sharing patient information on social media platforms

Question 111: Scenario: Mr. Smith, a 65-year-old patient, was administered the wrong medication due to a documentation error by the nurse. The patient experienced adverse effects as a result. The nurse responsible for the error immediately reported it to the supervisor. In this situation, which action best reflects a "just culture"?
A) The nurse is reprimanded and suspended without investigation.
B) The nurse is encouraged to cover up the error to avoid consequences.
C) The nurse is supported through an investigation to understand the root cause of the error.
D) The nurse is blamed for the error without considering system factors.

Question 112: In the context of change management, leadership, nursing teamwork, and collaboration, which best describes the role of 'Desire' in achieving success within a healthcare setting?
A) Desire is a superficial emotion that does not impact teamwork.
B) Desire fuels motivation and drives individuals to work towards common goals.
C) Desire is irrelevant in the healthcare setting as professionalism is the key.
D) Desire leads to conflicts among team members and should be avoided.

Question 113: Which of the following is a key component of a care bundle aimed at enhancing patient safety in medical-surgical settings?
A) Administering medications on time
B) Allowing longer rest periods for nursing staff
C) Increasing patient visitation hours
D) Using outdated medical equipment

Question 114: Which personal protective equipment (PPE) is essential for healthcare workers when caring for a patient on airborne precautions?
A) Gown and gloves
B) Surgical mask
C) N95 respirator
D) Face shield

Question 115: Which of the following is an essential component of standard precautions in infection control practices?
A) Wearing gloves only when touching blood or body fluids
B) Using a mask only when performing aerosol-generating procedures
C) Disinfecting equipment only if visibly soiled
D) Proper hand hygiene before and after patient contact

Question 116: Scenario: Mr. Johnson, a 65-year-old patient with a history of hypertension and diabetes, is prescribed multiple medications for his conditions. He discards his expired medications by flushing them down the toilet. As a CMSRN promoting stewardship in medication management, what action should you take?
A) Educate Mr. Johnson on the proper disposal of medications.
B) Instruct Mr. Johnson to continue flushing medications if expired.
C) Ignore Mr. Johnson's method of medication disposal.

D) Advise Mr. Johnson to throw medications in the regular trash.

Question 117: Which of the following equipment is essential for a Certified Medical Surgical Registered Nurse (CMSRN) to ensure a healthy practice environment?
A) Stethoscope
B) Hairdryer
C) Blender
D) Telescope

Question 118: Which of the following factors can contribute to financial implications for patients in the context of medication management and patient/care management?
A) Lack of insurance coverage for prescribed medications
B) Availability of generic medication options
C) Regular follow-up appointments with healthcare providers
D) Participation in a clinical trial for a new medication

Question 119: In the context of Nursing Teamwork and Collaboration, which leadership style focuses on making decisions based on input from the team members?
A) Autocratic leadership
B) Laissez-faire leadership
C) Transformational leadership
D) Democratic leadership

Question 120: In the context of patient safety assessments and reporting, which action by the nurse is most appropriate when suspecting abuse in a patient?
A) Ignore the signs and continue with routine care
B) Document the observations and report to the appropriate authority
C) Confront the suspected abuser immediately
D) Discuss the situation with colleagues but take no further action

Question 121: In the context of staffing for Certified Medical Surgical Registered Nurses (CMSRN), which factor is crucial for effective delegation and supervision?
A) Staffing based solely on budgetary considerations
B) Staffing without considering delegation and supervision needs
C) Staffing that promotes nursing teamwork and collaboration
D) Staffing without regard for teamwork dynamics

Question 122: Ms. Johnson, a 65-year-old patient, is admitted to the medical-surgical unit with a diagnosis of heart failure. The healthcare team is discussing the implementation of a new evidence-based practice guideline for heart failure management. Which action by the nurse best demonstrates adherence to evidence-based practice principles?
A) Continuing to use the previous outdated heart failure management protocol
B) Consulting the latest research studies and guidelines to update the patient's care plan
C) Relying solely on personal experience and anecdotal evidence for decision-making
D) Disregarding the need for evidence-based practice and following intuition in patient care

Question 123: Scenario: Mrs. Smith, a 65-year-old patient recovering from abdominal surgery, is scheduled for a dietary consultation. The nurse notes that Mrs. Smith has a history of diabetes and hypertension. During the consultation, Mrs. Smith expresses concerns about maintaining a balanced diet post-surgery to aid in her recovery. Which dietary recommendation would be most appropriate for Mrs. Smith post-abdominal surgery considering her medical history?
A) High-sodium diet to prevent electrolyte imbalances
B) High-carbohydrate diet to promote wound healing

C) Low-fat diet to manage diabetes and hypertension
D) High-protein diet to support tissue repair

Question 124: Scenario: Mr. Johnson, a 45-year-old patient admitted for a surgical procedure, has a history of depression and suicidal ideation. He has been expressing feelings of hopelessness and isolation since his admission. During a routine check, the nurse finds Mr. Johnson sitting alone in his room, staring blankly out of the window. He appears withdrawn and tearful. What should be the nurse's immediate action based on suicide prevention protocols?
A) Leave Mr. Johnson alone to give him space
B) Engage Mr. Johnson in a conversation about his feelings
C) Inform other staff members about Mr. Johnson's behavior
D) Provide Mr. Johnson with a sharp object for self-soothing

Question 125: Scenario: Mrs. Smith, a 65-year-old female, is admitted to the medical-surgical unit with a history of diabetes, hypertension, and recent pneumonia. During the health history assessment, the nurse notes discrepancies in the information provided by Mrs. Smith and her daughter. Mrs. Smith denies any recent illness, while her daughter reports that her mother has been experiencing cough and fever for the past week. What should be the nurse's initial action based on this situation?
A) Document the conflicting information and proceed with the assessment.
B) Confront Mrs. Smith about the inconsistencies in her health history.
C) Verify the information with other healthcare providers involved in Mrs. Smith's care.
D) Reassure Mrs. Smith and her daughter that the discrepancies will not affect her treatment.

Question 126: Scenario: Mr. Smith, a 65-year-old patient, is admitted to the medical-surgical unit for a scheduled surgery. During the pre-operative assessment, the healthcare team discusses the surgical procedure, potential risks, and post-operative care with Mr. Smith. The nurse ensures that Mr. Smith understands the information provided and encourages him to actively participate in decision-making regarding his care. Which action by the nurse best demonstrates the concept of shared decision-making in this scenario?
A) Providing Mr. Smith with a pamphlet about the surgery and leaving the room.
B) Explaining the surgical procedure to Mr. Smith without asking for his input.
C) Asking Mr. Smith about his preferences and involving him in the decision-making process.
D) Informing Mr. Smith that the healthcare team will make all decisions for him.

Question 127: Ms. Johnson, a 65-year-old patient, recently underwent a surgical procedure at a medical-surgical unit. The hospital administration decides to conduct a patient satisfaction survey to assess the quality of care provided. Which type of survey question would be most appropriate to gather specific feedback on Ms. Johnson's overall experience during her hospital stay?
A) "Did you find the hospital staff friendly?"
B) "How likely are you to recommend this hospital to a friend or family member?"
C) "Were you satisfied with the cleanliness of your room?"
D) "On a scale of 1 to 10, how would you rate your overall experience at the hospital?"

Question 128: Scenario: During the morning shift handover, a Certified Medical Surgical Registered Nurse (CMSRN)

overhears a colleague discussing a medication error made the previous night. The colleague mentions that they did not report the error to the charge nurse as they were afraid of getting into trouble. What should the CMSRN do in this situation?
A) Ignore the conversation and continue with their shift.
B) Confront the colleague in front of other staff members.
C) Report the incident to the charge nurse or nurse manager.
D) Advise the colleague to keep the error confidential.

Question 129: Which action by the nurse is most appropriate when suspecting abuse in a patient?
A) Ignore the signs and continue with routine care.
B) Document the findings and report to the appropriate authorities.
C) Confront the suspected abuser in front of the patient.
D) Discuss the suspicions with colleagues for gossip and validation.

Question 130: Scenario: Mr. Johnson, a 65-year-old patient, is admitted to the medical-surgical unit for a scheduled surgery. He expresses concerns about the upcoming procedure and requests to speak with the surgeon before giving consent. As the CMSRN, what action should you take to uphold the patient's rights and responsibilities?
A) Inform Mr. Johnson that speaking with the surgeon is not necessary for this procedure.
B) Respect Mr. Johnson's request and arrange for him to meet with the surgeon to address his concerns.
C) Disregard Mr. Johnson's concerns and proceed with obtaining consent from his family member.
D) Provide Mr. Johnson with a pamphlet about the surgery and ask him to sign the consent form immediately.

Question 131: Scenario: Mr. Johnson, a 65-year-old patient admitted for a surgical procedure, appears anxious and confused. He keeps asking repetitive questions about his upcoming surgery and seems distressed. As a CMSRN, how should you best address Mr. Johnson's concerns?
A) Provide him with detailed medical jargon to explain the procedure.
B) Listen actively, acknowledge his feelings, and offer clear, simple explanations.
C) Ignore his questions and focus on completing the necessary paperwork.
D) Tell him not to worry and that everything will be fine without further discussion.

Question 132: Scenario: Mrs. Thompson, a 78-year-old patient with advanced cancer, has been admitted to hospice care for palliative treatment. As the CMSRN, you understand the importance of providing holistic care to Mrs. Thompson during this critical time. Which intervention is most appropriate to ensure holistic patient care in the hospice setting?
A) Administering pain medication as per the prescribed schedule.
B) Encouraging Mrs. Thompson to engage in spiritual practices that are meaningful to her.
C) Limiting visits from family members to prevent emotional distress.
D) Focusing solely on physical symptoms and disregarding emotional and spiritual needs.

Question 133: Scenario: Mr. Johnson, a 65-year-old postoperative patient, is admitted to the medical-surgical unit following a hip replacement surgery. During the initial assessment, the nurse notes that Mr. Johnson is experiencing shortness of breath, tachycardia, and restlessness. His oxygen saturation is 88% on room air. The nurse suspects a possible pulmonary embolism and initiates appropriate interventions. Which action should the nurse prioritize to ensure patient safety in this situation?

A) Administering pain medication to keep the patient comfortable.
B) Notifying the healthcare provider about the patient's condition.
C) Documenting the vital signs and symptoms in the patient's chart.
D) Encouraging the patient to take deep breaths and cough.

Question 134: In a medical-surgical unit, a nurse receives critical information about a patient's deteriorating condition from the night shift nurse. What action should the nurse take to ensure effective communication and continuity of care?

A) Document the information in the patient's chart and wait for the next shift to inform the healthcare team.
B) Immediately inform the healthcare team and provide a detailed handover report.
C) Disregard the information as it is the responsibility of the night shift nurse to communicate with the healthcare team.
D) Discuss the information with the patient's family before informing the healthcare team.

Question 135: When providing care to a patient with limited English proficiency, the nurse should:

A) Use complex medical terminology to ensure accuracy.
B) Avoid the use of professional interpreters to maintain patient privacy.
C) Utilize family members as interpreters to establish rapport.
D) Use professional interpreters to ensure accurate communication.

Question 136: Which of the following best describes the role of a Certified Medical Surgical Registered Nurse (CMSRN) in relation to procedures within the scope of practice?

A) Performing surgical procedures independently
B) Assisting the surgeon during procedures
C) Administering anesthesia during procedures
D) Interpreting radiological images for procedural guidance

Question 137: In the hospital incident command structure, who is responsible for managing the overall incident response and ensuring coordination among all involved parties?

A) Chief Nursing Officer (CNO)
B) Charge Nurse on duty
C) Incident Commander
D) Head of Security

Question 138: Which communication barrier is commonly associated with physical and cognitive limitations in patients?

A) Language differences
B) Hearing impairment
C) Visual impairment
D) Cultural differences

Question 139: In the context of Care Coordination and Transition Management, which method best exemplifies effective interdisciplinary collaboration integration?

A) Holding separate team meetings for each discipline
B) Sharing patient information through secure electronic platforms
C) Restricting communication to written notes only
D) Avoiding discussions with other healthcare professionals

Question 140: Scenario: Mr. Smith, a 65-year-old patient, was recently admitted to the medical-surgical unit for post-operative care following a hip replacement surgery. While in the hospital, he developed a surgical site infection that required additional treatment. During a routine check, the nurse noticed that the wound dressing was not changed as per the protocol, leading to a delay in Mr. Smith's recovery

process. The nurse responsible for this oversight admitted to the error and expressed regret for the mistake. What principle of "just culture" is exemplified in this scenario?

A) Blame-free reporting
B) Punitive approach
C) Retributive justice
D) Non-punitive response

Question 141: Ms. Johnson, a 68-year-old patient, is admitted to the medical-surgical unit with a diagnosis of heart failure. She is receiving intravenous diuretics to manage her fluid overload. The nurse notes that Ms. Johnson has developed hypokalemia. Which intervention should the nurse prioritize in the care of this patient?

A) Administering potassium supplements orally
B) Monitoring serum magnesium levels
C) Increasing the rate of intravenous diuretics
D) Encouraging a high-sodium diet

Question 142: Scenario: Mrs. Smith, a 65-year-old patient, is being discharged from the medical-surgical unit following a successful surgical procedure. As the CMSRN overseeing her discharge, which action is most appropriate to ensure a smooth transition and continuity of care for Mrs. Smith?

A) Provide Mrs. Smith with a detailed list of community resources for post-discharge support.
B) Schedule a follow-up appointment with the primary care provider in three months.
C) Instruct Mrs. Smith to discontinue all medications prescribed during her hospital stay.
D) Advise Mrs. Smith to resume her normal activities immediately upon returning home.

Question 143: Which of the following best describes the goal of hospice care for patients with terminal illnesses?

A) To provide aggressive treatment to cure the illness
B) To focus on providing comfort and quality of life
C) To transfer the patient to a different healthcare facility
D) To encourage the patient to undergo experimental treatments

Question 144: Which regulatory body is responsible for overseeing compliance standards in healthcare facilities?

A) American Nurses Association (ANA)
B) Centers for Medicare & Medicaid Services (CMS)
C) Occupational Safety and Health Administration (OSHA)
D) National Council of State Boards of Nursing (NCSBN)

Question 145: In the context of 'Patient customer experience based on data results,' which of the following best defines the term 'Patient Satisfaction Surveys'?

A) Surveys conducted by hospital staff to evaluate patient satisfaction
B) Surveys completed by healthcare providers to assess their own performance
C) Questionnaires given to patients to gather feedback on their healthcare experience
D) Reports generated by insurance companies to measure hospital efficiency

Question 146: Scenario: During a shift change handoff, a Certified Medical Surgical Registered Nurse (CMSRN) notices that a colleague did not document a critical change in a patient's condition. The patient, Mr. Smith, was supposed to receive a specific medication due to this change, but it was missed. The nurse in question seems overwhelmed and mentions having a heavy workload. What should the CMSRN do in this situation?

A) Offer to document the missed information themselves

B) Inform the charge nurse about the missed documentation and medication
C) Ignore the situation as it is the responsibility of the nurse who missed the documentation
D) Confront the colleague in front of other staff members

Question 147: Scenario: Mr. Johnson, a 65-year-old patient admitted for a surgical procedure, is experiencing anxiety and restlessness. As a CMSRN, which non-pharmacological intervention would be most appropriate to address Mr. Johnson's symptoms?
A) Administering a sedative medication
B) Encouraging deep breathing exercises and relaxation techniques
C) Providing a higher dose of pain medication
D) Allowing unlimited visitation hours for family and friends

Question 148: Which of the following is an essential aspect of background information sharing in the context of a Certified Medical Surgical Registered Nurse (CMSRN)?
A) Sharing personal opinions
B) Providing only partial information
C) Communicating relevant facts and data
D) Withholding information from the team

Question 149: Scenario: Sarah, a dedicated and experienced nurse, has been feeling overwhelmed and stressed due to the high patient load and lack of support from her colleagues. She feels undervalued and unappreciated in her current workplace. Despite her passion for nursing, she is considering leaving her job to seek better opportunities elsewhere. As a nurse leader, what is the most effective strategy to address Sarah's concerns and improve retention?
A) Implement a recognition program to acknowledge Sarah's hard work and dedication.
B) Increase Sarah's workload to challenge her and help her grow professionally.
C) Ignore Sarah's concerns as they might be temporary and not significant.
D) Assign more night shifts to Sarah to accommodate staffing needs.

Question 150: Which of the following non-verbal communication cues is considered a positive indicator during a patient interaction for a Certified Medical Surgical Registered Nurse (CMSRN)?
A) Crossing arms
B) Maintaining eye contact
C) Turning away from the patient
D) Frowning

ANSWER WITH DETAILED EXPLANATION SET [2]

Question 1: Correct Answer: C) The patient's mobility status and any assistance needed
Rationale: During bedside report, it is crucial to prioritize information that directly impacts the patient's safety and care continuity. In this scenario, discussing the patient's mobility status and any assistance needed is essential as it ensures a smooth transition of care and helps prevent falls or other adverse events post-discharge. Options A, B, and D, although important for patient satisfaction and support, do not hold the same level of priority as ensuring the patient's mobility needs are clearly communicated to the oncoming staff.

Question 2: Correct Answer: C) Ensuring clarity and simplicity
Rationale: Effective written communication in healthcare requires clarity and simplicity to ensure that the message is easily understood by all parties involved. Using complex medical jargon (Option A) can lead to confusion and misinterpretation, hindering effective communication. Providing vague and ambiguous information (Option B) can result in misunderstandings and errors in patient care. Including personal opinions and biases (Option D) can compromise the objectivity and professionalism of the communication. Therefore, the correct approach is to prioritize clarity and simplicity in written communication to facilitate accurate and efficient exchange of information in the healthcare setting.

Question 3: Correct Answer: A) Local pharmacy for medication delivery service
Rationale: The correct answer is A) Local pharmacy for medication delivery service. This option aligns with the patient's specific needs for medication management post-surgery. The pharmacy can provide home delivery services for medications, ensuring Ms. Johnson has timely access to her prescribed drugs without the need for frequent trips outside. Option B) Senior center for social activities, Option C) Grocery store for meal delivery service, and Option D) Fitness center for exercise classes do not directly address Ms. Johnson's immediate requirements for wound care and medication assistance, making them less suitable community resources in this scenario.

Question 4: Correct Answer: D) The nurse should document vital signs every 4 hours.
Rationale: In this scenario, the correct answer is D) The nurse should document vital signs every 4 hours. Documentation of vital signs every 4 hours is crucial for postoperative patients to monitor their condition closely for any signs of deterioration. Option A is incorrect as vital signs should be documented more frequently than every 6 hours. Option B is incorrect as wound appearance should be assessed and documented more frequently than once a day to monitor for any signs of infection or delayed healing. Option C is incorrect as intake and output should be documented more frequently than every shift to ensure accurate fluid balance assessment.

Question 5: Correct Answer: A) Sterile gloves
Rationale: Sterile gloves are crucial during a dressing change to prevent contamination of the wound and reduce the risk of infection. Non-sterile gloves do not provide the same level of protection and can introduce harmful microorganisms to the wound site. Regular gauze pads are not sterile and can compromise the aseptic technique required for wound care. Alcohol wipes, although useful for cleaning the skin, do not substitute for the necessity of sterile gloves in maintaining a sterile field during a dressing change. Therefore, the correct answer is A) Sterile gloves.

Question 6: Correct Answer: D) Monitoring and documenting Mr. Smith's vital signs and intake and output.
Rationale: Option A is incorrect as adjusting medication dosages

should be done by the healthcare provider or under their direct supervision. Option B is outside the nurse's scope of practice as diet modifications should be done by a dietitian. Option C involves providing education, which is important but should be done by the appropriate healthcare provider. The correct answer, Option D, falls within the CMSRN's scope of practice as monitoring and documenting vital signs and intake and output are essential nursing responsibilities that ensure the patient's safety and well-being.

Question 7: Correct Answer: A) Providing the patient with a list of community resources before discharge.
Rationale: Effective care coordination involves ensuring a smooth transition for the patient from one healthcare setting to another. Providing the patient with a list of community resources before discharge facilitates continuity of care by connecting the patient with necessary support services post-discharge. Options B, C, and D are incorrect as they represent inadequate care coordination practices that can lead to gaps in care, medication errors, lack of follow-up care, and poor communication between healthcare providers, ultimately compromising patient outcomes.

Question 8: Correct Answer: A) Braden Scale
Rationale: The Braden Scale is specifically designed to assess a patient's risk of developing pressure ulcers. It evaluates factors such as sensory perception, moisture, activity, mobility, nutrition, and friction/shear. In Mr. Johnson's case, his limited mobility and poor nutritional status indicate a higher risk for pressure ulcers, making the Braden Scale the most suitable assessment tool. The Glasgow Coma Scale is used to assess level of consciousness, the Morse Fall Scale evaluates fall risk, and the Katz Index assesses activities of daily living, none of which directly address pressure ulcer risk in this scenario.

Question 9: Correct Answer: A) Ensuring the patient receives adequate pain management
Rationale: In the scenario provided, the most crucial aspect of postoperative care for Ms. Smith following hip replacement surgery would be ensuring she receives adequate pain management. Pain control is essential for patient comfort, early mobilization, and overall recovery. While monitoring vital signs like blood pressure (option B) and administering prescribed medications such as antibiotics (option C) are important components of care, they may not be as immediate and patient-specific as ensuring pain management. Providing a foot massage (option D) may offer comfort but is not a standard checklist item for postoperative care. Therefore, option A is the most appropriate and essential item to include in Ms. Smith's care checklist.

Question 10: Correct Answer: C) Anticoagulants
Rationale: Anticoagulants are medications frequently prescribed to surgical patients to prevent the formation of blood clots, which are a common risk postoperatively. Antibiotics (Option A) are used to treat infections, not prevent blood clots. Antihypertensives (Option B) are indicated for managing high blood pressure. Antidepressants (Option D) are prescribed for mood disorders and are not directly related to reducing the risk of blood clots in postoperative patients. Therefore, the correct answer is anticoagulants as they specifically target the prevention of blood clot formation in surgical patients, aligning with the focus on patient safety and risk factors in pharmacological management.

Question 11: Correct Answer: C) Collaborating with the healthcare team to provide comprehensive care to surgical patients
Rationale: The correct option is C because as a CMSRN, the nurse's scope of practice involves working collaboratively with the healthcare team to deliver holistic care to surgical patients. This includes coordinating care, implementing interventions, and

communicating effectively with other team members. Options A and B are incorrect as CMSRNs do not perform surgical procedures independently or prescribe medications without physician oversight. Option D is incorrect as healthcare decisions should be made in collaboration with other professionals to ensure the best outcomes for patients.

Question 12: Correct Answer: B) Notifying the healthcare provider

Rationale: In this scenario, the nurse's priority should be to notify the healthcare provider immediately. While administering antibiotics may be necessary, it should not be the first action without consulting the provider. Removing the central venous catheter may be required but should be done under the provider's guidance. Applying a warm compress is not appropriate for a site with purulent drainage as it can exacerbate the infection. Timely communication with the healthcare provider ensures prompt and appropriate treatment, reducing the risk of complications for the patient.

Question 13: Correct Answer: B) Obtain a 12-lead electrocardiogram (ECG) immediately.

Rationale: In this scenario, Mr. Johnson presents with symptoms suggestive of a cardiac event, such as chest pain, shortness of breath, hypertension, tachycardia, crackles in the lungs, and pedal edema. Given his history and clinical presentation, obtaining a 12-lead ECG is the priority to assess for possible myocardial infarction or other cardiac abnormalities. Administering oxygen, starting an IV line, or assisting with breathing exercises are important interventions but obtaining an ECG takes precedence in this critical situation to guide further management and interventions.

Question 14: Correct Answer: D) Reinforcement

Rationale: In the ADKAR model, the element of Reinforcement is crucial for ensuring that the change is sustained and integrated into the organizational culture effectively. While Awareness (A), Desire (B), and Knowledge (C) are essential stages in the change process, Reinforcement plays a vital role in solidifying the change and preventing regression to old behaviors. It involves consistently reinforcing the new behaviors, processes, and systems to make the change stick in the long term. Therefore, option D is the correct choice as it directly addresses the aspect of sustaining change through continuous reinforcement efforts.

Question 15: Correct Answer: D) Central Line Bundle algorithm

Rationale: The correct answer is D) Central Line Bundle algorithm. The Central Line Bundle algorithm is a set of evidence-based practices aimed at reducing CLABSIs. It includes components such as hand hygiene, maximal barrier precautions during insertion, chlorhexidine skin antisepsis, optimal catheter site selection, and daily assessment of line necessity with prompt removal of unnecessary lines. This algorithm has been proven effective in reducing CLABSIs significantly. Comparatively, options A, B, and C are machine learning algorithms not specifically designed for patient safety or care management in the context of CLABSIs. Random Forest and Support Vector Machine algorithms are used in data analysis and prediction tasks, while the Apriori algorithm is used for association rule mining in data sets. These algorithms do not directly address the prevention of CLABSIs as effectively as the Central Line Bundle algorithm does.

Question 16: Correct Answer: B) Explaining the billing process and insurance coverage to Mr. Johnson.

Rationale: In this scenario, the correct answer is B) Explaining the billing process and insurance coverage to Mr. Johnson. As a nurse, part of financial stewardship involves educating patients about the financial aspects of their care, including billing procedures and insurance coverage. This empowers patients to make informed decisions and understand their financial responsibilities. Option A is not the best choice as providing a detailed breakdown of hospital charges may overwhelm the patient. Option C is incorrect as suggesting alternative treatment options solely based on cost may compromise the quality of care. Option D is not the most appropriate as the nurse should first provide basic financial

information before referring to a financial counselor.

Question 17: Correct Answer: C) The mediator facilitates communication and negotiation between conflicting parties.

Rationale: In healthcare settings, a mediator plays a crucial role in facilitating communication and negotiation between conflicting parties, such as patients and healthcare providers. The mediator does not act as a judge (option A) but rather helps parties reach a mutually acceptable agreement. Providing legal advice (option B) or imposing solutions without input (option D) goes against the principles of mediation, which emphasize voluntary and collaborative problem-solving. By fostering dialogue and understanding, the mediator helps parties find common ground and work towards resolving disputes amicably.

Question 18: Correct Answer: A) Percutaneous endoscopic gastrostomy (PEG) tube

Rationale: The correct answer is A) Percutaneous endoscopic gastrostomy (PEG) tube. PEG tube placement is a common method for long-term enteral nutrition administration in patients who are unable to swallow. It is a minimally invasive procedure that allows for direct access to the stomach for feeding. Option B) Nasogastric (NG) tube is used for short-term enteral feeding and may not be suitable for long-term use. Option C) Dobhoff tube is a type of NG tube with a smaller diameter, often used for medication administration rather than nutrition. Option D) Jejunostomy tube is inserted into the jejunum and is typically used when feeding into the stomach is not feasible.

Question 19: Correct Answer: B) Request an interpreter who speaks Gujarati to assist with communication.

Rationale: Utilizing an interpreter who speaks the patient's native language, in this case, Gujarati, is crucial to ensure accurate communication and understanding of medical information. Using a language translation app may not capture nuances or provide accurate translations. Relying on family members for translation can lead to miscommunication or breaches in patient confidentiality. Speaking loudly and slowly in English does not address the language barrier effectively and may cause frustration for the patient. Therefore, the most appropriate action is to request an interpreter proficient in Gujarati to facilitate clear communication and promote holistic patient care.

Question 20: Correct Answer: B) Contact precautions

Rationale: Contact precautions are essential when caring for patients colonized or infected with multidrug-resistant organisms like MRSA. These precautions involve wearing gloves and gowns upon entering the patient's room and ensuring proper hand hygiene. Droplet precautions are used for diseases spread through respiratory droplets larger than 5 microns, such as influenza. Airborne precautions are for diseases transmitted through small droplet nuclei, like tuberculosis. Standard precautions are the basic level of infection control and should be followed for all patients to prevent the spread of infections. In this scenario, the correct answer is contact precautions as MRSA is primarily spread through direct contact.

Question 21: Correct Answer: B) Do Not Resuscitate

Rationale: The correct answer is B) Do Not Resuscitate. DNR is a medical order that instructs healthcare providers not to perform CPR if a patient's heart stops beating or if they stop breathing. Choosing DNR means that the patient does not wish to have cardiopulmonary resuscitation (CPR) attempted in the event of cardiac or respiratory arrest. Options A, C, and D are incorrect as they do not accurately represent the meaning of DNR in the context of code status discussions. It is crucial for healthcare professionals to understand and respect patients' end-of-life preferences, including their code status choices, to provide holistic and patient-centered care.

Question 22: Correct Answer: A) Conducting a risk assessment to identify potential issues

Rationale: In project development for quality management, conducting a risk assessment is crucial to identify potential issues that may impact patient care outcomes. By assessing risks proactively, the healthcare team can develop strategies to mitigate these risks and ensure patient safety. Skipping the pilot phase (option B) can lead to unforeseen challenges during full implementation. Ignoring feedback from frontline staff (option C) can result in overlooking valuable insights from those directly involved in patient care. Implementing changes without evaluating outcomes (option D) can hinder the ability to measure the effectiveness of the quality management initiative. Conducting a risk assessment is the foundational step to ensure a comprehensive approach to quality management in healthcare projects.

Question 23: Correct Answer: A) Providing medication education to the patient and family.

Rationale: Option A is the correct answer as providing medication education involves collaboration with the healthcare team, ensuring that all members are informed about the plan of care. This action promotes interprofessional collaboration and patient safety. Option B is incorrect as setting mobility goals without consulting the physical therapist disregards the expertise of team members. Option C is incorrect as making dietary decisions independently can lead to inadequate care and overlooks the input of other team members. Option D is incorrect as discharging the patient without involving the social worker may result in incomplete discharge planning and lack of necessary support post-discharge. Effective teamwork in healthcare involves communication, collaboration, and respect for each team member's expertise.

Question 24: Correct Answer: B) Providing individualized care based on patient's beliefs and values

Rationale: Providing individualized care based on a patient's beliefs and values is crucial in promoting diversity and inclusion in healthcare. This approach acknowledges and respects the unique cultural backgrounds, preferences, and values of each patient, leading to better patient outcomes and satisfaction. Ignoring cultural differences (Option A) can result in misunderstandings and inadequate care. Excluding family members (Option C) can hinder effective communication and support. Implementing a one-size-fits-all approach (Option D) overlooks the importance of personalized care in addressing diverse patient needs. Therefore, option B is the correct choice for promoting holistic patient care through diversity and inclusion.

Question 25: Correct Answer: C) Document all details promptly and accurately

Rationale: Adverse event reporting is crucial for quality management in healthcare. Option A is incorrect as delaying reporting can lead to crucial details being forgotten or overlooked. Option B is incorrect as all adverse events, regardless of severity, should be reported for comprehensive analysis. Option D is incorrect as relying on memory can result in inaccuracies. Prompt and accurate documentation (Option C) is essential to ensure all relevant information is captured, enabling effective analysis, identification of trends, and implementation of quality improvement measures.

Question 26: Correct Answer: C) Implement alternative measures such as frequent checks and diversional activities to prevent Mr. Johnson from attempting to get out of bed.

Rationale: The correct answer is to implement alternative measures such as frequent checks and diversional activities to prevent Mr. Johnson from attempting to get out of bed. Restraints should only be used as a last resort when all other options have been exhausted. Educating the patient and providing alternative methods to address the underlying reasons for the behavior are essential components of patient-centered care. Applying restraints without exploring less restrictive interventions first can lead to physical and psychological harm. Therefore, the focus should be on individualized care that promotes patient safety while respecting the patient's autonomy and dignity. Options A and D involve the use of restraints without considering less restrictive alternatives,

which can increase the risk of complications and violate the patient's rights. Option B, while addressing the issue of the IV line, does not address the root cause of Mr. Johnson's behavior and may not effectively prevent him from attempting to get out of bed.

Question 27: Correct Answer: B) Reporting a safety concern to the charge nurse

Rationale: Speaking up plays a crucial role in patient safety culture by promoting open communication and addressing potential risks. Reporting a safety concern to the charge nurse demonstrates advocacy for patient well-being and a commitment to maintaining high standards of care. In contrast, options A, C, and D involve actions that compromise patient safety by either overlooking errors or withholding vital information. Encouraging a culture where healthcare professionals feel empowered to voice concerns fosters a safer environment for patients and enhances overall quality of care.

Question 28: Correct Answer: B) Asking the patient about their preferences and any cultural considerations

Rationale: It is essential for CMSRNs to ask patients about their preferences and any cultural considerations when providing oral care. This approach demonstrates respect for diversity and ensures that care is tailored to meet the individual needs of each patient. Using standardized products for all patients (Option A) may not address specific cultural or linguistic needs. Avoiding oral care discussions (Option C) can lead to inadequate care and discomfort for the patient. Providing care without considering the patient's background (Option D) neglects the importance of holistic patient care and may result in suboptimal outcomes.

Question 29: Correct Answer: B) Maintaining a safe distance and personal space

Rationale: In de-escalation techniques, maintaining a safe distance and personal space is crucial to prevent the situation from escalating further. By respecting the patient's personal space, the nurse shows empathy and reduces the likelihood of the patient feeling threatened or overwhelmed. Raising voice to match the patient's tone can escalate the situation, making it harder to communicate effectively. Making direct threats or ignoring the patient's concerns are counterproductive and can lead to increased agitation and aggression. Therefore, maintaining a safe distance and personal space is the most appropriate action to take in de-escalating tense situations in a medical-surgical setting.

Question 30: Correct Answer: C) Patient safety and immediate needs

Rationale: During a crisis situation, the top priority for the CMSRN should always be patient safety and addressing immediate patient needs. This includes assessing and managing the patient's condition, ensuring necessary interventions are implemented promptly, and maintaining a safe environment. Administrative paperwork and personal breaks for the nursing team can be temporarily deferred during a crisis to focus on patient care. While staffing assignments are important, patient safety takes precedence during emergencies. By prioritizing patient safety and immediate needs, the CMSRN can effectively manage crisis situations and provide optimal care to patients in need.

Question 31: Correct Answer: C) Language barrier

Rationale: The correct answer is C) Language barrier. When patients and healthcare providers do not speak the same language, effective communication becomes challenging, impacting the quality of care. A language barrier can lead to misunderstandings, errors in treatment, and patient dissatisfaction. Option A) Physical barrier refers to obstacles that impede communication physically, such as noise or distance. Option B) Emotional barrier involves emotional factors hindering effective communication. Option D) Cultural barrier pertains to differences in beliefs and practices that may affect communication but is not the primary reason for the need for an interpreter or translator in healthcare settings.

Question 32: Correct Answer: A) Understanding and respecting the beliefs, values, and practices of individuals from diverse cultural backgrounds.

Rationale: Cultural competence in healthcare involves healthcare providers understanding and respecting the beliefs, values, and practices of individuals from diverse cultural backgrounds. This approach helps in providing patient-centered care that is sensitive to the cultural and linguistic needs of each individual. Option B is incorrect as ignoring cultural differences can lead to misunderstandings and hinder effective communication. Option C is incorrect as assuming all patients are the same disregards the importance of individualized care. Option D is incorrect as excluding patients based on cultural background goes against the principles of holistic and inclusive patient care.

Question 33: Correct Answer: A) Confirming the patient's identification and allergies before administering the medication.

Rationale: The correct answer demonstrates the 'check-back' concept by ensuring patient safety through the verification of the patient's identification and allergies before medication administration. This step helps prevent medication errors and adverse reactions. Option B is incorrect as administering medication without verifying patient information can lead to errors. Option C is incorrect as asking about allergies after administering the medication is not in line with the 'check-back' principle. Option D is incorrect as checking the patient's identification after medication administration does not align with the proactive approach of 'check-back' in ensuring patient safety.

Question 34: Correct Answer: A) Keep the call bell within the patient's reach

Rationale: In the scenario provided, the most appropriate intervention to ensure patient safety and prevent falls for a patient with COPD exacerbation is to keep the call bell within the patient's reach. This allows the patient to easily call for assistance if needed, reducing the risk of falls. Option B (Placing the patient's water pitcher on the bedside table) may promote hydration but does not directly address fall prevention. Option C (Ensuring the room temperature is comfortable) is important for patient comfort but does not specifically address fall risk. Option D (Providing reading materials) is beneficial for patient engagement but does not contribute to fall prevention in this context.

Question 35: Correct Answer: B) A medical error that was successfully intercepted before reaching the patient

Rationale: Near miss events refer to situations where an error in the healthcare process could have harmed the patient but did not reach them due to timely intervention or chance. Option A is incorrect as near misses do not result in patient harm. Option C is incorrect as near misses involve potential risks, not routine procedures. Option D is incorrect as a delay in medication administration does not necessarily constitute a near miss unless it posed a direct threat that was intercepted. The correct option, B, highlights the essence of near miss reporting in preventing harm by catching errors before they impact patients.

Question 36: Correct Answer: A) Competence and accountability

Rationale: Competence and accountability are crucial professional behaviors that promote effective nursing teamwork and collaboration. Competence ensures that nurses have the necessary skills and knowledge to contribute meaningfully to the team, while accountability fosters trust and reliability among team members. Autonomy and independence, although important, should be balanced with collaboration to achieve optimal patient outcomes. Conflict avoidance can hinder open communication and problem-solving within the team. Hierarchical communication may impede effective teamwork by limiting information flow and inhibiting input from all team members. Therefore, competence and accountability are the most vital professional behaviors for fostering successful nursing teamwork and collaboration.

Question 37: Correct Answer: A) Taking responsibility for one's actions and decisions

Rationale: Accountability in nursing practice is a fundamental professional concept that involves nurses taking responsibility for their actions, decisions, and the outcomes of their nursing interventions. It includes being answerable for one's actions and ensuring that nursing care is delivered safely and effectively. Option B is incorrect as nurses are encouraged to critically think and question orders to ensure patient safety. Option C is incorrect as blaming others is not a professional or ethical practice. Option D is incorrect as ignoring patient needs goes against the core principles of nursing care.

Question 38: Correct Answer: C) Physicians, nurses, pharmacists, and social workers

Rationale: Interprofessional rounding involves a team of healthcare professionals from various disciplines, including physicians, nurses, pharmacists, and social workers, working collaboratively to discuss and plan patient care. This approach ensures comprehensive and holistic patient management by incorporating diverse perspectives and expertise. Options A, B, and D are incorrect as they do not encompass the multidisciplinary nature of interprofessional rounding, which relies on the collective input of different healthcare professionals to optimize patient outcomes.

Question 39: Correct Answer: D) Documenting and reporting incidents of medication errors

Rationale: Documenting and reporting incidents of medication errors is crucial in patient safety assessments and reporting as it helps in identifying system weaknesses, implementing corrective measures, and preventing future errors. While ensuring timely administration of medications and implementing hand hygiene protocols are important aspects of patient safety, they do not directly relate to assessments and reporting. Conducting regular patient fall risk assessments is essential for preventing falls but is not specifically focused on reporting incidents related to medication errors, which have a significant impact on patient safety.

Question 40: Correct Answer: A) Vitamin C

Rationale: Vitamin C plays a crucial role in wound healing as it is necessary for collagen synthesis, which is essential for the formation of new tissue and skin repair. Sodium is an electrolyte important for fluid balance but does not directly impact wound healing. Iron is essential for red blood cell production but is not directly related to wound healing. Vitamin K is important for blood clotting but does not have a direct role in the wound healing process. Therefore, the correct answer is Vitamin C as it directly supports the healing of surgical wounds by promoting collagen formation.

Question 41: Correct Answer: D) Walker

Rationale: The correct answer is D) Walker. In this scenario, Mr. Johnson, a post-operative patient, requires a walker for ambulation to provide stability and support while walking. A wheelchair (option A) is not suitable for ambulation as it is used for transporting patients who cannot walk. Crutches (option B) and a cane (option C) are not ideal choices for a patient like Mr. Johnson who needs more support and stability post-surgery. Therefore, the most appropriate equipment for the nurse to ensure Mr. Johnson's safety during ambulation is a walker.

Question 42: Correct Answer: A) Physical therapy services

Rationale: Physical therapy services play a crucial role in promoting holistic patient care by focusing on the patient's physical rehabilitation and overall well-being post-surgery. This resource aids in restoring mobility, reducing pain, and enhancing the patient's quality of life. Option B, social media platforms, although can provide support, may not always offer personalized and professional guidance tailored to the patient's specific needs. Option C, hospital cafeteria menu, is important but not directly related to holistic care. Option D, hospital policy handbook, is essential for information but does not directly contribute to the patient's physical and emotional recovery like physical therapy services do.

Question 43: Correct Answer: D) Central Line Bundle

Rationale: The correct answer is D) Central Line Bundle. The Central Line Bundle is a set of evidence-based practices aimed at reducing CLABSIs, including hand hygiene, maximal barrier precautions during insertion, chlorhexidine skin antisepsis, optimal catheter site selection, and daily assessment of line necessity with prompt removal. Options A, B, and C are not specific to CLABSIs but focus on fall risk assessment, fire safety response, and communication techniques, respectively. The Central Line Bundle is a crucial algorithm in patient care management to enhance patient safety by preventing CLABSIs.

Question 44: Correct Answer: D) Engaging in one-on-one counseling sessions

Rationale: One-on-one counseling sessions are the most effective method for providing health information to meet the holistic needs of patients. This approach allows for personalized care, tailored information delivery, and the opportunity to address individual concerns and questions directly. In contrast, using only written materials (option A) may not cater to varying learning styles or provide the opportunity for immediate clarification. Group education sessions (option B) may lack individualized attention and may not address specific patient needs. While multimedia resources (option C) can be engaging, they may not allow for the same level of interaction and personalized guidance as one-on-one counseling sessions.

Question 45: Correct Answer: B) Opportunities for continuing education and professional growth

Rationale: Engaging in professional organizations offers nurses opportunities for continuing education, skill development, and networking with peers in the field. This involvement can lead to career advancement, staying updated on current practices, and enhancing teamwork and collaboration skills. Options A, C, and D are incorrect as they do not directly contribute to professional growth or development within the nursing field. It is crucial for CMSRNs to actively participate in professional organizations to stay informed, connected, and continuously improve their practice.

Question 46: Correct Answer: A) Offer to help the colleague with some of the tasks.

Rationale: The correct answer is to offer help to the struggling colleague as part of demonstrating professionalism in nursing teamwork and collaboration. By offering assistance, the CMSRN shows empathy, support, and teamwork, which are essential components of professional behavior. Option B is incorrect as ignoring the situation can lead to potential patient safety issues. Option C is not the best initial approach as reporting should be done after attempting to resolve the issue personally. Option D is inappropriate as confronting the colleague publicly can be embarrassing and counterproductive to fostering a positive work environment.

Question 47: Correct Answer: B) Providing emotional support and actively listening to the patient's concerns

Rationale: Holistic patient care involves addressing not only the physical needs of the patient but also their emotional, social, and spiritual well-being. Providing emotional support and actively listening to the patient's concerns are essential components of holistic care as they help establish a therapeutic relationship, build trust, and promote overall well-being. While administering medications, documenting vital signs, and maintaining hand hygiene are crucial aspects of nursing care, they primarily focus on the physical aspect of care and do not encompass the holistic approach that considers the patient as a whole.

Question 48: Correct Answer: B) Engage in regular aerobic exercise

Rationale: Engaging in regular aerobic exercise is a crucial health promotion goal for patients with COPD as it can help improve lung function, increase endurance, and enhance overall respiratory status. Options A, C, and D are incorrect as increasing caffeinated beverages can worsen COPD symptoms, limiting fluid intake can lead to dehydration and exacerbate respiratory issues, and avoiding prescribed inhalers can hinder proper management of COPD symptoms. Regular aerobic exercise is essential in promoting lung health and overall well-being in patients with COPD.

Question 49: Correct Answer: A) Provide Mrs. Smith with pill organizers labeled for each day of the week.

Rationale: Providing Mrs. Smith with pill organizers labeled for each day of the week is the most appropriate intervention to promote safe medication management at home. This strategy helps her organize and track her medications effectively, reducing the risk of missed doses or double dosing. Option B is incorrect as storing medications in one large container can lead to confusion and errors. Option C is incorrect as the bathroom is not an ideal place for medication storage due to humidity and temperature fluctuations. Option D is incorrect as sharing medications is unsafe and can lead to serious consequences.

Question 50: Correct Answer: C) Keeping the oxygen equipment away from potential ignition sources.

Rationale: Option A is incorrect as patients with COPD exacerbation are at risk of hyperthermia rather than hypothermia. Option B is incorrect as limiting access to water can lead to dehydration, which is detrimental to the patient's condition. Option D is incorrect as increasing humidity levels can exacerbate respiratory distress in patients with COPD. The correct answer is C because oxygen is a highly flammable substance, and keeping the equipment away from ignition sources reduces the risk of fire hazards, ensuring patient safety and effective care management.

Question 51: Correct Answer: C) Incident Commander

Rationale: The correct answer is C) Incident Commander. The Incident Commander plays a crucial role in managing the overall incident response within the hospital incident command structure. This individual is responsible for making strategic decisions, coordinating resources, and ensuring effective communication among all involved parties during an emergency or disaster situation. The Chief Nursing Officer (A) focuses on nursing leadership, the Charge Nurse on duty (B) oversees daily nursing operations, and the Head of Security (D) is responsible for security-related matters, but none of these roles hold the primary responsibility for managing the overall incident response and coordination as the Incident Commander does.

Question 52: Correct Answer: C) Providing education on dietary sodium restrictions

Rationale: Providing education on dietary sodium restrictions aligns with Standard V of the AMSN Scope and Standards, which emphasizes the nurse's responsibility to educate patients on self-care practices. This action promotes patient empowerment and supports the patient in managing their condition effectively. Options A, B, and D are incorrect as they do not reflect the ethical and professional responsibilities outlined in Standard V. Administering medications without verifying the patient's identity poses a safety risk, documenting vital signs only at the beginning of the shift neglects ongoing assessment, and ignoring the patient's call light goes against the principles of patient-centered care.

Question 53: Correct Answer: B) Acknowledging Sarah's hard work and dedication in a team meeting.

Rationale: Acknowledging Sarah's hard work and dedication in a team meeting is the best way to demonstrate employee engagement in this scenario. This action shows appreciation for Sarah's efforts, boosts her morale, and reinforces a positive work culture. Providing additional training on time management (Option A) may be helpful but does not directly address Sarah's need for recognition. Assigning Sarah to mentor a new nurse (Option C) could be beneficial for team development but may add to her stress. Increasing Sarah's workload (Option D) would likely exacerbate her feelings of being overwhelmed, rather than engaging her positively.

Question 54: Correct Answer: C) Use open-ended questions to encourage Mr. Johnson to share his thoughts and feelings.

Rationale: In this scenario, the most effective communication strategy is to use open-ended questions to encourage Mr. Johnson to express his concerns openly. Closed-ended questions may limit his ability to fully communicate his feelings, while providing written instructions may not address his underlying anxieties. Assuming understanding without clarification can lead to misunderstandings. Open-ended questions promote a therapeutic relationship, allowing Mr. Johnson to voice his worries and enabling better patient-centered care.

Question 55: Correct Answer: C) Empathy and compassion
Rationale: In the context of workplace safety, a healthy practice environment, and professional concepts, the most suitable emotional response for a CMSRN when encountering a difficult situation is to demonstrate empathy and compassion. Panic and anxiety (Option A) can hinder clear thinking and decision-making, while anger and frustration (Option B) may lead to conflict and negativity in the work environment. Indifference and apathy (Option D) are not conducive to providing quality patient care. By choosing empathy and compassion (Option C), the nurse can maintain a professional and caring demeanor, fostering a positive atmosphere and effective patient-centered care.

Question 56: Correct Answer: B) Making eye contact while listening
Rationale: Non-verbal communication plays a crucial role in conveying messages effectively. Making eye contact while listening demonstrates active engagement and shows the speaker that you are attentive and interested in what they are saying. This non-verbal cue encourages open communication and helps build trust between the nurse and the patient. Options A, C, and D are examples of verbal communication or documentation skills, which are important but do not specifically pertain to non-verbal communication skills essential for effective nurse-patient interactions.

Question 57: Correct Answer: B) In-person group workshops with role-playing exercises
Rationale: In-person group workshops with role-playing exercises are the most effective method for promoting Nursing Teamwork and Collaboration among CMSRNs. This approach allows nurses to actively engage with their peers, practice real-life scenarios, and enhance their communication and teamwork skills in a hands-on setting. Online modules may lack the interactive element essential for teamwork development. Self-directed study may not provide sufficient opportunities for real-time collaboration. Lecture-style presentations, while informative, do not offer the same level of active participation and skill-building as in-person workshops with role-playing exercises.

Question 58: Correct Answer: D) Encouraging interdisciplinary collaboration
Rationale: Encouraging interdisciplinary collaboration is crucial in improving documentation accuracy and comprehensiveness. This strategy promotes communication among healthcare team members, leading to a more holistic approach to patient care reflected in the documentation. Providing generic feedback (option A) may not address specific documentation issues, while conducting regular chart audits (option B) focuses more on identifying errors than improving overall quality. Offering rewards for quantity over quality (option C) can incentivize inappropriate documentation practices. In contrast, encouraging interdisciplinary collaboration fosters a team-based approach that enhances documentation accuracy and completeness.

Question 59: Correct Answer: D) Contact the hospital social worker to discuss the situation and seek guidance.
Rationale: In cases where human trafficking is suspected, it is crucial for healthcare providers to involve the appropriate resources such as social workers who are trained to handle such sensitive situations. Discharging the patient without further assessment or involving the social worker can put the patient at risk of further harm. Conducting a physical assessment, although important, should not take precedence over addressing the potential human trafficking situation. Asking the companion to step out may escalate the situation, and involving the social worker first is the most appropriate course of action to ensure the patient's safety and well-being.

Question 60: Correct Answer: C) Keeping medications in their original labeled containers
Rationale: Keeping medications in their original labeled containers is crucial for safe home medication management as it helps in proper identification of the medication, dosage, and expiry date. Storing medications in a bathroom medicine cabinet (Option A) is not ideal due to humidity and temperature changes. Sharing prescription medications with a family member (Option B) is unsafe and can lead to adverse reactions. Mixing different medications into a single container for convenience (Option D) can result in medication errors and interactions. Therefore, the correct option is C as it promotes safe medication practices at home.

Question 61: Correct Answer: C) The nurse collaborates with the physical therapist to develop a mobility plan for Mr. Smith.
Rationale: Effective interdisciplinary communication involves active collaboration and information sharing among team members to ensure holistic patient care. Option A is incorrect as updating the family without consulting the team may lead to fragmented care. Option B is incorrect as failing to communicate vital information to the team can result in missed interventions. Option D is incorrect as prescribing medications is outside the nurse's scope of practice and requires physician involvement. Option C is the correct answer as collaborating with the physical therapist promotes coordinated care and enhances patient outcomes through a comprehensive approach.

Question 62: Correct Answer: C) Utilizing professional medical interpreters
Rationale: Utilizing professional medical interpreters is the most appropriate approach when providing translated materials to patients with limited English proficiency. This ensures accurate communication, maintains patient confidentiality, and reduces the risk of misinterpretation or misunderstanding. Using free online translation tools (option A) may result in inaccuracies due to language nuances and medical terminology. Asking family members to interpret (option B) can lead to breaches in patient privacy and may not guarantee accurate communication. Providing written materials in English only (option D) disregards the patient's right to access information in their preferred language, hindering holistic patient care and inclusivity.

Question 63: Correct Answer: C) Request
Rationale: In the SBAR communication model, 'R' stands for 'Recommendation.' This component is crucial as it involves suggesting a course of action or a request for specific interventions based on the situation and assessment provided. The recommendation should be clear, concise, and relevant to ensure effective communication between healthcare team members. Options A, B, and D are incorrect as they do not align with the standard SBAR framework. Response (A) and Review (D) do not accurately represent the 'R' in SBAR, while Reflection (B) is not a typical component of this structured communication method.

Question 64: Correct Answer: B) Contact the surgeon who performed the procedure.
Rationale: In this scenario, the correct action for the nurse to take, following the chain of command principles, is to contact the surgeon who performed the procedure. When a postoperative patient shows signs of complications, it is crucial to involve the primary healthcare provider, in this case, the surgeon, as they are most familiar with the patient's surgical history and can provide immediate guidance on further assessment and intervention. Option A (Notify the charge nurse on the unit) may delay the necessary intervention as the charge nurse may not have the authority to make decisions regarding postoperative complications. Option C (Inform the nursing supervisor of the unit) is also not the

most appropriate action in this critical situation, as the supervisor may not have direct knowledge of the patient's surgical procedure. Option D (Call the patient's family to update them on the situation) is important but should not be the immediate action when the patient's condition is deteriorating, as the focus should be on timely medical intervention.

Question 65: Correct Answer: B) Use open-ended questions to encourage Mrs. Smith to share her concerns.

Rationale: In this scenario, the most appropriate approach to address Mrs. Smith's communication preferences is to use open-ended questions. This technique allows Mrs. Smith to express her concerns freely and helps the nurse understand her needs better. Option A may overwhelm Mrs. Smith with too much information. Option C may dismiss Mrs. Smith's concerns without addressing them effectively. Option D is not ideal as the nurse should prioritize direct communication with the patient to ensure patient-centered care.

Question 66: Correct Answer: B) Two-way communication where feedback is encouraged and essential

Rationale: In a closed-loop communication system, it is crucial for information to flow in both directions, ensuring that the sender's message is accurately received and understood by the receiver. This process involves active listening, seeking clarification, and providing feedback to confirm comprehension. Option A is incorrect as feedback is essential in closed-loop communication. Option C is incorrect as closed-loop communication involves all parties, including patients. Option D is incorrect as closed-loop communication aims to minimize misinterpretation through clarification and feedback, promoting effective information sharing and professional collaboration.

Question 67: Correct Answer: B) Enrolling in an accredited online medical-surgical nursing course

Rationale: Enrolling in an accredited online medical-surgical nursing course would be the most beneficial option for Sarah as it offers in-depth knowledge and skills specific to her field of interest. This educational resource will provide her with comprehensive information on medical-surgical nursing practices, patient care, and the latest advancements in the field. Attending a one-time seminar on general nursing topics, participating in a workshop on basic nursing skills, or reading general healthcare magazines, although informative, may not offer the specialized education and depth of knowledge that an accredited online course can provide.

Question 68: Correct Answer: C) Continuous improvement

Rationale: Total Quality Management (TQM) emphasizes continuous improvement as a fundamental principle. TQM focuses on involving all employees in the process of improving quality and efficiency within an organization. Option A is incorrect as TQM stresses teamwork and collective effort rather than individual performance. Option B is incorrect because TQM promotes a culture of shared responsibility and learning from mistakes rather than blaming individuals. Option D is incorrect as TQM encourages participatory decision-making processes rather than hierarchical structures, fostering a culture of collaboration and innovation.

Question 69: Correct Answer: B) Report the nurse's actions to the nursing manager or supervisor in a confidential manner.

Rationale: In the scenario described, the most appropriate action for Sarah, as a responsible CMSRN, is to report the nurse's consistent documentation errors to the nursing manager or supervisor in a confidential manner. This approach upholds patient safety and professional standards while maintaining the peer's dignity and privacy. Option A is incorrect as confronting the nurse publicly may lead to conflict and embarrassment. Option C is incorrect as patient safety is a collective responsibility of all healthcare professionals. Option D is incorrect as discussing the issue with colleagues may delay necessary intervention and resolution. Reporting to the appropriate authority ensures accountability and promotes a culture of safety and quality care.

Question 70: Correct Answer: C) The physical therapist and

dietitian work together to create a customized exercise and nutrition plan for the patient.

Rationale: In the context of interdisciplinary collaboration, option C is the most appropriate as it demonstrates effective teamwork between different healthcare professionals. Collaborating on a customized exercise and nutrition plan involves input from multiple disciplines, ensuring a holistic approach to the patient's care. Options A, B, and D are incorrect as they depict actions that do not promote collaboration or teamwork among the healthcare team members. Effective interdisciplinary collaboration involves active communication, shared decision-making, and coordinated efforts to achieve optimal patient outcomes.

Question 71: Correct Answer: B) Checking the patient's identification band

Rationale: Checking the patient's identification band is crucial during safety rounds as it helps in verifying the patient's identity before any procedures or medication administration, reducing the risk of errors. Documenting medication administration, updating the care plan, and reviewing dietary preferences are important tasks but may not directly impact immediate patient safety during safety rounds. Patient identification is a critical step to prevent medication errors, ensure correct procedures, and maintain overall patient safety.

Question 72: Correct Answer: D) Tunneled central venous catheter

Rationale: Tunneled central venous catheters are advanced access devices that are designed for long-term venous access. They are surgically inserted into a large central vein, tunneled under the skin, and have a Dacron cuff that promotes tissue ingrowth to secure the catheter in place for extended periods. Unlike peripheral IV catheters, midline catheters, and PICCs, tunneled central venous catheters are suitable for patients requiring long-term intravenous therapies such as chemotherapy, parenteral nutrition, or long-term antibiotic treatment. Therefore, the correct option is D.

Question 73: Correct Answer: C) Checking the compatibility of medications before mixing in the same IV line

Rationale: It is essential to check the compatibility of medications before mixing them in the same IV line to prevent potential drug interactions, precipitations, or incompatibilities that could harm the patient. Using an IV catheter that is larger than necessary can lead to complications such as phlebitis or infiltration. Administering medications rapidly can cause adverse effects or errors in dosage calculation. Skipping patient identification verification can result in medication errors and jeopardize patient safety. Therefore, ensuring compatibility of medications is a critical step in safe intravenous therapy administration.

Question 74: Correct Answer: A) Hemostat

Rationale: A hemostat is a surgical tool designed for clamping blood vessels or tissue to control bleeding during surgical procedures. The other options, such as the ophthalmoscope, stethoscope, and sphygmomanometer, are not used for grasping and holding tissues during surgeries. An ophthalmoscope is used to examine the eyes, a stethoscope is used for auscultation of sounds within the body, and a sphygmomanometer is used to measure blood pressure. Therefore, the correct answer is A) Hemostat, as it is specifically designed for the mentioned purpose in surgical settings.

Question 75: Correct Answer: C) The nurse uses the electronic system to directly input and save Ms. Smith's vital signs during the assessment.

Rationale: Option C is the correct answer as it demonstrates effective use of nursing informatics by utilizing the electronic system in real-time to input and save vital signs during the assessment. This approach ensures accurate and timely documentation, promoting efficient interprofessional care coordination. Options A and D involve inefficient manual documentation or neglecting electronic documentation, which can compromise data accuracy and patient safety. Option B is incorrect as it suggests passing off documentation responsibilities to another colleague, which is not in line with professional nursing practice standards.

Question 76: Correct Answer: C) Collaborating with the healthcare team to gather diverse perspectives.

Rationale: In the context of problem-solving, collaborating with the healthcare team to gather diverse perspectives is crucial for effective decision-making as a CMSRN. This approach allows for a comprehensive evaluation of the situation, consideration of various viewpoints, and integration of different expertise levels. Options A and D are incorrect as they promote impulsive decision-making, which can lead to errors in patient care. Option B is also incorrect as solely relying on past experiences may limit the nurse's ability to adapt to new challenges and advancements in medical practices. Collaborative problem-solving enhances critical thinking skills and promotes better patient outcomes.

Question 77: Correct Answer: B) Failure Mode and Effects Analysis (FMEA)

Rationale: Failure Mode and Effects Analysis (FMEA) is a systematic method used in healthcare to identify potential failure modes in processes, assess their impact, and prioritize actions to reduce risks. In contrast, SWOT analysis is more commonly used for strategic planning, Pareto analysis focuses on identifying the most significant factors contributing to a problem, and the Delphi technique involves expert consensus building. FMEA specifically targets patient safety and care management by proactively addressing potential failures, making it the most suitable risk assessment method in healthcare settings.

Question 78: Correct Answer: B) Ensuring Mr. Johnson's call bell is within reach at all times.

Rationale: Placing a "Fall Risk" sign on the door (Option A) is a reactive measure and does not actively prevent falls. Checking on the patient every hour (Option C) is important but may not prevent falls if the patient attempts to move independently. Applying physical restraints (Option D) should be avoided unless all other interventions have failed due to the risk of complications. Ensuring the call bell is within reach (Option B) is a proactive approach that allows the patient to easily request assistance, promoting safety and preventing falls.

Question 79: Correct Answer: B) Encouraging open communication and idea-sharing among colleagues

Rationale: Professional empowerment in nursing teamwork and collaboration involves fostering an environment where team members feel valued, respected, and encouraged to actively participate in decision-making processes. By encouraging open communication and idea-sharing among colleagues, Sarah is promoting a culture of collaboration and mutual respect, which ultimately leads to improved teamwork and job satisfaction. Assigning tasks without seeking input, making unilateral decisions, or micromanaging can hinder professional empowerment by limiting team members' autonomy and stifling their creativity and growth.

Question 80: Correct Answer: B) Recommending nicotine replacement therapy

Rationale: Nicotine replacement therapy (NRT) is a proven method to help individuals quit smoking by reducing withdrawal symptoms and cravings. While providing information on the harmful effects of smoking (Option A) is important, it may not directly aid in cessation. Joining a support group (Option C) can be beneficial but may not address the immediate need for nicotine replacement. Encouraging gradual reduction (Option D) is less effective than NRT in achieving successful smoking cessation. Therefore, recommending NRT is the most appropriate intervention to support Mrs. Smith in quitting smoking effectively.

Question 81: Correct Answer: B) An event that had the potential to cause harm but did not reach the patient

Rationale: Near miss events are incidents that had the potential to cause harm but were intercepted before reaching the patient. Option A is incorrect as near misses do not result in patient harm. Option C is incorrect as near misses are not routine procedures. Option D is incorrect as it describes an intercepted error, not a near miss where harm was avoided without intervention. Near miss reporting is crucial in improving patient safety by identifying system weaknesses and preventing future errors.

Question 82: Correct Answer: C) Offering guidance, support, and constructive feedback

Rationale: An effective mentor in nursing teamwork and collaboration should provide guidance, support, and constructive feedback to help the mentee grow and develop professionally. This approach fosters a positive learning environment, encourages open communication, and promotes continuous improvement. Options A and D are incorrect as they do not align with the supportive and developmental role of a mentor. Option B is also incorrect as being overly critical and discouraging can hinder the mentee's progress and confidence, rather than facilitating their professional growth.

Question 83: Correct Answer: C) Providing a professional interpreter to facilitate communication.

Rationale: In this scenario, the correct action that demonstrates an understanding of implicit bias is providing a professional interpreter to facilitate communication (Option C). Implicit bias can lead to assumptions or stereotypes based on a person's race, ethnicity, or language proficiency. By providing a professional interpreter, the nurse ensures effective communication, respects Ms. Rodriguez's autonomy, and avoids making unfounded assumptions. Options A, B, and D reflect potential biases or inadequate responses that may hinder effective patient care and violate principles of holistic patient care and diversity and inclusion.

Question 84: Correct Answer: C) Encouraging the patient to discuss their fears and concerns

Rationale: In end-of-life care, encouraging the patient to express their fears and concerns is crucial for providing holistic support. This approach allows the patient to address emotional, spiritual, and psychological needs, promoting comfort and dignity in their final days. Administering high-dose pain medication is important but does not address the holistic aspect of care. Initiating aggressive life-sustaining treatments may not align with the patient's wishes for comfort-focused care. Placing the patient in isolation contradicts the principles of holistic care, which emphasize emotional support and open communication.

Question 85: Correct Answer: C) Utilizing a professional medical interpreter to verbally translate the materials into Spanish.

Rationale: Utilizing a professional medical interpreter to verbally translate the materials into Spanish is the most appropriate option to ensure effective communication and understanding for Ms. Rodriguez. This approach maintains accuracy, confidentiality, and cultural sensitivity in conveying medical information. Option A is not ideal as online translation tools may not always provide accurate translations, leading to potential misunderstandings. Option B may delay the communication process and could result in misinterpretation. Option D, although involving a bilingual staff member, may not guarantee accurate and professional translation of complex medical information, which is crucial for Ms. Rodriguez's understanding and holistic care.

Question 86: Correct Answer: C) Early detection of clinical deterioration

Rationale: Telemonitoring technology plays a crucial role in early detection of clinical deterioration by continuously monitoring vital signs and symptoms remotely. This proactive approach enables timely interventions, preventing potential complications and reducing hospital readmissions. While improved patient satisfaction and enhanced communication are important aspects of healthcare delivery, the primary advantage of telemonitoring in this scenario is the ability to detect changes in Ms. Johnson's condition promptly. Cost savings, although a consideration, are secondary to the patient's well-being and clinical outcomes.

Question 87: Correct Answer: B) To verify patient identity, surgical site, and procedure

Rationale: A timeout before a procedure is crucial to ensure patient safety by verifying key elements such as patient identity, correct surgical site, and procedure to be performed. Option A is incorrect as the purpose of a timeout is not to delay the procedure but to enhance patient safety. Option C is incorrect as rushing through the checklist compromises safety protocols. Option D is incorrect as skipping safety steps can lead to serious errors and harm the patient. Therefore, the correct answer is B, emphasizing the importance of thorough verification during the timeout process.

Question 88: Correct Answer: B) Prepare the patient for an emergency appendectomy.

Rationale: In the scenario provided, the nurse's priority should be to prepare the patient for an emergency appendectomy. Appendicitis is a surgical emergency that requires prompt intervention to prevent complications such as perforation and peritonitis. Administering pain medication (Option A) may provide temporary relief but does not address the underlying cause. Inserting a nasogastric tube (Option C) may be necessary postoperatively but is not the immediate priority. Initiating IV fluid therapy (Option D) is important for hydration but does not address the urgent need for surgical intervention in appendicitis. Therefore, preparing the patient for an emergency appendectomy is the most critical action to ensure Mr. Johnson's timely and appropriate care.

Question 89: Correct Answer: C) Checklists help standardize care processes and improve patient outcomes.

Rationale: Checklists play a crucial role in enhancing patient safety and care management by standardizing procedures, reducing variability, and ensuring essential steps are consistently followed. They are designed to prevent errors, enhance communication among healthcare team members, and improve overall quality of care. Research has shown that the implementation of checklists leads to a decrease in adverse events and complications, ultimately resulting in better patient outcomes. Therefore, option C is the correct choice as it aligns with the significant benefits of utilizing checklists in healthcare settings. Options A, B, and D are incorrect as they do not reflect the proven advantages of checklists in patient care.

Question 90: Correct Answer: B) Immediately assess the patient, initiate appropriate interventions, and notify the healthcare provider.

Rationale: In this scenario, the correct response is to prioritize patient care and safety by promptly assessing the unstable patient, initiating necessary interventions such as administering oxygen or medications, and promptly notifying the healthcare provider for further orders or transfer to a higher level of care. Option A is incorrect as the charge nurse should not delegate a critical situation like this. Option C is incorrect as waiting for the primary nurse can delay potentially life-saving interventions. Option D is incorrect as documenting should not take precedence over immediate patient care in an emergency situation.

Question 91: Correct Answer: B) Reflective practice is a structured process that involves looking back on experiences to learn and improve.

Rationale: Reflective practice in nursing involves a structured approach where individuals analyze their experiences, actions, and decisions to gain insights for improvement. Option A is incorrect as reflective practice extends beyond personal goals to encompass professional development. Option C is inaccurate as reflective practice requires active engagement to identify areas for growth. Option D is misleading as reflective practice is an ongoing process that fosters continuous learning and development, contributing significantly to professional growth and enhancing patient care outcomes.

Question 92: Correct Answer: A) Checking the patient's identification band before administering medication.

Rationale: Patient safety is paramount in healthcare settings, and checking the patient's identification band before administering medication is a crucial step to prevent medication errors. Verifying the patient's identity helps ensure that the right medication is given to the right patient, reducing the risk of adverse events. Options B, C, and D are incorrect as they all pose potential risks to patient safety. Skipping hand hygiene with gloves on can lead to the spread of infections, ignoring a patient's call light compromises timely care, and administering medication without checking for allergies can result in severe allergic reactions.

Question 93: Correct Answer: C) Decreased empathy towards patients

Rationale: Burnout can lead to decreased empathy towards patients as nurses experiencing burnout may feel emotionally exhausted, leading to a reduced ability to connect with patients on an emotional level. This can impact the quality of care provided and the overall patient experience. Options A, B, and D are incorrect as burnout typically results in decreased job satisfaction, poorer patient outcomes, and impaired teamwork due to the emotional and physical exhaustion experienced by nurses. It is crucial to address burnout proactively to prevent such negative consequences and maintain a healthy practice environment.

Question 94: Correct Answer: B) Double-checking the patient's allergies before administering a new medication

Rationale: Adhering to patient safety protocols is crucial in preventing medication errors and ensuring patient well-being. Double-checking a patient's allergies before administering a new medication is a fundamental step in medication safety to prevent adverse reactions. Option A is incorrect as administering medication without verifying the patient's identity can lead to serious errors. Option C is incorrect as hand hygiene is essential to prevent the spread of infections. Option D is incorrect as ignoring a patient's call light compromises patient care and safety. Double-checking allergies aligns with patient safety best practices and is a key aspect of patient-centered care.

Question 95: Correct Answer: B) Verifying the patient's identity and surgical site with another nurse

Rationale: Verifying the patient's identity and surgical site with another nurse is a crucial pre-procedural action to prevent wrong-site surgery and ensure patient safety, aligning with pre-procedural unit standards. Administering aspirin for pain relief is contraindicated due to its anticoagulant effects. Allowing the patient to eat a heavy meal the night before surgery increases the risk of aspiration during anesthesia induction. Skipping the pre-operative checklist compromises patient safety and violates unit standards by omitting essential verification steps. Therefore, option B is the correct choice as it adheres to pre-procedural unit standards and prioritizes patient safety.

Question 96: Correct Answer: A) The importance of deep breathing exercises post-surgery

Rationale: The correct answer is A) The importance of deep breathing exercises post-surgery. Pre-operative education plays a crucial role in preparing patients for surgery and promoting positive post-operative outcomes. Deep breathing exercises help prevent complications such as pneumonia, improve lung function, and aid in the recovery process. Option B is incorrect as focusing on the history of surgical procedures is not directly beneficial for Ms. Johnson's immediate care. Option C is irrelevant to Ms. Johnson's pre-operative education. Option D is inappropriate as the nurse's personal experiences should not be shared with the patient as it may not be professional or evidence-based.

Question 97: Correct Answer: B) Encourage her to practice relaxation techniques such as deep breathing exercises.

Rationale: The correct answer is to encourage Ms. Smith to practice relaxation techniques such as deep breathing exercises. This option focuses on non-pharmacological interventions that can help manage her emotional distress effectively. Providing a list of community support groups (Option A) may be beneficial but should not be the initial action. Administering sedative medication (Option C) should only be considered after non-pharmacological interventions have been attempted. Referring her to a mental health professional (Option D) may be necessary if her emotional distress persists or worsens despite initial interventions.

Question 98: Correct Answer: B) A patient who is experiencing chest pain and shortness of breath.

Rationale: Prioritizing care is crucial in the medical-surgical setting to ensure patient safety and optimal outcomes. In this scenario, the patient experiencing chest pain and shortness of breath requires immediate attention as these symptoms could indicate a life-threatening condition such as a myocardial infarction or pulmonary embolism. Addressing this patient's needs promptly aligns with the principle of prioritizing care based on the urgency and severity of the situation. The other options, including a stable patient, a patient requesting hygiene assistance, and a patient awaiting discharge instructions, can be attended to after addressing the emergent situation to ensure comprehensive care delivery.

Question 99: Correct Answer: B) Notify the healthcare provider immediately.

Rationale: In this scenario, the patient is displaying signs and symptoms of a surgical site infection, such as warmth, redness, swelling, purulent drainage, fever, and systemic symptoms like chills. These findings indicate a potential serious complication that requires prompt intervention by the healthcare provider. Administering acetaminophen or applying a warm compress may temporarily alleviate symptoms but will not address the underlying issue. Increasing IV fluids may not be appropriate without further assessment. Therefore, the priority action is to notify the healthcare provider for timely evaluation and management of the surgical site infection.

Question 100: Correct Answer: B) Using written notes or gestures to supplement verbal communication.

Rationale: In this scenario, the most appropriate action for the nurse to facilitate effective communication with Mr. Johnson, who has a hearing impairment, is to use written notes or gestures to supplement verbal communication. Speaking loudly may not be helpful and can be perceived as insensitive. Asking the family to interpret may breach patient confidentiality and autonomy. Limiting communication to essential information only may lead to inadequate patient understanding. Using written notes or gestures enhances communication by providing visual cues to aid comprehension, ensuring effective interaction with the patient.

Question 101: Correct Answer: A) Attend training sessions on how to use the new electronic health record system.

Rationale: Option A is the correct answer as actively participating in training sessions will equip the nurse with the necessary skills to effectively utilize the new electronic health record system, ensuring seamless integration into daily practice. This demonstrates adaptability and willingness to embrace change for the benefit of patient care. Option B is incorrect as ignoring the change can lead to errors in documentation and hinder efficient patient care delivery. Option C is a distractor as providing feedback is essential, but attending training sessions is more immediate and directly supports the team. Option D is incorrect as encouraging resistance to change can create division within the nursing team and impede progress towards improved patient outcomes.

Question 102: Correct Answer: A) Recognize personal biases and work to minimize their impact on patient care.

Rationale: Self-regulation in nursing practice involves acknowledging personal biases and actively working to mitigate their influence on patient care. Option A is correct as it aligns with the core principle of self-awareness and continuous improvement. Options B, C, and D are incorrect as they promote behaviors contrary to self-regulation. Ignoring feedback, relying solely on intuition, and disregarding ethical principles can compromise patient safety and quality of care. Nurses must prioritize self-reflection, critical thinking, and adherence to professional standards to uphold the highest standards of practice.

Question 103: Correct Answer: C) Transportation access

Rationale: Transportation access is the most likely social determinant impacting Mrs. Smith's situation as it directly affects her ability to attend follow-up appointments and access healthcare services. While socioeconomic status (option A) and social support (option D) can also influence health outcomes, in this scenario, the primary concern is Mrs. Smith's transportation barriers. Health literacy (option B) is important but not the primary factor affecting her current situation. By addressing transportation issues, healthcare providers can help improve Mrs. Smith's access to care and overall well-being.

Question 104: Correct Answer: B) Opportunities for interprofessional collaboration

Rationale: Participating in a professional organization offers nurses like Sarah the chance to engage in interprofessional collaboration, which can lead to improved patient outcomes through shared knowledge and expertise. Option A is incorrect as the primary benefit is not related to discounted supplies. Option C is incorrect as increased administrative responsibilities are not a typical benefit of joining a professional organization. Option D is incorrect as mandatory overtime shifts are not a direct benefit of professional organization participation.

Question 105: Correct Answer: B) Comprehensive patient education materials

Rationale: Comprehensive patient education materials play a crucial role in promoting patient-centered care by empowering patients with knowledge about their conditions, treatments, and self-care practices. These resources enhance patient engagement, improve health literacy, and foster shared decision-making between healthcare providers and patients. While advanced medical equipment, increased nurse-to-patient ratio, and updated hospital policies are important in delivering quality care, they do not directly contribute to the patient's active involvement in their care or decision-making process, unlike patient education materials.

Question 106: Correct Answer: C) Seeking assistance from other healthcare team members when needed

Rationale: In this scenario, the nurse facing staffing challenges demonstrates effective resource allocation by seeking assistance from other healthcare team members when needed. This action ensures that all patients, including Mr. Johnson, receive the necessary care despite the staffing shortage. Prioritizing medication administration, delaying mobility assistance, or decreasing communication with the patient would compromise the quality of care provided. By collaborating with other team members, the nurse optimizes resource utilization and maintains a healthy practice environment, reflecting professional nursing concepts.

Question 107: Correct Answer: D) Serum transferrin level of 150 mg/dL

Rationale: Serum transferrin is a more sensitive indicator of protein-energy malnutrition than albumin or prealbumin. In malnutrition, serum transferrin levels decrease due to decreased protein synthesis. BMI alone may not accurately reflect malnutrition as it does not differentiate between muscle mass and fat mass. Albumin level may be influenced by factors other than malnutrition, such as inflammation. Hemoglobin level is more indicative of anemia rather than malnutrition. Therefore, in the context of malnutrition assessment, a low serum transferrin level is a more reliable indicator.

Question 108: Correct Answer: C) Collecting patient data

Rationale: During the assessment phase of the nursing process, the nurse's primary focus is on collecting comprehensive and accurate patient data. This step involves gathering information through various methods such as patient interviews, physical assessments, medical records review, and consultation with other healthcare team members. By collecting relevant data, the nurse can identify the patient's needs, health status, and potential risks, which forms the foundation for the subsequent steps of diagnosis, planning, implementation, and evaluation. Administering medications (Option A) is part of the implementation phase, developing a care plan (Option B) occurs after data collection in the planning phase, and implementing interventions (Option D) follows the planning phase.

Question 109: Correct Answer: B) Conduct a comprehensive medication review and deprescribe unnecessary medications.
Rationale: The correct answer is to conduct a comprehensive medication review and deprescribe unnecessary medications (Option B). Polypharmacy, the concurrent use of multiple medications, can lead to adverse drug reactions, drug interactions, and medication non-adherence, especially in older adults like Mrs. Smith. Deprescribing unnecessary medications can help simplify her regimen, reduce the risk of adverse effects, and improve her overall health outcomes. Options A, C, and D are incorrect as they do not address the root cause of polypharmacy and may potentially worsen Mrs. Smith's condition by either causing abrupt discontinuation of essential medications or adding to the existing medication burden.

Question 110: Correct Answer: C) Using a secure hospital communication system
Rationale: Sharing patient information through a secure hospital communication system is the most appropriate method as it ensures confidentiality and privacy are maintained. Options A, B, and D are incorrect as they all pose significant risks to patient privacy and confidentiality. Sending patient details via unsecured email can lead to unauthorized access, discussing patient information in a crowded hallway can breach confidentiality, and sharing patient information on social media platforms is a clear violation of privacy laws. Therefore, using a secure hospital communication system is the best practice for information sharing among healthcare team members.

Question 111: Correct Answer: C) The nurse is supported through an investigation to understand the root cause of the error.
Rationale: In a "just culture," the focus is on system improvement rather than individual blame. Option C is the correct choice as it aligns with the principles of a just culture by promoting open reporting, learning from errors, and addressing system issues to prevent future occurrences. Options A and D promote blame and punishment, which are contrary to the principles of a just culture. Option B encourages dishonesty and covering up errors, which undermines patient safety and organizational transparency.

Question 112: Correct Answer: B) Desire fuels motivation and drives individuals to work towards common goals.
Rationale: Desire plays a crucial role in the success of healthcare teams. It acts as a powerful motivator, inspiring individuals to strive for excellence and work collaboratively towards achieving shared objectives. Unlike the notion that desire is superficial or leads to conflicts, in reality, a strong desire to excel fosters a positive work environment, enhances teamwork, and promotes effective leadership. Professionalism is essential, but coupled with a genuine desire to make a difference, it propels healthcare professionals to overcome challenges, adapt to change, and deliver high-quality patient care.

Question 113: Correct Answer: A) Administering medications on time
Rationale: Care bundles are a set of evidence-based practices that, when implemented together, have been shown to improve patient outcomes. Administering medications on time is crucial in preventing medication errors and ensuring optimal patient care. The other options, such as allowing longer rest periods for nursing staff, increasing patient visitation hours, and using outdated medical equipment, do not directly contribute to patient safety or care management as effectively as timely medication administration. Patient safety is paramount in medical-surgical settings, and adherence to care bundles, including timely medication administration, plays a vital role in achieving this goal.

Question 114: Correct Answer: C) N95 respirator
Rationale: When caring for a patient on airborne precautions, healthcare workers must wear an N95 respirator to protect themselves from inhaling infectious airborne particles. Options A, B, and D are not sufficient for airborne precautions. A gown and gloves (Option A) are typically used for contact precautions, a surgical mask (Option B) is used for droplet precautions, and a face shield (Option D) may be used in conjunction with other PPE but is not specific to airborne precautions. The N95 respirator creates a seal around the nose and mouth, filtering out at least 95% of airborne particles, making it the correct choice for this scenario.

Question 115: Correct Answer: D) Proper hand hygiene before and after patient contact
Rationale: Proper hand hygiene is a fundamental aspect of standard precautions in infection control to prevent the spread of microorganisms. Options A, B, and C are incorrect as they do not encompass the comprehensive approach required by standard precautions. Wearing gloves only when touching blood or body fluids, using a mask only during aerosol-generating procedures, and disinfecting equipment only if visibly soiled are all limited practices that do not provide adequate protection against the transmission of infections in healthcare settings.

Question 116: Correct Answer: A) Educate Mr. Johnson on the proper disposal of medications.
Rationale: The correct answer is to educate Mr. Johnson on the proper disposal of medications. Flushing medications can lead to environmental contamination and is not a recommended method of disposal. Option B is incorrect as flushing medications is not safe. Option C is incorrect as ignoring the incorrect disposal method goes against the principles of stewardship. Option D is incorrect as throwing medications in the regular trash can also have negative environmental impacts. Proper disposal methods, such as using drug take-back programs or mixing medications with undesirable substances before disposal, should be emphasized to ensure safe drug management and disposal in line with stewardship principles.

Question 117: Correct Answer: A) Stethoscope
Rationale: A stethoscope is a crucial tool for a CMSRN to assess heart, lung, and bowel sounds, making it essential for patient assessment and monitoring in a medical-surgical setting. The stethoscope aids in identifying abnormal sounds, crucial for early detection of health issues. Options B, C, and D (Hairdryer, Blender, Telescope) are not relevant to medical-surgical nursing practice and do not contribute to a healthy practice environment. Therefore, the correct answer is A) Stethoscope, as it directly aligns with the professional concept of utilizing appropriate equipment for patient care and assessment.

Question 118: Correct Answer: A) Lack of insurance coverage for prescribed medications
Rationale: Lack of insurance coverage for prescribed medications can significantly impact patients financially as they may have to bear the full cost of expensive medications out-of-pocket. This can lead to financial strain, non-adherence to prescribed treatment plans, and potential negative health outcomes. Options B, C, and D are not directly related to the financial implications for patients. Availability of generic medication options (Option B) can actually help reduce costs for patients. Regular follow-up appointments (Option C) and participation in clinical trials (Option D) may have other implications but are not directly linked to financial burden on patients.

Question 119: Correct Answer: D) Democratic leadership
Rationale: Democratic leadership style in nursing teamwork and collaboration encourages active participation from all team members in decision-making processes. This approach fosters open communication, mutual respect, and shared responsibility within the team. In contrast, autocratic leadership involves making decisions without consulting the team, which can lead to decreased morale and motivation. Laissez-faire leadership allows team

members to make decisions independently, which may result in lack of direction and coordination. Transformational leadership focuses on inspiring and motivating team members towards a shared vision, but it may not always involve collaborative decision-making as in democratic leadership.

Question 120: Correct Answer: B) Document the observations and report to the appropriate authority

Rationale: When suspecting abuse in a patient, the nurse's primary responsibility is to ensure the safety and well-being of the patient. Documenting the observations and reporting to the appropriate authority, such as the nurse manager or social worker, is crucial in protecting the patient from harm. Ignoring the signs (Option A) can lead to further harm to the patient. Confronting the suspected abuser immediately (Option C) may escalate the situation and jeopardize the patient's safety. Discussing the situation with colleagues but taking no further action (Option D) delays the necessary intervention and protection for the patient. Reporting to the appropriate authority ensures a timely and effective response to address the abuse and safeguard the patient.

Question 121: Correct Answer: C) Staffing that promotes nursing teamwork and collaboration

Rationale: Staffing decisions in medical-surgical settings should prioritize nursing teamwork and collaboration to ensure optimal patient care outcomes. While budgetary considerations are important, staffing decisions solely based on budgets (option A) may compromise patient safety and quality of care. Staffing without considering delegation and supervision needs (option B) can lead to inefficiencies and errors. Similarly, staffing without regard for teamwork dynamics (option D) can result in communication breakdowns and decreased patient satisfaction. Therefore, the correct approach is to prioritize staffing that fosters nursing teamwork and collaboration, enhancing overall patient care delivery.

Question 122: Correct Answer: B) Consulting the latest research studies and guidelines to update the patient's care plan

Rationale: Adhering to evidence-based practice principles involves integrating the best available research evidence with clinical expertise and patient values. In this scenario, option B is the correct choice as it demonstrates the nurse's commitment to staying current with evidence-based guidelines for optimal patient care. Options A, C, and D are incorrect as they do not align with evidence-based practice principles. Option A reflects resistance to change and outdated practices, option C relies on subjective experiences rather than empirical evidence, and option D disregards the importance of evidence-based practice in favor of intuition.

Question 123: Correct Answer: D) High-protein diet to support tissue repair

Rationale: Mrs. Smith, being a post-abdominal surgery patient with diabetes and hypertension, would benefit most from a high-protein diet to support tissue repair and aid in her recovery. Protein is essential for wound healing and tissue regeneration. Option A is incorrect as a high-sodium diet would not be suitable for a patient with hypertension. Option B is incorrect as excessive carbohydrates may negatively impact blood sugar levels in a diabetic patient. Option C is incorrect as a low-fat diet alone may not provide adequate nutrients for post-surgery recovery, especially in a patient with increased protein needs.

Question 124: Correct Answer: B) Engage Mr. Johnson in a conversation about his feelings

Rationale: Engaging Mr. Johnson in a conversation about his feelings is the correct immediate action based on suicide prevention protocols. This approach allows the nurse to assess Mr. Johnson's current mental state, provide emotional support, and potentially prevent any self-harm. Leaving him alone may exacerbate his feelings of isolation and hopelessness. Informing other staff members is important but not the immediate action. Providing a sharp object goes against suicide prevention protocols

and puts the patient at risk. By engaging in a conversation, the nurse can actively listen, assess the situation, and provide appropriate support to address Mr. Johnson's emotional distress.

Question 125: Correct Answer: C) Verify the information with other healthcare providers involved in Mrs. Smith's care.

Rationale: In this scenario, the nurse should verify the information with other healthcare providers involved in Mrs. Smith's care to ensure accurate and comprehensive health history assessment. Option A is incorrect as simply documenting the discrepancies without verification may lead to incomplete information. Option B is inappropriate as confronting the patient may cause distress and hinder trust. Option D is incorrect as reassuring without clarification may compromise patient safety. Verifying information with other healthcare providers ensures a collaborative approach and enhances care coordination, aligning with the principles of interprofessional care.

Question 126: Correct Answer: C) Asking Mr. Smith about his preferences and involving him in the decision-making process.

Rationale: Shared decision-making involves actively involving patients in their care by discussing treatment options, considering patient preferences, and making decisions collaboratively. Option A is incorrect as simply providing information without engaging in a discussion does not promote shared decision-making. Option B is incorrect as it does not involve Mr. Smith in the decision-making process. Option D is incorrect as it goes against the principle of shared decision-making, which emphasizes patient autonomy and involvement in decision-making. Option C is the correct answer as it demonstrates the nurse's effort to engage Mr. Smith in the decision-making process, respecting his preferences and promoting shared decision-making.

Question 127: Correct Answer: D) "On a scale of 1 to 10, how would you rate your overall experience at the hospital?"

Rationale: Option D is the most appropriate question for gathering specific feedback on Ms. Johnson's overall experience during her hospital stay. This type of question allows for a quantitative assessment of satisfaction, providing a clear and measurable indicator of the patient's perception. Options A, B, and C are more general in nature and may not capture the nuanced details of Ms. Johnson's experience. Option A focuses on staff friendliness, B on likelihood of recommendation, and C on room cleanliness, which are important but do not provide a comprehensive view of the overall patient experience.

Question 128: Correct Answer: C) Report the incident to the charge nurse or nurse manager.

Rationale: In this scenario, the correct course of action for the CMSRN is to report the medication error incident to the charge nurse or nurse manager. This action aligns with professional reporting and resources, scope of practice and ethics, and professional concepts. Reporting errors is crucial for patient safety and quality care delivery. Option A is incorrect as ignoring the conversation would not address the issue of patient safety. Option B is inappropriate as confronting the colleague publicly may not be professional or effective. Option D is incorrect as advising to keep the error confidential goes against ethical principles of transparency and accountability in healthcare practice.

Question 129: Correct Answer: B) Document the findings and report to the appropriate authorities.

Rationale: When abuse is suspected in a patient, the most crucial step is to document the findings accurately and report them to the appropriate authorities, such as the hospital's patient safety team or social services. Ignoring the signs (Option A) can lead to serious consequences for the patient. Confronting the suspected abuser in front of the patient (Option C) can escalate the situation and compromise the patient's safety. Discussing suspicions with colleagues for gossip and validation (Option D) violates patient confidentiality and does not address the issue effectively. Reporting to the appropriate authorities ensures that the patient's safety is prioritized and that necessary interventions are implemented promptly.

Question 130: Correct Answer: B) Respect Mr. Johnson's request and arrange for him to meet with the surgeon to address his concerns.

Rationale: Upholding patients' rights and responsibilities includes respecting their autonomy and ensuring informed consent. In this scenario, it is crucial to honor Mr. Johnson's request to speak with the surgeon as part of the informed consent process. Option A is incorrect as patient autonomy should be respected. Option C is incorrect as obtaining consent from a family member without addressing the patient's concerns directly violates the patient's rights. Option D is incorrect as providing information and obtaining consent should be done after addressing the patient's concerns, not rushed.

Question 131: Correct Answer: B) Listen actively, acknowledge his feelings, and offer clear, simple explanations.

Rationale: Option B is the correct answer as effective communication in healthcare involves active listening, acknowledging the patient's emotions, and providing clear, simple explanations to address their concerns. This approach helps build trust, reduce anxiety, and ensure the patient feels informed and supported. Options A, C, and D are incorrect as they neglect the patient's emotional state, fail to provide appropriate information, and may lead to increased distress and misunderstanding. Effective communication is essential in nursing practice to promote patient-centered care and positive outcomes.

Question 132: Correct Answer: B) Encouraging Mrs. Thompson to engage in spiritual practices that are meaningful to her.

Rationale: In the hospice setting, holistic care is essential to address the physical, emotional, social, and spiritual needs of the patient. Encouraging Mrs. Thompson to engage in spiritual practices that are meaningful to her promotes holistic well-being. Option A is important but focuses only on the physical aspect of care. Option C is incorrect as family support is crucial in hospice care. Option D is incorrect as holistic care involves addressing all aspects of the patient's well-being, not just physical symptoms.

Question 133: Correct Answer: B) Notifying the healthcare provider about the patient's condition.

Rationale: In this scenario, the correct action to prioritize patient safety is to notify the healthcare provider about the patient's condition. Shortness of breath, tachycardia, and low oxygen saturation are concerning signs that may indicate a pulmonary embolism, a life-threatening condition. Prompt communication with the healthcare provider is crucial to ensure timely evaluation and appropriate management. Administering pain medication (Option A) may mask symptoms and delay necessary interventions. Documenting vital signs (Option C) is important but not as urgent as notifying the healthcare provider. Encouraging deep breathing and coughing (Option D) may worsen the patient's condition if a pulmonary embolism is present.

Question 134: Correct Answer: B) Immediately inform the healthcare team and provide a detailed handover report.

Rationale: Effective communication is crucial in ensuring patient safety and continuity of care. Option B is the correct choice as it aligns with professional standards of information sharing in a timely manner to the healthcare team, allowing for prompt intervention and appropriate care planning. Options A, C, and D are incorrect as they either delay crucial communication, ignore the responsibility of the nurse, or breach patient confidentiality by discussing sensitive information with unauthorized individuals.

Question 135: Correct Answer: D) Use professional interpreters to ensure accurate communication.

Rationale: It is crucial to use professional interpreters when caring for patients with limited English proficiency to ensure accurate communication and understanding of medical information. Using complex medical terminology may lead to misunderstandings. Avoiding professional interpreters compromises patient confidentiality. While utilizing family members as interpreters may seem convenient, it can result in misinterpretation of information, breaches in confidentiality, and potential conflicts of interest. Therefore, the best practice is to use trained interpreters to provide safe, effective, and patient-centered care.

Question 136: Correct Answer: B) Assisting the surgeon during procedures

Rationale: As a Certified Medical Surgical Registered Nurse (CMSRN), the primary role related to procedures within the scope of practice is to assist the surgeon during various surgical and procedural interventions. This involves tasks such as preparing the patient, ensuring the sterile field, passing instruments, and providing support to the surgical team. While CMSRNs play a crucial role in the perioperative care of patients, they do not perform surgical procedures independently (Option A), administer anesthesia (Option C), or interpret radiological images (Option D) during procedures. The focus is on collaborative patient care and assisting in the smooth execution of procedures under the guidance of the surgical team.

Question 137: Correct Answer: C) Incident Commander

Rationale: The correct answer is C) Incident Commander. The Incident Commander plays a crucial role in managing the overall incident response within the hospital incident command structure. This individual is responsible for making strategic decisions, coordinating resources, and ensuring effective communication among all involved parties during an emergency or disaster situation. The Chief Nursing Officer (A) focuses on nursing leadership, the Charge Nurse on duty (B) oversees daily nursing operations, and the Head of Security (D) is responsible for security-related matters, but none of these roles hold the primary responsibility for managing the overall incident response and coordination as the Incident Commander does.

Question 138: Correct Answer: B) Hearing impairment

Rationale: Hearing impairment is a prevalent communication barrier in patients with physical and cognitive limitations. Patients with hearing impairments may struggle to understand verbal instructions or conversations, leading to potential misunderstandings in a healthcare setting. While language differences (option A) and cultural differences (option D) can also pose communication challenges, they are not directly related to physical or cognitive limitations. Visual impairment (option C) can hinder communication but is distinct from the auditory challenges faced by individuals with hearing impairments. Therefore, the correct answer is B) Hearing impairment, as it directly impacts effective communication in patients with physical and cognitive limitations.

Question 139: Correct Answer: B) Sharing patient information through secure electronic platforms

Rationale: Effective interdisciplinary collaboration integration involves seamless communication and sharing of patient information among healthcare professionals from different disciplines. Option B, sharing patient information through secure electronic platforms, facilitates real-time updates, enhances coordination, and ensures all team members are informed about the patient's care plan. In contrast, options A, C, and D hinder effective collaboration by either isolating disciplines, limiting communication channels, or avoiding interaction altogether, which can lead to fragmented care and compromised patient outcomes.

Question 140: Correct Answer: A) Blame-free reporting

Rationale: In the scenario described, the principle of blame-free reporting is demonstrated. This principle of "just culture" encourages open and honest reporting of errors without fear of retribution. The nurse admitting the oversight without facing punitive measures reflects a culture that prioritizes learning from mistakes rather than assigning blame. Options B, C, and D are incorrect as they involve punitive measures, retribution, and non-learning approaches, which are contrary to the concept of "just culture" that focuses on system improvement and error prevention through open communication and shared accountability.

Question 141: Correct Answer: A) Administering potassium supplements orally

Rationale: In the scenario provided, the nurse should prioritize administering potassium supplements orally to address the hypokalemia in the patient with heart failure receiving diuretics. Hypokalemia is a common electrolyte imbalance associated with diuretic therapy, and potassium supplementation is essential to prevent complications such as cardiac dysrhythmias. Monitoring serum magnesium levels (Option B) is important but not the priority in this case. Increasing the rate of intravenous diuretics (Option C) can exacerbate electrolyte imbalances. Encouraging a high-sodium diet (Option D) is contraindicated in heart failure management due to its association with fluid retention and worsening of the condition.

Question 142: Correct Answer: A) Provide Mrs. Smith with a detailed list of community resources for post-discharge support.

Rationale: Option A is the correct answer as providing Mrs. Smith with a detailed list of community resources for post-discharge support is essential for ensuring a smooth transition and continuity of care. This action helps Mrs. Smith access necessary services such as home health care, physical therapy, or support groups, promoting her recovery and well-being post-discharge. Options B, C, and D are incorrect as scheduling a follow-up appointment, discontinuing medications abruptly, and resuming normal activities without proper guidance can lead to gaps in care, medication errors, and potential complications, respectively. It is crucial for CMSRNs to facilitate a comprehensive discharge plan to optimize patient outcomes and prevent readmissions.

Question 143: Correct Answer: B) To focus on providing comfort and quality of life

Rationale: Hospice care aims to enhance the quality of life for patients with terminal illnesses by focusing on symptom management, pain relief, emotional support, and spiritual care rather than aggressive treatments aimed at curing the illness. This approach emphasizes comfort and dignity for the patient during their end-of-life journey. Options A, C, and D are incorrect as they do not align with the philosophy of hospice care, which prioritizes holistic patient-centered support rather than curative interventions or transfers to other facilities.

Question 144: Correct Answer: B) Centers for Medicare & Medicaid Services (CMS)

Rationale: The correct answer is B) Centers for Medicare & Medicaid Services (CMS). CMS is a federal agency within the U.S. Department of Health and Human Services that administers the Medicare program and works in partnership with state governments to administer Medicaid. CMS sets and enforces regulations for healthcare facilities participating in these programs to ensure compliance with quality and safety standards. Options A, C, and D are incorrect as they do not have the primary responsibility for overseeing compliance standards in healthcare facilities. The ANA focuses on nursing practice standards, OSHA on workplace safety, and NCSBN on nursing licensure.

Question 145: Correct Answer: C) Questionnaires given to patients to gather feedback on their healthcare experience

Rationale: Patient Satisfaction Surveys are tools used to collect feedback directly from patients regarding their healthcare experience. These surveys help healthcare facilities assess the quality of care provided, identify areas for improvement, and enhance patient-centered care. Option A is incorrect as the surveys are typically completed by patients themselves. Option B is incorrect as these surveys are not for healthcare providers to assess themselves. Option D is incorrect as Patient Satisfaction Surveys focus on patient experience, not hospital efficiency.

Question 146: Correct Answer: B) Inform the charge nurse about the missed documentation and medication

Rationale: It is crucial for the CMSRN to prioritize patient safety and advocate for the best interest of the patient. In this scenario, the correct course of action is to inform the charge nurse about the missed documentation and medication to ensure that appropriate measures are taken to address the situation promptly. Option A may not address the root cause of the issue and could potentially lead to errors. Option C is not in line with professional accountability and patient safety. Option D could embarrass the colleague and is not the most professional approach to resolving the issue.

Question 147: Correct Answer: B) Encouraging deep breathing exercises and relaxation techniques

Rationale: Non-pharmacological interventions play a crucial role in managing anxiety and restlessness in patients. Option B is the correct choice as deep breathing exercises and relaxation techniques are effective in promoting relaxation, reducing anxiety, and improving overall well-being without the use of medications. Options A and C involve pharmacological interventions, which are not the first-line approach for managing anxiety in this scenario. Option D, while supportive, may not directly address Mr. Johnson's symptoms of anxiety and restlessness. Therefore, option B is the most appropriate non-pharmacological intervention for Mr. Johnson.

Question 148: Correct Answer: C) Communicating relevant facts and data

Rationale: Background information sharing is crucial for effective communication and collaboration among healthcare teams. By choosing option C, which emphasizes communicating relevant facts and data, the CMSRN ensures that all team members are well-informed and can make informed decisions regarding patient care. Options A, B, and D are incorrect as they promote behaviors that can hinder teamwork, compromise patient safety, and lead to misunderstandings. Effective background information sharing involves transparent communication of pertinent details to facilitate optimal patient outcomes and professional collaboration.

Question 149: Correct Answer: A) Implement a recognition program to acknowledge Sarah's hard work and dedication.

Rationale: Option A is the correct answer as implementing a recognition program can help boost Sarah's morale, show appreciation for her efforts, and make her feel valued within the team. This strategy can improve retention by enhancing job satisfaction and motivation. Option B is incorrect as increasing Sarah's workload without support can lead to burnout and further dissatisfaction. Option C is incorrect as ignoring Sarah's concerns can result in her leaving the job, impacting retention negatively. Option D is incorrect as forcing more night shifts on Sarah without considering her well-being can worsen her situation and lead to further disengagement.

Question 150: Correct Answer: B) Maintaining eye contact

Rationale: Maintaining eye contact is a crucial non-verbal communication cue that signifies attentiveness, empathy, and active listening during patient interactions. It helps establish trust and rapport between the nurse and the patient, enhancing the quality of care provided. In contrast, options A, C, and D can convey negative messages or lack of interest. Crossing arms may indicate defensiveness or closed-off attitude, turning away suggests disinterest, and frowning can be perceived as judgmental or unfriendly. Therefore, among the options provided, maintaining eye contact is the most appropriate and effective non-verbal communication cue for a CMSRN.

CMSRN Exam Practice Questions [SET 3]

Question 1: Which of the following is a common symptom of compassion fatigue among medical surgical registered nurses?
A) Increased empathy towards patients
B) Decreased job satisfaction
C) Enhanced sense of personal accomplishment
D) Improved work-life balance

Question 2: Ms. Johnson, a 65-year-old patient, is being discharged from the hospital after undergoing a surgical procedure. As the Certified Medical Surgical Registered Nurse (CMSRN) responsible for her care coordination and transition, which action is most crucial to ensure a smooth transition and continuity of care for Ms. Johnson?
A) Providing her with a list of community resources for post-operative care
B) Ensuring she has a follow-up appointment scheduled with her primary care physician
C) Giving her a detailed explanation of her medications and their side effects
D) Recommending a new diet plan for her recovery period

Question 3: Which of the following is a pertinent potential complication in surgical patients that requires immediate intervention by the Certified Medical Surgical Registered Nurse (CMSRN)?
A) Postoperative nausea and vomiting
B) Delayed wound healing
C) Urinary tract infection
D) Pulmonary embolism

Question 4: In the context of ethics for Certified Medical Surgical Registered Nurses (CMSRNs), which action best demonstrates professional integrity?
A) Falsifying patient records to cover up a mistake
B) Reporting a colleague for unethical behavior
C) Ignoring a patient's request for pain medication
D) Sharing confidential patient information with friends

Question 5: Scenario: As a medical-surgical nurse, you are caring for a patient who has been recently diagnosed with a terminal illness. The patient expresses a desire to discontinue treatment and requests to be kept comfortable until the end. The patient's family, however, insists on aggressive treatment despite the patient's wishes. What action should the nurse take based on the Code of Ethics for Nurses with Interpretive Statements?
A) Respect the patient's autonomy and advocate for the patient's wishes.
B) Follow the family's wishes as they are legally responsible for the patient.
C) Proceed with aggressive treatment to satisfy the family's demands.
D) Seek guidance from the healthcare provider without involving the patient or family.

Question 6: Scenario: Mr. Johnson, a 65-year-old patient admitted for a surgical procedure, is prescribed multiple medications. The nurse is preparing to administer medications to Mr. Johnson. Which action by the nurse demonstrates safe medication administration practice?
A) Crushing a sustained-release tablet for easier swallowing
B) Administering medications without checking the patient's identification

C) Using an electronic medication administration record (eMAR) to document medication administration
D) Combining all medications into one cup for simultaneous administration

Question 7: Scenario: Ms. Smith, a postoperative patient, requires frequent wound dressing changes due to a surgical site infection. The nurse is considering the most cost-effective approach to managing Ms. Smith's wound care while maintaining quality standards. Which action by the nurse demonstrates fiscal efficiency in this situation?
A) Using sterile gloves for each dressing change
B) Changing the wound dressing more frequently than ordered
C) Applying a new dressing without assessing the wound site
D) Utilizing a transparent dressing to allow for visual wound assessment

Question 8: Scenario: Ms. Johnson, a 65-year-old postoperative patient, is admitted to the medical-surgical unit following a total knee replacement surgery. The nurse is preparing to implement a checklist to ensure all necessary care bundles are completed for Ms. Johnson's postoperative care. Which item is most likely to be included in the checklist for Ms. Johnson's care bundles?
A) Administering pain medication every 6 hours
B) Encouraging early ambulation and deep breathing exercises
C) Providing a daily back massage for pain relief
D) Applying heat packs to the surgical site every hour

Question 9: Which of the following is an example of a standard precaution for infection control in a healthcare setting?
A) Wearing gloves only when directly handling bodily fluids
B) Using a mask only when performing aerosol-generating procedures
C) Proper hand hygiene before and after patient contact
D) Wearing a gown only during surgical procedures

Question 10: Scenario: Mr. Smith, a 65-year-old patient, is admitted to the medical-surgical unit for post-operative care following a hip replacement surgery. During morning rounds, the nurse notices that Mr. Smith appears agitated and frustrated. When asked about his discomfort, Mr. Smith expresses dissatisfaction with the level of pain relief provided by the current medication regimen. He feels that his pain is not adequately managed and demands stronger pain medication immediately. Which of the following responses by the nurse demonstrates effective conflict resolution skills in this situation?
A) Explaining to Mr. Smith that he must follow the prescribed pain medication regimen as ordered by the physician.
B) Acknowledging Mr. Smith's concerns, assessing his pain level thoroughly, and discussing alternative pain management options with the healthcare team.
C) Dismissing Mr. Smith's complaints as common post-operative discomfort and reassuring him that his pain will improve with time.
D) Ignoring Mr. Smith's requests for stronger pain medication and informing him that no changes can be made to his current treatment plan.

Question 11: In Root Cause Analysis (RCA), which step involves identifying contributing factors that led to the

adverse event?
A) Implementing corrective actions
B) Reporting the adverse event to the supervisor
C) Analyzing the immediate cause of the event
D) Identifying contributing factors

Question 12: In the context of licensed and unlicensed team members, which statement regarding delegation is accurate?
A) Unlicensed assistive personnel (UAP) can perform tasks that require nursing judgment.
B) Licensed practical nurses (LPN) can delegate tasks to registered nurses (RN).
C) Registered nurses (RN) can delegate tasks that are within the scope of practice of the UAP.
D) Delegation relieves the delegating nurse of accountability for the task.

Question 13: Which of the following is an essential component of current evidence-based practice for infection control and prevention procedures in the context of Patient/Care Management?
A) Routine use of antibiotics for all patients
B) Proper hand hygiene practices
C) Reusing disposable gloves after disinfection
D) Ignoring isolation precautions for infectious patients

Question 14: A nurse is working in a local hospital and encounters a situation where a patient's family member requests confidential information about the patient's condition. What action should the nurse take based on the scope of practice and code of ethics for nurses per local and regional nursing bodies?
A) Provide the family member with the requested information to maintain transparency.
B) Politely decline to share the information and explain the importance of patient confidentiality.
C) Ask the family member to sign a waiver before disclosing any information.
D) Direct the family member to the hospital administration for information.

Question 15: Scenario: During a busy shift on the medical-surgical unit, a conflict arises between two nurses regarding the delegation of tasks for a patient named Mr. Smith, who requires urgent care. Nurse A believes that Nurse B is not prioritizing Mr. Smith's needs appropriately, while Nurse B feels overwhelmed with multiple tasks at hand. Nurse A confronts Nurse B in front of other team members, leading to a tense situation. Which action by the charge nurse demonstrates effective conflict management in this scenario?
A) The charge nurse takes Nurse A and Nurse B aside separately to discuss the issue privately.
B) The charge nurse publicly reprimands Nurse A for confronting Nurse B in front of others.
C) The charge nurse ignores the conflict and allows Nurse A and Nurse B to resolve it on their own.
D) The charge nurse immediately assigns Mr. Smith's care to another nurse to avoid further conflict.

Question 16: Scenario: Mr. Johnson, a 65-year-old male patient, is admitted to the medical-surgical unit with a history of hypertension, diabetes, and obesity. He is scheduled for a cholecystectomy due to symptomatic gallstones. During the preoperative assessment, the nurse identifies several risk factors that may impact Mr. Johnson's surgical outcome. Which of the following risk factors is most likely to increase the postoperative complications for Mr. Johnson?
A) Controlled diabetes

B) Hypertension managed with medication
C) Obesity with a BMI of 32
D) Regular exercise routine

Question 17: In the context of 'Service recovery' within Quality Management and Professional Concepts, which action is NOT recommended when addressing a patient's complaint?
A) Acknowledge the issue and apologize sincerely
B) Blame the patient for the misunderstanding
C) Listen actively to the patient's concerns
D) Offer a solution or compensation to rectify the situation

Question 18: Which of the following is a characteristic of enteral nutrition administration?
A) It involves delivering nutrients directly into the bloodstream.
B) It bypasses the gastrointestinal tract.
C) It is suitable for patients with functional gastrointestinal systems.
D) It is primarily used for short-term nutritional support.

Question 19: During hourly rounding, the nurse finds a patient complaining of pain. What is the most appropriate action for the nurse to take?
A) Document the complaint and inform the next shift nurse.
B) Administer pain medication immediately without further assessment.
C) Assess the patient's pain using a pain scale, notify the healthcare provider if necessary, and provide comfort measures.
D) Ignore the complaint as it is common for patients to experience pain in the hospital setting.

Question 20: In the context of 'Care Coordination and Transition Management' within the 'Elements of Interprofessional Care,' which action is a key component of effective care coordination for a patient being discharged from the hospital?
A) Providing the patient with a list of medications without explanation
B) Scheduling a follow-up appointment with a primary care provider within a month
C) Discharging the patient without informing the primary care provider
D) Advising the patient to manage their post-discharge care on their own

Question 21: Scenario: Mr. Johnson, a 65-year-old patient admitted for post-operative care following a hip replacement surgery, is experiencing shortness of breath and chest pain. At the same time, another patient, Mrs. Smith, requires assistance with ambulation to prevent falls. The nursing team is short-staffed, and you are the charge nurse on duty. Which task should the Certified Medical Surgical Registered Nurse prioritize in this situation?
A) Assisting Mr. Johnson with shortness of breath and chest pain
B) Assisting Mrs. Smith with ambulation to prevent falls
C) Delegating the tasks to the available nursing staff
D) Notifying the physician about Mr. Johnson's condition

Question 22: In the context of nursing teamwork and collaboration, which statement best describes the role of a mentor in career development relationships?
A) A mentor provides direct patient care alongside the mentee.
B) A mentor offers guidance, support, and advice to help the mentee grow professionally.
C) A mentor focuses solely on their own career advancement without assisting others.
D) A mentor competes with the mentee for career opportunities within the healthcare facility.

Question 23: Which of the following is a crucial aspect of discharge procedures for patients in the context of Care Coordination and Transition Management?
A) Providing detailed medication reconciliation
B) Ensuring the patient has a comfortable room temperature
C) Offering a variety of magazines for patient entertainment
D) Scheduling a follow-up appointment for the healthcare provider

Question 24: Which of the following is the most effective method for preventing healthcare-associated infections in a medical-surgical unit?
A) Wearing gloves only when performing invasive procedures
B) Using alcohol-based hand sanitizer before and after patient contact
C) Reusing disposable isolation gowns if not visibly soiled
D) Placing used needles in a puncture-resistant container immediately after use

Question 25: In Failure Mode and Effects Analysis (FMEA), which step involves assigning a numerical value to the frequency of occurrence, likelihood of detection, and severity of the potential failure mode?
A) Step 1: Define the scope and boundaries of the analysis
B) Step 2: Identify potential failure modes
C) Step 3: Assign a numerical value to occurrence, detection, and severity
D) Step 4: Calculate the Risk Priority Number (RPN)

Question 26: In the context of a medical-surgical setting, which inference can be drawn from a patient's sudden increase in blood pressure and heart rate during a routine check-up?
A) The patient may be experiencing anxiety.
B) The patient's blood pressure and heart rate are normal.
C) The patient is dehydrated.
D) The patient is not following the prescribed medication regimen.

Question 27: Scenario: Sarah, a CMSRN, is leading a nursing team in a busy medical-surgical unit. She believes in fostering a culture of open communication, mutual respect, and shared decision-making among the team members. One day, a new nurse, Emily, expresses concerns about a patient's deteriorating condition. Sarah listens attentively, acknowledges Emily's observations, and collaborates with her to develop a plan of action. Which nursing philosophy principle is Sarah demonstrating in this scenario?
A) Autonomy
B) Paternalism
C) Advocacy
D) Collaborative Leadership

Question 28: Scenario: Mr. Patel, a 65-year-old male patient of Indian descent, is admitted to the medical-surgical unit with a diagnosis of pneumonia. As a CMSRN providing care to Mr. Patel, which action best demonstrates holistic patient care in terms of diversity and inclusion?
A) Providing culturally sensitive care by respecting Mr. Patel's dietary preferences and religious practices.
B) Assigning a nurse of the same ethnicity as Mr. Patel to care for him exclusively.
C) Ignoring Mr. Patel's cultural background and focusing solely on his medical needs.
D) Restricting communication with Mr. Patel to only essential medical information.

Question 29: Scenario: Mr. Johnson, a 65-year-old patient recovering from abdominal surgery, is on strict bed rest. The nurse is preparing to assist him with ambulation using a walker. Which equipment is essential for the nurse to ensure patient safety during this activity?
A) Wheelchair
B) Crutches
C) Cane
D) Walker

Question 30: When considering budgetary considerations in medical-surgical nursing, which supply management approach helps in controlling costs while ensuring adequate resources for patient care?
A) Just-in-time inventory system
B) Stockpiling supplies in excess
C) Ordering supplies in bulk without assessing usage
D) Using disposable supplies for single patient encounters

Question 31: Which of the following is an essential component of active listening in the context of communication skills for a Certified Medical Surgical Registered Nurse (CMSRN)?
A) Interrupting the speaker to provide immediate solutions
B) Demonstrating empathy and understanding
C) Focusing on formulating your response while the speaker is talking
D) Avoiding eye contact to reduce distractions

Question 32: Scenario: Ms. Johnson, a 55-year-old patient, has recently undergone a surgical procedure. The healthcare team has implemented a new change management strategy focusing on reinforcing the importance of the ADKAR model (Awareness, Desire, Knowledge, Ability, Reinforcement) to aid in her recovery process. Ms. Johnson seems hesitant to engage in the new approach and expresses doubts about its effectiveness. Which of the following actions by the nurse best demonstrates the 'Reinforcement' stage of the ADKAR model in this scenario?
A) Providing Ms. Johnson with educational materials on the benefits of the new strategy.
B) Encouraging Ms. Johnson to attend a support group session to discuss the change.
C) Regularly checking in with Ms. Johnson to review her progress and offer positive feedback.
D) Explaining to Ms. Johnson the step-by-step process of the new change management strategy.

Question 33: Scenario: Mr. Smith, a 65-year-old patient, is admitted to the medical-surgical unit with severe malnutrition and an inability to tolerate oral intake due to a recent surgery. The healthcare team decides to initiate parenteral nutrition to meet his nutritional needs. As the CMSRN, you are responsible for monitoring Mr. Smith's parenteral nutrition therapy closely. Which of the following statements regarding parenteral nutrition is accurate?
A) Parenteral nutrition is always administered through the gastrointestinal tract.
B) Parenteral nutrition is the preferred route for nutrition administration in patients with intact gastrointestinal function.
C) Parenteral nutrition bypasses the gastrointestinal tract and delivers nutrients directly into the bloodstream.
D) Parenteral nutrition is primarily used for patients who can tolerate oral intake adequately.

Question 34: Which of the following statements regarding suicide risk assessment in medical-surgical patients is accurate?
A) Patients with a history of suicide attempts are not at increased risk for future attempts.
B) Patients who express suicidal thoughts should not be taken seriously unless they have a specific plan.

C) Patients with a diagnosis of depression are not at risk for suicide.
D) Patients with access to lethal means are at higher risk for suicide.

Question 35: Scenario: Mrs. Smith, a 68-year-old patient with a history of heart failure and diabetes, was recently discharged from the hospital after a congestive heart failure exacerbation. She lives alone and has limited family support. Mrs. Smith has difficulty affording her medications and struggles to follow a low-sodium diet. She has been readmitted to the hospital multiple times in the past year due to medication non-compliance and poor disease management. As a CMSRN, which intervention is most crucial to prevent readmissions for Mrs. Smith?
A) Providing Mrs. Smith with a detailed list of community resources for medication assistance.
B) Educating Mrs. Smith on the importance of a low-sodium diet and providing easy-to-follow meal plans.
C) Scheduling a follow-up appointment with a social worker to address Mrs. Smith's financial concerns.
D) Arranging for a home health nurse to visit Mrs. Smith regularly to monitor her condition and medication adherence.

Question 36: Scenario: Mrs. Smith, a 65-year-old patient, is admitted to the medical-surgical unit with a diagnosis of postoperative pain following a total knee replacement surgery. She expresses her concerns about managing her pain effectively during her recovery period. Which statement by Mrs. Smith indicates a realistic expectation regarding pain management?
A) "I expect to have no pain at all after taking pain medication."
B) "I understand that complete pain relief may not always be possible, but I hope to have manageable pain."
C) "I demand immediate relief from pain as soon as I request medication."
D) "I believe that pain is a normal part of the recovery process, and I should endure it without any medication."

Question 37: Scenario: During the night shift, Nurse Sarah is preparing medication for her patient, Mr. Johnson, who is admitted for post-operative care following a knee replacement surgery. While checking the medication, she notices that the dosage of the pain medication prescribed seems unusually high for Mr. Johnson's weight and medical history. Nurse Sarah recalls the hospital's policy on near miss reporting and realizes this situation falls under that category. Which action should Nurse Sarah take next in this scenario?
A) Administer the medication as prescribed to avoid any delays in pain management for the patient.
B) Consult with the charge nurse or pharmacist to verify the medication dosage before administering it.
C) Disregard her concerns and administer the medication as per the doctor's orders.
D) Document the incident in the patient's chart without reporting it as a near miss.

Question 38: Scenario: Mr. Johnson, a 58-year-old patient, is admitted to the medical-surgical unit following a lumbar laminectomy. He has an epidural catheter in place for postoperative pain management. The nurse notes that the epidural infusion is not providing adequate pain relief, and Mr. Johnson is experiencing increased discomfort. On assessment, the nurse observes that the catheter is intact and properly secured. Mr. Johnson is alert and oriented, with stable vital signs. What is the nurse's priority action in this situation?
A) Check the infusion pump settings and ensure proper medication

delivery.
B) Reposition the patient to see if pain relief improves.
C) Administer an oral pain medication as a supplement to the epidural infusion.
D) Notify the healthcare provider for further orders.

Question 39: Which of the following actions by a nurse best demonstrates adherence to patient safety protocols in a medical-surgical setting?
A) Administering medication without checking the patient's identification band
B) Double-checking the patient's identification before administering medication
C) Skipping hand hygiene before and after patient contact
D) Disregarding the expiration date of medical supplies during patient care

Question 40: Scenario: Ms. Smith, a postoperative patient, requires frequent wound dressing changes due to a surgical site infection. The nurse is considering using a specific type of advanced wound dressing that is more expensive but promotes faster healing. The nurse is aware of the budgetary constraints on the unit. What action should the nurse take regarding the wound dressing choice for Ms. Smith?
A) Use the advanced wound dressing without considering the cost implications.
B) Consult with the healthcare team to discuss the cost-effectiveness of the advanced wound dressing.
C) Opt for a traditional wound dressing to stay within budget limits.
D) Use the advanced wound dressing regardless of the cost, as patient outcomes are the priority.

Question 41: Ms. Patel, a 65-year-old female patient from India, is admitted to the medical-surgical unit for post-operative care following a gastrointestinal surgery. She speaks limited English and prefers to communicate in her native language, Gujarati. During the assessment, the nurse notices that Ms. Patel is experiencing dry mouth and difficulty speaking. Which intervention is most appropriate to address Ms. Patel's oral care needs while considering cultural and linguistic preferences?
A) Provide a pamphlet on oral care written in English.
B) Offer Ms. Patel a mint-flavored mouthwash.
C) Consult with an interpreter to explain oral care instructions in Gujarati.
D) Demonstrate proper oral care techniques without verbal instructions.

Question 42: Scenario: Mr. Smith, a 68-year-old male patient with a history of terminal cancer, was under palliative care at a hospice facility. He passed away peacefully in his sleep during the night. The nurse on duty discovered him in the morning and confirmed his death. The coroner was called to the facility to examine the body. As a CMSRN, what is the appropriate action regarding reporting Mr. Smith's death?
A) Notify the coroner immediately upon discovering the patient's death.
B) Wait for the family to arrive before contacting the coroner.
C) Contact the hospice physician first and then inform the coroner.
D) Follow facility protocol for reporting deaths to the coroner.

Question 43: Scenario: Mrs. Rodriguez, a 65-year-old Hispanic female, is admitted to the medical-surgical unit with complaints of severe abdominal pain. She speaks limited English and appears to be struggling to communicate her symptoms to the healthcare team. As a CMSRN, what is the most appropriate action to take in this situation?
A) Use basic English words and gestures to try to understand her

symptoms.

B) Ask the patient's family members who are present to interpret for her.

C) Utilize a professional medical interpreter to facilitate communication.

D) Proceed with the assessment without addressing the language barrier.

Question 44: Scenario: Mrs. Smith, a 65-year-old postoperative patient recovering from abdominal surgery, expresses interest in using aromatherapy for pain management. She asks the nurse about the potential benefits of lavender essential oil. Which statement by the nurse is most appropriate regarding the use of lavender essential oil in aromatherapy for pain relief?

A) Lavender essential oil is contraindicated for postoperative pain management.

B) Lavender essential oil may help reduce postoperative pain and promote relaxation.

C) Lavender essential oil should be applied directly to the surgical incision site.

D) Lavender essential oil is only effective when ingested orally.

Question 45: A patient is scheduled for a surgical procedure and is receiving preoperative teaching. Which statement by the patient indicates a need for further education regarding postoperative care?

A) "I will use the incentive spirometer every hour to help with my breathing."

B) "I will keep the surgical site dry and clean to prevent infection."

C) "I will apply heat to the surgical incision to promote healing."

D) "I will report any signs of infection, such as increased redness or drainage, to my healthcare provider."

Question 46: Which of the following is a key component of patient safety assessments and reporting in the context of Patient Safety and Patient/Care Management?

A) Ensuring timely administration of medications

B) Proper documentation of patient care interventions

C) Minimizing patient interaction with healthcare team

D) Disregarding patient concerns and complaints

Question 47: In a healthcare setting, which action best demonstrates sensitivity to cultural and linguistic needs?

A) Providing written instructions only

B) Using a professional medical interpreter when needed

C) Ignoring the patient's cultural background

D) Speaking loudly to ensure understanding

Question 48: In the context of 'Professional Concepts,' which statement best describes critical thinking for a Certified Medical Surgical Registered Nurse (CMSRN)?

A) Critical thinking involves making quick decisions without considering all available information.

B) Critical thinking is a linear process that does not require reflection or evaluation.

C) Critical thinking includes analyzing information objectively and making informed decisions.

D) Critical thinking relies solely on intuition and personal beliefs.

Question 49: During bedside report, the nurse should:

A) Discuss patient's personal information with other healthcare staff.

B) Ensure patient privacy and confidentiality are maintained.

C) Skip medication reconciliation to save time.

D) Use medical jargon that the patient may not understand.

Question 50: Scenario: Mrs. Smith, a 65-year-old patient, is

being discharged from the hospital after undergoing a surgical procedure. As part of the continuum of care, which action by the nurse demonstrates effective care coordination and transition management for Mrs. Smith?

A) Providing Mrs. Smith with a list of community resources for post-operative care.

B) Ensuring Mrs. Smith has a follow-up appointment with her primary care physician within a week.

C) Instructing Mrs. Smith to manage her wound care at home without any further guidance.

D) Advising Mrs. Smith to resume her normal activities immediately upon discharge.

Question 51: Scenario: Sarah, a newly hired nurse, is about to start her orientation on a busy medical-surgical unit. As her preceptor, you are discussing the importance of effective orientation planning. Which of the following statements best reflects a key aspect of orientation planning and preceptor best practices?

A) Providing minimal guidance to encourage independence

B) Allowing the orientee to skip certain training modules

C) Tailoring the orientation process to the individual's learning needs

D) Assigning complex tasks without proper supervision

Question 52: Scenario: During the morning shift handover, a Certified Medical Surgical Registered Nurse (CMSRN) is assigned to supervise a group of nursing assistants caring for a postoperative patient, Mr. Smith, who underwent abdominal surgery yesterday. The patient is stable but requires frequent monitoring of vital signs and wound care. One of the nursing assistants approaches the CMSRN and asks if they can remove the patient's surgical dressing. Which action should the CMSRN take in this situation?

A) Allow the nursing assistant to remove the dressing under direct supervision.

B) Instruct the nursing assistant to remove the dressing independently.

C) Delegate the task of dressing removal to another nursing assistant.

D) Perform the dressing removal personally.

Question 53: Scenario: During a disaster drill in the hospital, a patient named Mr. Smith is brought in with severe burns on his arms and face. As a CMSRN, what is the priority action in managing Mr. Smith's burns?

A) Administering pain medication

B) Assessing the patient's airway and breathing

C) Applying cold compress to the burns

D) Notifying the family about the situation

Question 54: Which of the following actions by a Certified Medical Surgical Registered Nurse (CMSRN) best demonstrates safe medication management in patient care?

A) Administering a medication without checking the patient's identification band.

B) Crushing a sustained-release medication for easier administration.

C) Verifying the medication with another nurse before administration.

D) Using an outdated drug reference guide for medication information.

Question 55: When documenting patient care, which element is crucial for ensuring accurate and comprehensive record-keeping?

A) Using abbreviations and acronyms to save time

B) Delaying documentation until the end of the shift

C) Recording information as soon as possible after providing care
D) Relying on memory for undocumented details

Question 56: Scenario: Sarah, a newly certified Medical Surgical Registered Nurse, is eager to advance her career and explore various career development resources. She is particularly interested in enhancing her nursing teamwork and collaboration skills. Which of the following resources would be most beneficial for Sarah in achieving her career goals?
A) Attending a workshop on conflict resolution within healthcare teams.
B) Subscribing to a nursing journal focusing on career advancement.
C) Participating in a social media group for nurses.
D) Watching online tutorials on basic nursing skills.

Question 57: Which of the following is a key principle of workplace safety for Certified Medical Surgical Registered Nurses (CMSRNs)?
A) Ignoring safety protocols to save time
B) Using personal protective equipment (PPE) only when convenient
C) Reporting any unsafe conditions or practices promptly
D) Disregarding ergonomic principles during patient care

Question 58: Scenario: Mr. Johnson, a 65-year-old patient, is admitted to the medical-surgical unit with complaints of severe abdominal pain, nausea, and vomiting. His vital signs are stable, but he appears restless and uncomfortable. Upon assessment, you notice that his abdomen is distended and tender to touch. Mr. Johnson mentions that the pain started suddenly and is worsening. What should be the nurse's immediate action based on critical thinking?
A) Administer pain medication as ordered
B) Notify the healthcare provider immediately
C) Offer Mr. Johnson some antacids for relief
D) Document the assessment findings in the chart

Question 59: Ms. Johnson, a 65-year-old patient, is admitted to the medical-surgical unit with a stage IV pressure ulcer on her sacrum. The wound is deep, with visible bone and signs of infection. The healthcare team has initiated aggressive wound care management. Which of the following interventions is the highest priority in the care of Ms. Johnson's pressure ulcer?
A) Applying a hydrocolloid dressing to the wound
B) Administering oral antibiotics for the infection
C) Turning and repositioning the patient every two hours
D) Implementing a pressure redistribution mattress on the bed

Question 60: Scenario: Ms. Smith, a CMSRN, is caring for a postoperative patient who is experiencing severe pain. The patient requests a specific pain medication that is not ordered by the physician. Ms. Smith knows that administering this medication without a physician's order is against hospital policy. What should Ms. Smith do in this situation?
A) Administer the requested medication to alleviate the patient's pain.
B) Inform the patient that the medication cannot be given without a physician's order.
C) Consult with the charge nurse to seek guidance on the situation.
D) Ask the patient to wait until the physician rounds to discuss the pain management.

Question 61: Scenario: During a busy shift, a Certified Medical Surgical Registered Nurse (CMSRN) notices that one of the nursing assistants, Sarah, is being unfairly assigned a disproportionately high number of patients compared to others. The nurse observes Sarah looking overwhelmed and stressed. What should the CMSRN do in this situation to advocate for staff well-being and fair workload distribution?
A) Approach the charge nurse privately to discuss the issue and request a fair redistribution of patients.
B) Ignore the situation as it is not the CMSRN's responsibility to intervene in staff assignments.
C) Confront Sarah directly and advise her to manage her workload better.
D) Report the issue to the hospital administration without discussing it with anyone else.

Question 62: During safety rounds on the medical-surgical unit, the nurse finds a patient, Mr. Johnson, who is confused and attempting to get out of bed unassisted. Which action should the nurse prioritize to ensure patient safety during this situation?
A) Administering a sedative to calm the patient
B) Calling for assistance to help reorient and safely transfer the patient back to bed
C) Documenting the incident in the patient's chart for future reference
D) Ignoring the behavior as it is common in confused patients

Question 63: Scenario: Mr. Smith, a 55-year-old patient with a history of chronic illness, is admitted to the medical-surgical unit for management of his condition. He requires long-term intravenous therapy and the healthcare team decides to use a central venous catheter for his treatment. Which of the following is a characteristic of a peripherally inserted central catheter (PICC) that differentiates it from other central venous access devices?
A) Subcutaneous port for medication administration
B) External catheter that exits the body
C) Inserted through a peripheral vein with tip placement in the central venous system
D) Used for short-term intravenous therapy

Question 64: In the context of patient-centered care, seeking a second opinion can be beneficial for patients facing complex medical decisions because it:
A) Provides a fresh perspective and additional expertise.
B) Increases the cost of healthcare unnecessarily.
C) Delays the treatment process and causes confusion.
D) Indicates a lack of trust in the primary healthcare provider.

Question 65: In the context of a "just culture" within patient safety, which of the following best defines the term?
A) Blaming individuals for errors
B) Encouraging open communication about errors
C) Punishing healthcare providers for system failures
D) Ignoring errors to maintain harmony

Question 66: Scenario: Mr. Johnson, a 65-year-old patient, is admitted to the medical-surgical unit with a history of chronic lower back pain due to degenerative disc disease. He reports his pain level as 8/10 on the pain scale. The healthcare provider prescribes a combination of acetaminophen and oxycodone for pain management. Mr. Johnson has a past medical history of liver cirrhosis. Which intervention should the nurse prioritize when managing Mr. Johnson's pain?
A) Administering the prescribed acetaminophen and oxycodone as ordered
B) Suggesting non-pharmacological pain management techniques such as heat therapy
C) Consulting with the healthcare provider to adjust the pain medication due to liver cirrhosis
D) Recommending physical therapy for long-term pain management

Question 67: Scenario: Mr. Johnson, a 65-year-old patient, has been admitted to the medical-surgical unit with a diagnosis of congestive heart failure. During the interdisciplinary team meeting, the nurse notices that the physical therapist suggests a more aggressive rehabilitation plan, while the cardiologist recommends adjusting the medication regimen. The nurse, understanding the importance of effective communication skills, decides to:
A) Advocate for the physical therapist's rehabilitation plan.
B) Implement the cardiologist's medication regimen without question.
C) Coordinate a meeting to discuss and integrate both recommendations.
D) Disregard both recommendations and follow personal judgment.

Question 68: Which non-pharmacological intervention is most effective for managing acute pain in postoperative patients?
A) Heat therapy
B) Massage therapy
C) Distraction techniques
D) Cold therapy

Question 69: Which of the following actions is most appropriate for a Certified Medical Surgical Registered Nurse (CMSRN) when caring for a patient at risk for suicide?
A) Allowing the patient to be alone in their room for extended periods.
B) Removing potentially harmful objects from the patient's environment.
C) Providing the patient with sharp objects for personal use under supervision.
D) Discussing suicide methods in detail with the patient to understand their perspective.

Question 70: Which nonpharmacological intervention is commonly used in chronic pain management to promote relaxation and reduce stress?
A) Acupuncture
B) Massage therapy
C) Herbal supplements
D) Electrotherapy

Question 71: Which communication skill is essential for a Certified Medical Surgical Registered Nurse (CMSRN) when working within an interdisciplinary team?
A) Active listening
B) Interrupting others
C) Avoiding eye contact
D) Speaking over colleagues

Question 72: Scenario: Mr. Johnson, a 65-year-old patient, is admitted to the medical-surgical unit with a history of hypertension, diabetes, and recent myocardial infarction. During the initial assessment, the nurse notes that Mr. Johnson is experiencing shortness of breath and chest pain. Which risk assessment method would be most appropriate for the nurse to utilize in this situation?
A) Braden Scale
B) Morse Fall Scale
C) Glasgow Coma Scale
D) Modified Early Warning Score (MEWS)

Question 73: When discussing end-of-life preferences with a patient, which action by the nurse best demonstrates holistic patient care?
A) Providing information solely based on medical interventions.
B) Ignoring the patient's emotional and spiritual needs.

C) Involving the patient in decision-making and respecting their values.
D) Making decisions for the patient without their input.

Question 74: Mr. Smith, a 65-year-old patient, is admitted to the medical-surgical unit with a diagnosis of heart failure. The healthcare team includes nurses, physicians, physical therapists, and dietitians. Which action best demonstrates interprofessional care for Mr. Smith?
A) The nurse independently adjusts the diuretic dosage based on the patient's weight.
B) The physician prescribes a new medication without consulting other team members.
C) The physical therapist collaborates with the nurse to develop a mobility plan for Mr. Smith.
D) The dietitian provides dietary recommendations without considering the patient's preferences.

Question 75: Scenario: During the morning shift handover, the nurse receives report about a postoperative patient, Mr. Johnson, who is scheduled for discharge later in the day. The nurse notices that the patient's vital signs are stable, the surgical site is clean and dry, and the patient reports minimal pain. However, the patient's daughter expresses concerns about her father's ability to manage his medications at home due to his forgetfulness. The nurse decides to involve the healthcare team in addressing this issue. Which action by the nurse best demonstrates effective nursing teamwork and collaboration in this situation?
A) Providing the daughter with written instructions on medication administration.
B) Scheduling a follow-up appointment with the primary care physician.
C) Consulting with the pharmacist to simplify the medication regimen.
D) Initiating a multidisciplinary team meeting to discuss the patient's discharge plan.

Question 76: Scenario: Mr. Johnson, a 65-year-old postoperative patient, has a surgical wound on his abdomen following a cholecystectomy. The nurse is providing care for Mr. Johnson and is implementing infection control measures. Which action by the nurse demonstrates adherence to current evidence-based practice for infection prevention in surgical wound care?
A) Changing the wound dressing daily using sterile technique.
B) Cleaning the wound with hydrogen peroxide during each dressing change.
C) Applying antibiotic ointment to the wound at every dressing change.
D) Using alcohol-based hand rub before and after wound care procedures.

Question 77: Scenario: Mr. Smith, a 55-year-old patient, is admitted to the medical-surgical unit with a diagnosis of sepsis. He has a triple lumen central venous catheter in place for intravenous access. The nurse notes redness, warmth, and tenderness at the catheter site. On further assessment, the nurse observes purulent drainage at the insertion site and a temperature of 38.9 蜎 (102 蚌). Mr. Smith is hemodynamically stable. What is the most appropriate initial nursing action in this situation?
A) Notify the healthcare provider immediately
B) Administer a broad-spectrum antibiotic through the central line
C) Remove the central line and send the tip for culture
D) Apply a warm compress to the insertion site

Question 78: Which technology trend in health care allows for

remote monitoring of patients' vital signs and health status?
A) Electronic Health Records (EHR)
B) Telemedicine
C) Artificial Intelligence (AI) in Diagnostics
D) Virtual Reality (VR)

Question 79: Scenario: Mr. Johnson, a 65-year-old patient, is admitted to the medical-surgical unit with a history of heart failure. As the CMSRN, you are reviewing his plan of care. Which action by the nurse reflects adherence to regulatory requirements and standards of practice?
A) Administering a medication without checking the patient's identification band.
B) Documenting vital signs in the electronic health record without assessing the patient.
C) Verifying the patient's identity using two unique identifiers before administering medication.
D) Allowing a family member to make decisions without the patient's consent.

Question 80: In the context of 'unsafe practice' related to Professional reporting and resources, Scope of Practice and Ethics, and Professional Concepts, which action by a medical surgical registered nurse (MSRN) would be considered unsafe?
A) Reporting a medication error immediately to the supervisor
B) Providing care outside the scope of practice without proper training
C) Following evidence-based practice guidelines for patient care
D) Collaborating with the healthcare team for effective patient outcomes

Question 81: Which action is a regulatory requirement for reporting death in the context of Palliative/End-of-Life Care and Holistic Patient Care?
A) Notify the primary care physician only
B) Document the time and date of death in the patient's medical record
C) Inform the family before documenting the death
D) Delay reporting the death until the next shift

Question 82: Scenario: Mr. Smith, a 65-year-old male patient, is admitted to the medical-surgical unit with complaints of chest pain and shortness of breath. During the assessment, the nurse notes that Mr. Smith is diaphoretic, pale, and clutching his chest. He rates his chest pain as 8/10 on the pain scale. His vital signs are: BP 160/90 mmHg, HR 110 bpm, RR 24/min, and SpO2 92% on room air. What should be the nurse's immediate action based on this assessment?
A) Administer oxygen at 2 L/min via nasal cannula
B) Perform a 12-lead ECG and notify the healthcare provider
C) Offer Mr. Smith a warm blanket to make him comfortable
D) Document the findings and continue routine assessments

Question 83: Which of the following is an example of an unintended consequence in the context of a healthy practice environment for Certified Medical Surgical Registered Nurses (CMSRNs)?
A) Implementing a new electronic health record system that leads to increased documentation errors
B) Providing additional training opportunities that improve staff competency
C) Introducing a new shift schedule that enhances work-life balance for nurses
D) Offering flexible work hours that result in decreased staff satisfaction

Question 84: Which action by the nurse best demonstrates

patient advocacy in the context of pain management?
A) Administering pain medication as ordered without verifying the patient's pain level
B) Encouraging the patient to endure severe pain without requesting any pain relief
C) Advocating for the patient to receive pain medication based on the patient's self-report
D) Disregarding the patient's pain complaints and focusing solely on completing tasks

Question 85: In the context of the Nursing professional practice model, which element emphasizes the importance of continuous improvement and innovation in delivering quality patient care?
A) Evidence-based practice
B) Cost-effective care
C) Patient-centered care
D) Traditional nursing care

Question 86: Scenario: Mrs. Smith, a 78-year-old patient with advanced cancer, expresses her wish to discontinue aggressive treatments and focus on comfort care measures. She mentions her desire to spend her remaining time at home surrounded by her family. Mrs. Smith is experiencing increased pain and shortness of breath despite medication adjustments. As her CMSRN, what is the most appropriate action to take based on her end-of-life preferences?
A) Initiate discussions about hospice care options with Mrs. Smith and her family.
B) Increase the dosage of pain medications to manage her symptoms more effectively.
C) Recommend a new chemotherapy regimen to target the advanced cancer.
D) Transfer Mrs. Smith to the intensive care unit for closer monitoring.

Question 87: Scenario: Mr. Johnson, a 65-year-old patient, is admitted to the medical-surgical unit with a diagnosis of pneumonia. The primary nurse, Sarah, is discussing the patient's condition with the nursing team during the shift handover. Sarah mentions that Mr. Johnson has a history of COPD and is currently receiving oxygen therapy at 2 liters per minute via nasal cannula. She also informs the team that his oxygen saturation levels have been fluctuating between 88-92% despite the oxygen therapy. Which action by the nursing team is most appropriate in this situation?
A) Increase the oxygen flow rate to 4 liters per minute.
B) Place Mr. Johnson on a non-rebreather mask at 15 liters per minute.
C) Notify the healthcare provider about the fluctuating oxygen saturation levels.
D) Discontinue the oxygen therapy and monitor Mr. Johnson closely.

Question 88: Scenario: Mr. Patel, a 65-year-old patient admitted to the medical-surgical unit, speaks Gujarati as his primary language. He is experiencing severe abdominal pain and is unable to communicate effectively in English. As a CMSRN, what is the most appropriate action to ensure effective communication with Mr. Patel regarding his pain assessment?
A) Use a language translation app on a smartphone to communicate with Mr. Patel.
B) Ask Mr. Patel's family members to interpret his symptoms and pain level.
C) Utilize written materials in English to explain the pain assessment process to Mr. Patel.
D) Request a professional medical interpreter fluent in Gujarati to

assist with the pain assessment.

Question 89: Scenario: During a busy shift at the medical-surgical unit, a Certified Medical Surgical Registered Nurse (CMSRN) encounters a patient, Mr. Smith, who has been readmitted for the third time in two months due to complications from diabetes. Mr. Smith is frustrated and expresses his concerns about his health and the impact on his family. The nurse has been providing care for Mr. Smith since his first admission and has developed a strong bond with him. Despite feeling emotionally drained and overwhelmed by the workload, the nurse continues to provide compassionate care to Mr. Smith. Which of the following best describes the concept illustrated in this scenario?
A) Burnout
B) Empathy
C) Compassion fatigue
D) Sympathy

Question 90: Which assessment finding is indicative of severe malnutrition in a patient?
A) BMI of 25
B) Albumin level of 4.0 g/dL
C) Hemoglobin level of 12 g/dL
D) Prealbumin level of 10 mg/dL

Question 91: In interprofessional collaboration, which element is essential for successful collaborative problem-solving?
A) Autonomy
B) Competition
C) Communication
D) Isolation

Question 92: Which of the following is a key characteristic of a healthy practice environment for Certified Medical Surgical Registered Nurses (CMSRNs)?
A) High nurse-to-patient ratios
B) Lack of interprofessional collaboration
C) Limited access to professional development opportunities
D) Supportive nurse leadership and management

Question 93: Scenario: During a busy shift in the medical-surgical unit, a Certified Medical Surgical Registered Nurse (CMSRN) notices a spill of medication on the floor in a high-traffic area. The nurse observes several staff members walking near the spill without noticing it. What should the nurse do first to ensure workplace safety?
A) Quickly clean up the spill using available supplies
B) Place a caution sign near the spill and notify the unit manager
C) Ask a nursing assistant to clean up the spill
D) Ignore the spill and continue with patient care

Question 94: Ms. Johnson, a 65-year-old patient with multiple chronic conditions, is prescribed a new medication for her heart condition. Due to financial constraints, she expresses concerns about the cost of the medication. As a CMSRN, what is the most appropriate action to take in this situation?
A) Provide information on patient assistance programs offered by pharmaceutical companies.
B) Advise the patient to skip doses to make the medication last longer.
C) Suggest the patient switch to an over-the-counter alternative.
D) Recommend the patient to stop taking the medication altogether.

Question 95: During a crisis situation in a medical-surgical unit, the nurse should prioritize which action first?
A) Documenting the events

B) Ensuring patient safety
C) Contacting the family members
D) Administering medications

Question 96: Scenario: Mr. Smith, a 55-year-old patient, is scheduled for a minor surgical procedure requiring moderate sedation. As the CMSRN overseeing the sedation process, which of the following actions is most appropriate during the pre-procedural phase?
A) Administering the sedative medication without informing the patient about potential side effects.
B) Obtaining informed consent from the patient after explaining the procedure, risks, benefits, and alternatives.
C) Skipping the patient assessment as it is a minor procedure.
D) Allowing the patient's family member to sign the consent form on behalf of the patient.

Question 97: Scenario: Mrs. Smith, a 65-year-old postoperative patient, is scheduled for a complex surgical procedure. As the CMSRN, you notice that the nursing team is experiencing challenges in adapting to the new postoperative care protocols. Mrs. Smith's recovery is dependent on effective teamwork and collaboration among the healthcare providers. What action should you take to address this situation?
A) Implement a top-down approach to enforce the new protocols.
B) Organize a team meeting to discuss the importance of teamwork in patient care.
C) Assign blame to individual team members for the lack of compliance.
D) Ignore the situation and hope that the team adapts on their own.

Question 98: In the context of Nursing Teamwork and Collaboration, which action by a nurse best demonstrates effective collaboration with the healthcare team?
A) Providing patient care without consulting other team members
B) Attending interdisciplinary team meetings regularly
C) Ignoring input from other healthcare professionals
D) Making decisions independently without considering team opinions

Question 99: In the context of early warning systems for crisis situations, what is the primary purpose of implementing such systems in a healthcare setting?
A) To create unnecessary panic among healthcare staff
B) To provide timely alerts and notifications for potential crises
C) To increase workload for healthcare professionals
D) To delay response time in emergency situations

Question 100: When planning an orientation for a newly hired nurse, what is a crucial aspect of preceptor best practices to ensure successful integration into the healthcare team?
A) Assigning multiple preceptors to provide diverse perspectives
B) Allowing the preceptor to focus solely on clinical skills training
C) Encouraging the preceptor to provide constructive feedback and support
D) Minimizing communication between the preceptor and the orientee

Question 101: Scenario: Mr. Johnson, a 65-year-old patient, is admitted to the medical-surgical unit for post-operative care following a hip replacement surgery. While performing the initial assessment, the nurse notes that the patient is experiencing shortness of breath, tachycardia, and confusion. The oxygen saturation level is 88%. The nurse suspects a potential complication and initiates appropriate interventions. Which action should the nurse prioritize to ensure patient safety in this situation?

A) Administering pain medication to alleviate discomfort
B) Notifying the healthcare provider immediately
C) Documenting the findings in the patient's chart
D) Providing the patient with a warm blanket

Question 102: Which action by the nurse best demonstrates effective patient-centered care in the context of Patient/Care Management?
A) Providing the patient with a detailed explanation of the treatment plan.
B) Making decisions for the patient based on the nurse's judgment.
C) Disregarding the patient's preferences and concerns during care planning.
D) Implementing interventions without considering the patient's cultural beliefs.

Question 103: Which personal protective equipment (PPE) is essential for healthcare workers to wear when caring for a patient on airborne precautions?
A) Gown and gloves
B) Surgical mask
C) N95 respirator
D) Face shield

Question 104: Which vital sign is crucial to monitor frequently in a patient undergoing a surgical procedure in the post-anesthesia care unit (PACU)?
A) Blood pressure
B) Temperature
C) Respiratory rate
D) Capillary refill time

Question 105: Which of the following is an example of a physical communication barrier?
A) Language differences
B) Cultural differences
C) Noise in the environment
D) Lack of trust between sender and receiver

Question 106: Scenario: Mr. Smith, a 65-year-old patient with a history of diabetes and hypertension, is admitted to the medical-surgical unit for a scheduled knee replacement surgery. During the pre-operative assessment, the nurse identifies a potential risk of infection due to the patient's comorbidities. As part of the risk assessment process, the healthcare team decides to conduct a Failure Mode and Effects Analysis (FMEA) to prevent any adverse events during the perioperative period. Which of the following best describes the purpose of conducting an FMEA in this scenario?
A) To identify potential failure points in the surgical equipment
B) To evaluate the effectiveness of post-operative pain management
C) To assess the risk of infection associated with the patient's comorbidities
D) To review the patient's medical history for surgical clearance

Question 107: Which of the following is a key component of a care bundle aimed at enhancing patient safety in medical-surgical settings?
A) Administering medications on time
B) Ensuring patient privacy during rounds
C) Providing extra blankets for patient comfort
D) Allowing family members to stay overnight

Question 108: Which of the following best defines health literacy in the context of education of patients and families for holistic patient care?

A) The ability to understand and use healthcare information to make informed decisions.
B) The number of medical terms a patient can memorize.
C) The speed at which a patient can read medical documents.
D) The level of medical training a patient has received.

Question 109: Which communication approach is most aligned with the principles of patient-centered care in the context of holistic patient care?
A) Using medical jargon to convey information
B) Speaking in a calm and empathetic tone
C) Providing minimal information to avoid overwhelming the patient
D) Rushing through explanations to save time

Question 110: A patient who has undergone abdominal surgery is experiencing moderate pain. Which expectation regarding pain management should the Certified Medical Surgical Registered Nurse (CMSRN) prioritize?
A) Administering pain medication only upon patient request
B) Implementing non-pharmacological pain management techniques
C) Delaying pain medication administration until pain becomes severe
D) Providing timely pain medication as prescribed by the healthcare provider

Question 111: Which of the following is a key characteristic of evidence-based practice in nursing?
A) Relying solely on tradition and personal experience
B) Making decisions based on outdated research
C) Incorporating the best available evidence with clinical expertise and patient preferences
D) Disregarding patient values and beliefs

Question 112: Scenario: Mr. Smith, a 65-year-old patient, is admitted to the medical-surgical unit with a history of hypertension and diabetes. He is currently receiving intravenous fluids for dehydration. During your assessment, you notice that Mr. Smith is restless, tachypneic, and his oxygen saturation is dropping. He appears confused and his blood pressure is dropping. What action should the nurse take first based on the early warning system principles?
A) Notify the healthcare provider immediately
B) Increase the rate of intravenous fluids
C) Administer oxygen therapy
D) Perform a thorough head-to-toe assessment

Question 113: Ms. Johnson, a 65-year-old patient, is admitted to the medical-surgical unit with a diagnosis of pneumonia. The healthcare team has been utilizing the electronic health record (EHR) system for documenting her care. Which aspect of EHR documentation is crucial for ensuring effective interprofessional care coordination?
A) Including detailed information on the patient's social history
B) Ensuring timely and accurate entry of vital signs
C) Documenting the patient's dietary preferences
D) Recording the healthcare team's communication notes

Question 114: In the context of resource allocation in a medical-surgical unit, which principle should guide the nurse's decision-making process?
A) Equal distribution of resources to all patients
B) Prioritizing patients based on their insurance coverage
C) Allocating resources based on acuity and need
D) Providing resources first come, first served

Question 115: Ms. Patel, a 65-year-old Indian American woman, is admitted to the hospital with advanced cancer. She

expresses her desire for traditional Ayurvedic treatments alongside conventional medical care. As her nurse, what is the most appropriate action to take to support Ms. Patel's cultural beliefs and preferences?
A) Encourage Ms. Patel to solely focus on conventional medical treatments.
B) Respect Ms. Patel's wishes and work with the healthcare team to integrate Ayurvedic treatments into her care plan.
C) Disregard Ms. Patel's cultural beliefs and provide care based solely on Western medical practices.
D) Suggest alternative treatments without considering Ayurvedic practices.

Question 116: Which of the following is a potential complication associated with central lines?
A) Phlebitis
B) Hypertension
C) Hyperglycemia
D) Bradycardia

Question 117: Which of the following is the most appropriate method for safe disposal of unused or expired medications?
A) Flushing them down the toilet
B) Throwing them in the household trash
C) Returning them to a pharmacy or authorized collection site
D) Burying them in the backyard

Question 118: Scenario: Sarah, a dedicated Medical Surgical Registered Nurse, has been working long hours due to short staffing at the hospital. She often finds herself making difficult decisions that challenge her moral compass. Despite her best efforts, she feels overwhelmed and emotionally drained. Sarah is experiencing:
A) Burnout
B) Compassion fatigue
C) Moral distress
D) Moral resilience

Question 119: In the context of Continuous Quality and Process Improvement, which of the following tools is commonly used to display trends and variations in a process over time?
A) Pareto Chart
B) Scatter Diagram
C) Control Chart
D) Fishbone Diagram

Question 120: During the assessment phase of the nursing process, the nurse should prioritize which action?
A) Administering medications
B) Developing a care plan
C) Collecting patient data
D) Evaluating patient outcomes

Question 121: Which of the following is considered a nursing sensitive indicator based on evidence-based guidelines for quality management in medical-surgical nursing?
A) Patient falls
B) Hospital readmission rates
C) Physician satisfaction scores
D) Hospital revenue generation

Question 122: Scenario: Mr. Johnson, a 65-year-old patient, is admitted to the medical-surgical unit with complaints of chest pain and shortness of breath. During your assessment, he appears anxious and is having difficulty expressing himself clearly due to his distress. As a CMSRN, which of the following responses demonstrates active listening?

A) Interrupting Mr. Johnson to ask direct questions about his symptoms.
B) Nodding your head while looking at the computer to document his vital signs.
C) Placing a hand on Mr. Johnson's shoulder and saying, "I can see you're feeling worried. Can you tell me more about your chest pain?"
D) Checking the IV infusion rate while Mr. Johnson speaks about his medical history.

Question 123: Scenario: Mr. Johnson, a 65-year-old patient recovering from a surgical procedure, expresses dissatisfaction with the nursing care he received due to prolonged wait times for pain medication administration. As a CMSRN, how should you handle this situation to ensure effective service recovery?
A) Apologize to Mr. Johnson and explain the reasons for the delay in pain medication administration.
B) Dismiss Mr. Johnson's concerns and assure him that delays are common in healthcare settings.
C) Ignore Mr. Johnson's complaints and continue with the standard care protocol.
D) Offer Mr. Johnson a discount on his hospital bill to compensate for the inconvenience.

Question 124: Scenario: Mrs. Smith, a 65-year-old patient, was admitted to a high accountable organization for a surgical procedure. During her stay, the nursing staff noticed a discrepancy in her medication chart. Despite being busy, the nurse promptly investigated the issue, identified the error, and rectified it before administering the medication to Mrs. Smith. This action reflects the organization's commitment to patient safety culture and effective patient management. Which of the following best describes the action taken by the nurse in this scenario?
A) Ignoring the error and proceeding with medication administration.
B) Reporting the error at the end of the shift.
C) Investigating, identifying, and rectifying the medication error promptly.
D) Seeking assistance from another nurse without addressing the error.

Question 125: Ms. Johnson, a 65-year-old patient, has recently been diagnosed with hypertension. She is eager to learn more about managing her condition effectively. As a CMSRN, which of the following actions would be most appropriate to provide health information to meet Ms. Johnson's needs?
A) Provide written materials in medical jargon for detailed understanding.
B) Use simple language and visual aids to explain hypertension management.
C) Recommend online resources without further explanation.
D) Discuss advanced treatment options without assessing her readiness.

Question 126: In disaster planning and management, which action is a priority for the medical surgical nurse in ensuring effective teamwork and collaboration during a crisis situation?
A) Assigning tasks based on individual preferences
B) Communicating clearly and regularly with team members
C) Working independently to expedite patient care
D) Ignoring input from other healthcare professionals

Question 127: In the context of 'Leadership, Nursing Teamwork, and Collaboration,' which statement best describes shared decision-making?
A) Shared decision-making involves healthcare providers making

decisions without involving patients.

B) Shared decision-making is a process where only the most senior healthcare provider makes decisions for the patient.

C) Shared decision-making is a collaborative process between healthcare providers and patients to make healthcare decisions together.

D) Shared decision-making is a process where patients are not informed about their treatment options.

Question 128: In the context of 'Interprofessional roles and responsibilities' related to Care Coordination and Transition Management, which action best exemplifies effective interprofessional collaboration?

A) Providing care without consulting other healthcare team members

B) Communicating patient updates only within the nursing team

C) Attending interprofessional team meetings to discuss patient care

D) Making decisions independently without considering input from other disciplines

Question 129: Scenario: Mr. Johnson, a 55-year-old patient, is admitted to the medical-surgical unit with a history of aggressive behavior. He becomes agitated when his pain is not adequately managed. As the nurse, you notice Mr. Johnson clenching his fists and pacing the room. He starts yelling, "I need my pain medication now!" What is the most appropriate verbal intervention technique to use in this situation?

A) Raise your voice to match his intensity and demand compliance.

B) Approach Mr. Johnson calmly and maintain a non-threatening posture.

C) Ignore his behavior and walk out of the room to give him space.

D) Threaten to withhold his pain medication if he does not calm down.

Question 130: Scenario: Mr. Johnson, a 68-year-old patient, is admitted to the medical-surgical unit following a hip replacement surgery. The healthcare team is focused on promoting his mobility and preventing complications associated with immobility. As the CMSRN, you are responsible for assessing Mr. Johnson's mobility status and implementing appropriate interventions. Which intervention is most crucial in promoting mobility for Mr. Johnson post hip replacement surgery?

A) Encouraging passive range of motion exercises

B) Limiting weight-bearing activities on the affected hip

C) Implementing early ambulation with assistive devices

D) Keeping the patient on strict bed rest for 48 hours

Question 131: In the context of care coordination and transition management, which action is essential for an effective interprofessional care team?

A) Working in silos without communication

B) Delaying sharing of patient information

C) Collaborating and sharing information openly

D) Ignoring input from other team members

Question 132: Which disease process is characterized by the body's inability to produce or respond to insulin, leading to abnormal carbohydrate metabolism?

A) Hypothyroidism

B) Celiac disease

C) Diabetes mellitus

D) Chronic obstructive pulmonary disease

Question 133: Which of the following factors is NOT a significant predictor for patients at risk for readmissions?

A) Lack of social support

B) History of non-compliance with medications

C) Regular follow-up appointments with healthcare provider

D) Limited health literacy

Question 134: Scenario: During a surgical procedure, the circulating nurse initiates a timeout procedure. The patient, Mr. Smith, is already on the operating table, and the surgical team is ready to begin. The circulating nurse states the patient's name, date of birth, and the procedure to be performed. The surgeon confirms the information, and the anesthesia provider acknowledges. Suddenly, the scrub nurse interrupts, stating that a crucial instrument is missing from the sterile field. What is the most appropriate action for the circulating nurse to take next?

A) Proceed with the surgery as planned

B) Pause the procedure, conduct a thorough search for the missing instrument

C) Ask another team member to locate the missing instrument

D) Inform the surgeon that the instrument is missing but continue with the surgery

Question 135: Scenario: Mr. Smith, a 65-year-old patient admitted for a surgical procedure, has a history of diabetes mellitus type 2 and hypertension. He is prescribed a diabetic diet and low-sodium diet. The nurse notes that Mr. Smith has poor appetite and is experiencing nausea post-surgery. Which intervention is most appropriate to address Mr. Smith's nutritional needs?

A) Initiate enteral nutrition via nasogastric tube

B) Offer small, frequent meals with foods he enjoys within his dietary restrictions

C) Administer total parenteral nutrition (TPN)

D) Provide a high-calorie, high-protein diet regardless of his preferences

Question 136: Scenario: Ms. Smith, a 65-year-old patient, is admitted to the medical-surgical unit with a diagnosis of heart failure. The nurse caring for Ms. Smith is implementing a nursing professional practice model. Which of the following best describes the key focus of a nursing professional practice model in this scenario?

A) Ensuring adequate staffing levels

B) Promoting evidence-based practice

C) Providing patient education on heart failure

D) Administering medications as ordered

Question 137: Which of the following is an essential component of active listening in the context of patient-centered care?

A) Interrupting the patient to save time

B) Providing unsolicited advice during the conversation

C) Demonstrating empathy and understanding

D) Focusing on formulating responses while the patient speaks

Question 138: Which of the following is an indication for alternate nutrition administration in a patient?

A) Dysphagia

B) Hypertension

C) Urinary tract infection

D) Skin rash

Question 139: Which of the following is a correct application of heat therapy for a patient in a medical-surgical setting?

A) Placing a heating pad on a patient with acute inflammation

B) Applying a warm compress to a fresh post-operative incision

C) Using a warm blanket on a patient with peripheral vascular disease

D) Administering a warm water bottle to a patient with an open wound

Question 140: Scenario: Mr. Johnson, a 65-year-old male patient, is admitted to the medical-surgical unit with complaints of severe abdominal pain, nausea, and vomiting. His vital signs are as follows: temperature 38.5 蜕, heart rate 110 bpm, blood pressure 140/90 mmHg, and respiratory rate 22 breaths/min. Laboratory results show an elevated white blood cell count. The nurse notes that Mr. Johnson's abdomen is distended and tender to palpation. Which interpretation should the nurse make based on Mr. Johnson's clinical presentation?
A) Mr. Johnson is likely experiencing an acute myocardial infarction.
B) Mr. Johnson may have a urinary tract infection.
C) Mr. Johnson is exhibiting signs of acute pancreatitis.
D) Mr. Johnson is at risk for developing deep vein thrombosis.

Question 141: Which of the following is a key principle of quality management in healthcare settings?
A) Cost reduction at the expense of quality
B) Reactive approach to problem-solving
C) Emphasis on individual blame
D) Continuous quality improvement

Question 142: Scenario: Mrs. Smith, a 65-year-old patient recovering from a recent stroke, is experiencing difficulty swallowing and requires speech consultation for evaluation of her ability to safely consume food and liquids. As a CMSRN, you understand the importance of assessing her swallowing function to prevent aspiration pneumonia and ensure adequate nutrition intake. Which of the following is the primary goal of speech consultation in this scenario?
A) To recommend a strict oral intake restriction to prevent any risk of aspiration.
B) To assess Mrs. Smith's swallowing function and recommend appropriate diet modifications.
C) To immediately initiate tube feeding to ensure adequate nutrition intake.
D) To advise Mrs. Smith to resume her regular diet without any modifications.

Question 143: Which of the following activities best exemplifies health promotion in the context of holistic patient care?
A) Administering prescribed medications
B) Encouraging regular exercise and physical activity
C) Monitoring vital signs every hour
D) Providing wound care dressing changes

Question 144: Scenario: Mr. Johnson, a 65-year-old patient, is admitted to the medical-surgical unit for post-operative care following a hip replacement surgery. The nurse observes that the patient is experiencing shortness of breath and increased heart rate. Upon further assessment, the nurse notices that Mr. Johnson's oxygen saturation levels are dropping. Despite informing the physician, there is a delay in implementing the prescribed oxygen therapy. Which action by the nurse best demonstrates a commitment to patient safety culture in this scenario?
A) Notifying the charge nurse about the situation.
B) Documenting the vital signs accurately in the patient's chart.
C) Advocating for the prompt initiation of oxygen therapy for Mr. Johnson.
D) Administering pain medication as ordered to keep the patient comfortable.

Question 145: Scenario: During a busy shift on the medical-surgical unit, a Certified Medical Surgical Registered Nurse (CMSRN) notices that a patient's vital signs are deteriorating rapidly. The nurse immediately informs the nursing team and requests assistance. The team collaborates efficiently to stabilize the patient and escalate care as needed. What professional behavior and skill is exemplified in this scenario?
A) Effective Communication and Collaboration
B) Time Management and Prioritization
C) Patient Advocacy and Empowerment
D) Clinical Judgment and Decision Making

Question 146: In the context of patient safety and care management, which of the following is a key purpose of utilizing checklists in care bundles?
A) To increase healthcare costs
B) To decrease adherence to evidence-based practices
C) To improve communication among healthcare team members
D) To reduce patient engagement in their own care

Question 147: Scenario: Sarah, a Certified Medical Surgical Registered Nurse, notices a medication error made by a colleague that could potentially harm the patient. Despite feeling hesitant, Sarah knows the importance of advocating for patient safety. What action should Sarah take to address this situation effectively?
A) Confront the colleague publicly to ensure immediate correction.
B) Report the error to the charge nurse or supervisor privately.
C) Ignore the error and hope it does not cause harm to the patient.
D) Discuss the error with the patient's family to seek their opinion.

Question 148: Ms. Thompson, a 68-year-old patient with advanced cancer, expresses her concerns about managing her symptoms and emotional distress as she approaches the end of life. As a CMSRN providing holistic care, which resource would be most appropriate to recommend to Ms. Thompson and her family for comprehensive support during this challenging time?
A) Hospice care services
B) Chemotherapy treatment centers
C) Weight loss clinics
D) Cosmetic surgery facilities

Question 149: Scenario: Mrs. Smith, a 65-year-old female patient, is admitted to the medical-surgical unit with a history of hypertension, diabetes, and obesity. During the assessment, the nurse notes that Mrs. Smith is a smoker and lives alone. Which demographic factor poses the highest risk for Mrs. Smith's health status?
A) Age
B) Smoking status
C) Living alone
D) Medical history

Question 150: Which of the following interventions is most effective in preventing patient falls in a medical-surgical unit?
A) Placing the call bell within the patient's reach
B) Keeping the patient's room well-lit during the night
C) Using bed and chair alarms for high-risk patients
D) Administering sedative medications to promote sleep

ANSWER WITH DETAILED EXPLANATION SET [3]

Question 1: Correct Answer: B) Decreased job satisfaction
Rationale: Compassion fatigue is characterized by emotional and physical exhaustion leading to a reduced ability to empathize with patients. Decreased job satisfaction is a common symptom as nurses may feel overwhelmed, detached, and emotionally drained. Options A, C, and D are incorrect as they do not align with the concept of compassion fatigue. Increased empathy towards patients (Option A) would not be indicative of compassion fatigue, while enhanced sense of personal accomplishment (Option C) and improved work-life balance (Option D) are more associated with job satisfaction and well-being rather than symptoms of compassion fatigue.

Question 2: Correct Answer: B) Ensuring she has a follow-up appointment scheduled with her primary care physician
Rationale: In the scenario provided, the most critical action for the CMSRN to take to facilitate a smooth transition and continuity of care for Ms. Johnson is to ensure she has a follow-up appointment scheduled with her primary care physician. This step is essential to monitor her recovery progress, address any post-operative concerns, and coordinate ongoing care. Option A is important but may not be as immediate as ensuring a follow-up appointment. Option C is crucial but should ideally be done in conjunction with the primary care physician. Option D, while relevant, is not as urgent or directly related to continuity of care as ensuring a follow-up appointment with the primary care provider.

Question 3: Correct Answer: D) Pulmonary embolism
Rationale: Pulmonary embolism is a life-threatening complication that can occur postoperatively in surgical patients. It requires immediate recognition and intervention by the CMSRN to prevent further complications such as respiratory distress, hypoxia, and even death. Postoperative nausea and vomiting, delayed wound healing, and urinary tract infections are common complications in surgical patients but do not pose the same level of immediate threat as a pulmonary embolism. Recognizing the signs and symptoms of pulmonary embolism, such as sudden shortness of breath, chest pain, and tachycardia, is crucial for the CMSRN to initiate prompt treatment and prevent adverse outcomes.

Question 4: Correct Answer: B) Reporting a colleague for unethical behavior
Rationale: Reporting a colleague for unethical behavior is the most appropriate action that demonstrates professional integrity. This choice aligns with the CMSRN's duty to uphold ethical standards and prioritize patient safety. Falsifying patient records, ignoring patient needs, and sharing confidential information are all violations of professional ethics and compromise patient care. By choosing to report unethical behavior, the nurse upholds the values of honesty, accountability, and patient advocacy, which are essential components of professional integrity in the healthcare setting.

Question 5: Correct Answer: A) Respect the patient's autonomy and advocate for the patient's wishes.
Rationale: Option A is the correct answer as per the Code of Ethics for Nurses with Interpretive Statements, which emphasizes the nurse's duty to respect the patient's autonomy and advocate for their wishes, even if they differ from the family's preferences. This principle upholds the patient's right to self-determination and informed decision-making regarding their healthcare. Options B, C, and D are incorrect as they do not align with the ethical responsibility of prioritizing the patient's autonomy and best interests over familial pressures or personal opinions. It is crucial for nurses to uphold ethical standards and advocate for patient-centered care in challenging situations like this.

Question 6: Correct Answer: C) Using an electronic medication administration record (eMAR) to document medication administration
Rationale: Option A is incorrect as crushing sustained-release tablets can alter their intended effect and lead to potential harm. Option B is incorrect as checking the patient's identification is crucial to ensure the right patient receives the right medication. Option D is incorrect as combining medications into one cup can result in drug interactions or errors. Option C is the correct answer as using an eMAR enhances accuracy, reduces errors, and ensures proper documentation of medication administration, promoting patient safety and effective care management.

Question 7: Correct Answer: D) Utilizing a transparent dressing to allow for visual wound assessment
Rationale: In the scenario provided, the most fiscally efficient approach is option D, utilizing a transparent dressing. This option allows for visual wound assessment without the need for frequent dressing changes, thus reducing material costs and nursing time. Option A is not cost-effective as it increases the use of supplies. Option B is wasteful and may lead to increased costs without improving patient outcomes. Option C is not in line with best practices as wound assessment is crucial for effective care. Therefore, option D is the most appropriate choice for maintaining fiscal efficiency while ensuring quality care for the patient.

Question 8: Correct Answer: B) Encouraging early ambulation and deep breathing exercises
Rationale: In the context of postoperative care bundles for a patient like Ms. Johnson, encouraging early ambulation and deep breathing exercises is crucial to prevent complications such as pneumonia and deep vein thrombosis. This intervention promotes circulation, prevents respiratory complications, and aids in the patient's overall recovery. Administering pain medication is important but should be based on the patient's pain level rather than a fixed schedule. Providing a daily back massage may offer comfort but is not a standard care bundle item. Applying heat packs every hour may not be recommended postoperatively due to the risk of burns and altered sensation in the surgical area.

Question 9: Correct Answer: C) Proper hand hygiene before and after patient contact
Rationale: Proper hand hygiene is a fundamental standard precaution in infection control to prevent the spread of microorganisms. Options A, B, and D are incorrect as they represent limited or specific precautions that do not encompass the comprehensive approach of standard precautions. Hand hygiene is crucial in reducing healthcare-associated infections by removing transient flora and reducing the risk of cross-contamination between patients and healthcare workers. It is a basic yet essential practice that all healthcare professionals must adhere to consistently to maintain a safe patient care environment

Question 10: Correct Answer: B) Acknowledging Mr. Smith's concerns, assessing his pain level thoroughly, and discussing alternative pain management options with the healthcare team.
Rationale: Option A is incorrect because simply instructing Mr. Smith to follow the prescribed regimen without addressing his concerns may escalate the conflict. Option C is incorrect as it dismisses Mr. Smith's pain and fails to offer a proactive solution. Option D is incorrect as ignoring the patient's requests can lead to further dissatisfaction and breakdown in communication. Option B is the correct answer as it demonstrates active listening, empathy, and a collaborative approach to resolving the conflict. By acknowledging Mr. Smith's concerns, assessing his pain, and exploring alternative options, the nurse shows a patient-centered approach to conflict resolution, fostering trust and effective communication.

Question 11: Correct Answer: D) Identifying contributing factors

Rationale: In Root Cause Analysis (RCA), the step that involves identifying contributing factors that led to the adverse event is crucial in understanding the underlying causes. While implementing corrective actions (Option A) is important for preventing future occurrences, reporting the adverse event to the supervisor (Option B) is an initial step but not directly related to identifying contributing factors. Analyzing the immediate cause of the event (Option C) focuses on the surface-level reason and does not delve into the deeper contributing factors that RCA aims to uncover. Therefore, the correct answer is D) Identifying contributing factors.

Question 12: Correct Answer: C) Registered nurses (RN) can delegate tasks that are within the scope of practice of the UAP.
Rationale: Delegation is a critical aspect of nursing teamwork and collaboration. The correct option, C, highlights the importance of delegating tasks that fall within the scope of practice of the unlicensed assistive personnel (UAP). This ensures safe and effective patient care delivery. Option A is incorrect as tasks requiring nursing judgment should be performed by licensed nurses. Option B is incorrect as LPNs cannot delegate tasks to RNs due to differences in their scopes of practice. Option D is incorrect as the delegating nurse retains accountability for the delegated task.

Question 13: Correct Answer: B) Proper hand hygiene practices
Rationale: Proper hand hygiene practices are a fundamental aspect of infection control and prevention in healthcare settings. It is crucial for healthcare providers to wash their hands regularly using soap and water or alcohol-based hand sanitizers to prevent the spread of infections. Routine use of antibiotics for all patients is not recommended due to the risk of antibiotic resistance. Reusing disposable gloves after disinfection can lead to cross-contamination. Ignoring isolation precautions for infectious patients can result in the transmission of infections to other patients and healthcare workers. Therefore, the correct answer is B) Proper hand hygiene practices, which is supported by current evidence-based guidelines for infection control and prevention.

Question 14: Correct Answer: B) Politely decline to share the information and explain the importance of patient confidentiality.
Rationale: Option B is the correct answer as per the scope of practice and code of ethics for nurses. Nurses are bound by ethical standards to maintain patient confidentiality at all times. Sharing patient information without proper authorization violates the patient's rights and breaches confidentiality. Options A, C, and D are incorrect as they go against the principles of patient confidentiality and could lead to legal and ethical consequences for the nurse. It is essential for nurses to prioritize patient privacy and confidentiality in all interactions to uphold professional standards and trust in the healthcare system.

Question 15: Correct Answer: A) The charge nurse takes Nurse A and Nurse B aside separately to discuss the issue privately.
Rationale: Option A is the correct answer as it demonstrates effective conflict management by addressing the issue privately, allowing both nurses to express their concerns without escalating the conflict further. This approach promotes open communication, maintains professionalism, and respects the dignity of all team members involved. In contrast, Option B could worsen the conflict by publicly shaming Nurse A, Option C neglects the responsibility of the charge nurse to intervene and facilitate resolution, and Option D avoids addressing the underlying conflict and may lead to resentment among team members.

Question 16: Correct Answer: C) Obesity with a BMI of 32
Rationale: Obesity, especially with a BMI of 30 or higher, is a significant risk factor for postoperative complications such as wound infections, deep vein thrombosis, and respiratory issues. While controlled diabetes and hypertension managed with medication are important considerations, obesity poses a higher risk due to its association with increased surgical site infections, delayed wound healing, and challenges in anesthesia

administration. Regular exercise, although beneficial for overall health, may not directly impact the immediate postoperative complications related to obesity in this scenario.

Question 17: Correct Answer: B) Blame the patient for the misunderstanding
Rationale: Blaming the patient for the misunderstanding is not recommended in service recovery as it can escalate the situation and damage the patient-provider relationship. Instead, acknowledging the issue, apologizing sincerely, actively listening to the patient's concerns, and offering a solution or compensation are essential steps in resolving complaints effectively. By taking responsibility, showing empathy, and providing a resolution, healthcare providers can demonstrate their commitment to patient-centered care and quality service delivery.

Question 18: Correct Answer: C) It is suitable for patients with functional gastrointestinal systems.
Rationale: Enteral nutrition administration refers to the delivery of nutrients directly into the gastrointestinal tract. This method is preferred for patients with functional gastrointestinal systems as it helps maintain gut integrity, supports the immune system, and prevents complications associated with prolonged fasting. Options A and B are incorrect as they describe parenteral nutrition, which involves delivering nutrients directly into the bloodstream and bypassing the gastrointestinal tract. Option D is incorrect as enteral nutrition can be used for both short-term and long-term nutritional support, depending on the patient's condition.

Question 19: Correct Answer: C) Assess the patient's pain using a pain scale, notify the healthcare provider if necessary, and provide comfort measures.
Rationale: During hourly rounding, it is crucial for the nurse to assess the patient's pain promptly and effectively. By using a pain scale, the nurse can accurately evaluate the intensity of the pain and take appropriate actions. Administering pain medication without proper assessment can be dangerous and ineffective. Documenting the complaint and informing the next shift nurse may lead to delays in pain management. Ignoring the complaint goes against patient safety protocols and can result in inadequate care. Therefore, assessing the patient's pain, notifying the healthcare provider if needed, and providing comfort measures are the best course of action to ensure patient safety and well-being.

Question 20: Correct Answer: B) Scheduling a follow-up appointment with a primary care provider within a month
Rationale: Effective care coordination involves ensuring a smooth transition for the patient from the hospital to home. Scheduling a follow-up appointment with a primary care provider within a month is crucial as it allows for continued monitoring of the patient's health post-discharge, facilitates communication between healthcare providers, and helps prevent readmissions. Providing a list of medications without explanation (Option A) can lead to confusion and medication errors. Discharging the patient without informing the primary care provider (Option C) hinders continuity of care. Advising the patient to manage their post-discharge care on their own (Option D) can result in inadequate follow-up and potential complications.

Question 21: Correct Answer: A) Assisting Mr. Johnson with shortness of breath and chest pain
Rationale: In this scenario, the priority for the nurse should be to address Mr. Johnson's shortness of breath and chest pain as these symptoms could indicate a medical emergency such as a pulmonary embolism or cardiac issue. Immediate assessment and intervention are crucial to ensure patient safety and prevent further complications. While assisting Mrs. Smith with ambulation is important for fall prevention, it is not as urgent as addressing a potentially life-threatening condition in Mr. Johnson. Delegating tasks or notifying the physician can be done after ensuring the immediate needs of the patient experiencing distress are met. Prioritization skills in nursing involve identifying and addressing the most critical issues first to provide safe and effective patient care.

Question 22: Correct Answer: B) A mentor offers guidance, support, and advice to help the mentee grow professionally.
Rationale: A mentor plays a crucial role in career development relationships by providing valuable guidance, support, and advice to the mentee. This assistance helps the mentee navigate their career path, develop new skills, and achieve professional growth. Option A is incorrect as mentors typically focus on mentorship rather than direct patient care with the mentee. Option C is incorrect as mentors are expected to support and assist others in their career development, not solely focus on their own advancement. Option D is incorrect as mentors should not compete with mentees but rather facilitate their career progression.

Question 23: Correct Answer: A) Providing detailed medication reconciliation
Rationale: Providing detailed medication reconciliation is a critical component of discharge procedures as it ensures that the patient understands their medications, dosages, and schedules post-discharge, reducing the risk of medication errors and improving adherence. Option B is not directly related to the discharge process. Option C, offering magazines, is not a priority compared to medication reconciliation. Option D, scheduling a follow-up appointment, is important but does not encompass the entirety of discharge procedures like medication reconciliation does.

Question 24: Correct Answer: B) Using alcohol-based hand sanitizer before and after patient contact
Rationale: Alcohol-based hand sanitizers are crucial in infection prevention as they effectively reduce the number of microorganisms on hands. Wearing gloves only during invasive procedures (Option A) is not sufficient, as hand hygiene should be practiced consistently. Reusing disposable isolation gowns (Option C) can lead to cross-contamination and should be avoided. Placing used needles in a puncture-resistant container (Option D) is important but does not directly address the prevention of healthcare-associated infections through hand hygiene. Therefore, using alcohol-based hand sanitizer before and after patient contact is the most effective method for infection prevention in a medical-surgical unit.

Question 25: Correct Answer: C) Step 3: Assign a numerical value to occurrence, detection, and severity
Rationale: In FMEA, Step 3 involves assigning a numerical value to the frequency of occurrence, likelihood of detection, and severity of the potential failure mode. This step is crucial as it helps in quantifying the risks associated with each potential failure mode. Options A, B, and D are incorrect as they do not specifically address the process of assigning numerical values to occurrence, detection, and severity, which is a key aspect of FMEA.

Question 26: Correct Answer: A) The patient may be experiencing anxiety.
Rationale: In a medical-surgical setting, sudden increases in blood pressure and heart rate during a routine check-up can often be attributed to anxiety. Patients may feel nervous or stressed during medical appointments, leading to physiological responses such as elevated blood pressure and heart rate. Options B, C, and D are less likely in this scenario as they do not directly correlate with the common response of anxiety during medical assessments. It is crucial for medical-surgical nurses to consider the psychological aspect of patient care and recognize the potential impact of anxiety on vital signs.

Question 27: Correct Answer: D) Collaborative Leadership
Rationale: Collaborative leadership involves working together with team members to achieve common goals, promote open communication, and foster a supportive environment. In the scenario, Sarah demonstrates collaborative leadership by actively involving Emily in decision-making and valuing her input. Option A, Autonomy, focuses on respecting individuals' rights to make decisions about their care, which is not the primary focus of the scenario. Option B, Paternalism, involves making decisions for others without their input, which contrasts with Sarah's approach.

Option C, Advocacy, entails speaking up for patients' rights and needs, which is important but not the central theme of Sarah's leadership style in this scenario.

Question 28: Correct Answer: A) Providing culturally sensitive care by respecting Mr. Patel's dietary preferences and religious practices.
Rationale: Option A is the correct answer as it aligns with the principles of holistic patient care, which emphasize considering the patient's cultural background, beliefs, and preferences in the care plan. By respecting Mr. Patel's dietary preferences and religious practices, the nurse demonstrates cultural sensitivity and inclusion, promoting a therapeutic relationship and enhancing patient outcomes. Options B, C, and D are incorrect as they do not address the importance of cultural competence and may lead to inadequate care delivery, potentially compromising the patient's well-being.

Question 29: Correct Answer: D) Walker
Rationale: In this scenario, the correct equipment for the nurse to ensure patient safety during ambulation for Mr. Johnson, who is recovering from abdominal surgery and on strict bed rest, is a walker. A walker provides the most stability and support for patients who need assistance with walking, especially those who are recovering from surgery and may have limited mobility. Comparing the other options: - Wheelchair (Option A): While a wheelchair may be used for patient transport, it does not provide the support and stability needed for ambulation during the recovery process. - Crutches (Option B): Crutches are typically used for patients who can bear weight on their lower extremities but need assistance with balance and mobility. In this scenario, a walker would be more appropriate for a patient on strict bed rest. - Cane (Option C): A cane is used for patients who need minimal support and assistance with balance. However, for a patient recovering from surgery and on strict bed rest, a walker would offer better stability and support during ambulation.

Question 30: Correct Answer: A) Just-in-time inventory system
Rationale: Just-in-time inventory system is the most cost-effective approach as it involves ordering supplies only as needed, reducing excess inventory costs and minimizing waste. Stockpiling supplies in excess (option B) can lead to increased expenses due to storage and expiration of unused items. Ordering supplies in bulk without assessing usage (option C) may result in unnecessary expenses and wastage. Using disposable supplies for single patient encounters (option D) can be costly and unsustainable in the long run, impacting the budget negatively. Therefore, the most efficient method for managing supplies within budget constraints is the just-in-time inventory system.

Question 31: Correct Answer: B) Demonstrating empathy and understanding
Rationale: Active listening is a crucial skill for CMSRNs, and demonstrating empathy and understanding is a key component. Option A is incorrect as interrupting the speaker hinders effective communication. Option C is incorrect because active listening involves focusing on the speaker, not formulating responses. Option D is incorrect as maintaining eye contact shows respect and engagement in the conversation, essential for active listening. By choosing option B, the nurse can establish rapport, build trust, and better comprehend the patient's needs, leading to improved patient outcomes.

Question 32: Correct Answer: C) Regularly checking in with Ms. Johnson to review her progress and offer positive feedback.
Rationale: In the context of the ADKAR model, the 'Reinforcement' stage involves providing ongoing support, feedback, and encouragement to individuals to sustain the change. Option C is the correct answer as it aligns with the reinforcement phase by emphasizing the importance of regularly checking in with Ms. Johnson to review her progress and offer positive feedback. Options A, B, and D focus more on the Knowledge and Desire stages of the model, rather than the specific reinforcement needed

to support Ms. Johnson through the change process.

Question 33: Correct Answer: C) Parenteral nutrition bypasses the gastrointestinal tract and delivers nutrients directly into the bloodstream.

Rationale: The correct answer is C) Parenteral nutrition bypasses the gastrointestinal tract and delivers nutrients directly into the bloodstream. This route is essential for patients like Mr. Smith who cannot tolerate oral intake or have gastrointestinal issues. Option A is incorrect as parenteral nutrition is administered outside the gastrointestinal tract. Option B is incorrect as enteral nutrition is usually preferred when the gastrointestinal tract is functional. Option D is incorrect as parenteral nutrition is indicated for patients who cannot tolerate oral intake, making it a crucial alternative route for meeting nutritional needs.

Question 34: Correct Answer: D) Patients with access to lethal means are at higher risk for suicide.

Rationale: Patients with access to lethal means, such as firearms or medications, are at a significantly higher risk for completing suicide. This is a crucial aspect of suicide risk assessment as it directly impacts patient safety. Options A, B, and C are incorrect as they provide inaccurate information that could potentially lead to overlooking serious warning signs. Understanding the correlation between access to lethal means and suicide risk is essential for healthcare providers to implement appropriate patient safety protocols and interventions.

Question 35: Correct Answer: D) Arranging for a home health nurse to visit Mrs. Smith regularly to monitor her condition and medication adherence.

Rationale: The most crucial intervention to prevent readmissions for Mrs. Smith, a high-risk patient with heart failure and diabetes, is arranging for a home health nurse to provide regular monitoring of her condition and medication adherence. While options A, B, and C are important aspects of care coordination and transition management, the direct oversight and support provided by a home health nurse are essential for patients like Mrs. Smith who have complex care needs, limited support, and a history of frequent readmissions. Regular monitoring can help identify issues early, provide education, and ensure continuity of care, ultimately reducing the risk of hospital readmissions.

Question 36: Correct Answer: B) "I understand that complete pain relief may not always be possible, but I hope to have manageable pain."

Rationale: Mrs. Smith's statement in option B reflects a realistic expectation regarding pain management. It acknowledges the possibility that complete pain relief may not always be achievable but emphasizes the importance of having pain at a manageable level. This approach aligns with the principles of effective pain management, which aim to control pain to a tolerable level rather than completely eliminating it. Options A, C, and D present unrealistic expectations by either expecting total pain elimination, demanding immediate relief without considering medical protocols, or advocating for enduring pain without appropriate intervention, respectively. Mrs. Smith's understanding in option B demonstrates a balanced perspective on pain management expectations, focusing on achieving a tolerable level of pain during her recovery.

Question 37: Correct Answer: B) Consult with the charge nurse or pharmacist to verify the medication dosage before administering it.

Rationale: In this scenario, the correct course of action for Nurse Sarah is to consult with the charge nurse or pharmacist to verify the medication dosage before administering it. This aligns with the principles of patient safety culture and near miss reporting, where healthcare professionals are encouraged to speak up and address potential errors or near misses to prevent harm to patients. Option A is incorrect as administering the medication without verification could pose a risk to the patient's safety. Option C is incorrect as disregarding concerns goes against the principles of patient safety. Option D is incorrect as documenting the incident without reporting it does not address the potential risk to the patient and misses the

opportunity for improvement in the system.

Question 38: Correct Answer: A) Check the infusion pump settings and ensure proper medication delivery.

Rationale: In this scenario, the nurse's priority action should be to check the infusion pump settings and ensure proper medication delivery through the epidural catheter. This step is crucial to verify that the epidural infusion is functioning correctly and delivering the prescribed medication at the appropriate rate. Repositioning the patient or administering oral pain medication may not address the underlying issue of inadequate pain relief from the epidural infusion. Notifying the healthcare provider should be done after ensuring the pump settings are correct, as the provider may need this information to make further decisions.

Question 39: Correct Answer: B) Double-checking the patient's identification before administering medication

Rationale: Patient safety is paramount in healthcare, and one crucial aspect is medication administration. Double-checking the patient's identification before giving medication helps ensure that the right medication is given to the right patient, reducing the risk of medication errors. Options A, C, and D all pose significant threats to patient safety by increasing the likelihood of medication errors, infections, and compromised care quality. Therefore, option B is the correct choice as it aligns with patient safety protocols and best practices in healthcare.

Question 40: Correct Answer: B) Consult with the healthcare team to discuss the cost-effectiveness of the advanced wound dressing.

Rationale: Option B is the correct answer as it demonstrates the nurse's understanding of the importance of budgetary considerations in healthcare while also prioritizing patient care. By consulting with the healthcare team, the nurse can gather input on the cost-effectiveness of the advanced wound dressing and make an informed decision that balances quality patient care with financial constraints. Options A and D are incorrect as they overlook the budgetary implications, potentially leading to resource wastage. Option C, while considering budget limits, does not involve a collaborative approach or consideration of the patient's specific needs, making it a less optimal choice in this scenario.

Question 41: Correct Answer: C) Consult with an interpreter to explain oral care instructions in Gujarati.

Rationale: Providing culturally sensitive care involves respecting the patient's language preferences. In this scenario, Ms. Patel's preferred language is Gujarati, so using an interpreter to explain oral care instructions ensures effective communication. Option A is incorrect as providing information in English may not be understood by the patient. Option B is not the best choice as the patient's dry mouth may require more than just a mint-flavored mouthwash. Option D, while non-verbal demonstration is helpful, verbal instructions in the patient's language are crucial for understanding and compliance.

Question 42: Correct Answer: D) Follow facility protocol for reporting deaths to the coroner.

Rationale: In this scenario, the correct action for the CMSRN is to follow the facility's protocol for reporting deaths to the coroner. It is essential to adhere to established procedures to ensure legal and regulatory requirements are met. Option A is incorrect as notifying the coroner immediately may not be in line with the facility's specific protocols. Option B is incorrect because waiting for the family to arrive before contacting the coroner could delay the necessary procedures. Option C is incorrect as the primary step should be to report the death to the appropriate authorities as per facility guidelines. Therefore, option D is the most appropriate course of action in this situation.

Question 43: Correct Answer: C) Utilize a professional medical interpreter to facilitate communication.

Rationale: In this scenario, the most appropriate action for the CMSRN to take is to utilize a professional medical interpreter to facilitate effective communication with Mrs. Rodriguez. Option A is incorrect as using basic English words and gestures may lead to misinterpretation of symptoms. Option B is not recommended as family members may not accurately convey medical information. Option D is inappropriate as ignoring the language barrier can compromise patient care and safety. Utilizing a professional medical interpreter ensures accurate communication, promotes patient understanding, and upholds ethical standards of care.

Question 44: Correct Answer: B) Lavender essential oil may help reduce postoperative pain and promote relaxation.

Rationale: Option A is incorrect as lavender essential oil is generally safe for postoperative pain and has been shown to have analgesic and anxiolytic effects. Option C is incorrect as essential oils should never be applied directly to surgical incision sites due to the risk of irritation or infection. Option D is incorrect as essential oils should not be ingested orally without proper guidance. Option B is the correct answer as lavender essential oil is commonly used in aromatherapy for its calming and pain-relieving properties, making it a suitable option for Mrs. Smith's postoperative pain management.

Question 45: Correct Answer: C) "I will apply heat to the surgical incision to promote healing."

Rationale: Option C is incorrect because applying heat to a surgical incision can increase the risk of infection and delay healing. The correct postoperative care includes keeping the surgical site clean and dry, monitoring for signs of infection, and using techniques like deep breathing exercises with an incentive spirometer to prevent respiratory complications. Heat application can lead to vasodilation, which may increase the risk of bleeding and infection at the surgical site. Therefore, it is essential for the patient to avoid applying heat to the incision site postoperatively.

Question 46: Correct Answer: B) Proper documentation of patient care interventions

Rationale: Proper documentation of patient care interventions is crucial for patient safety assessments and reporting as it provides a detailed record of the care provided, any changes in the patient's condition, and the outcomes of interventions. This documentation helps in tracking the patient's progress, identifying any potential safety issues, and ensuring continuity of care among healthcare team members. Options A, C, and D are incorrect as they do not align with the principles of patient safety, which emphasize effective communication, collaboration, and responsiveness to patient needs and concerns.

Question 47: Correct Answer: B) Using a professional medical interpreter when needed

Rationale: Utilizing a professional medical interpreter when needed is crucial in addressing cultural and linguistic needs effectively. Option A is incorrect as relying solely on written instructions may not be sufficient for patients with language barriers. Option C is incorrect as ignoring a patient's cultural background can lead to misunderstandings and hinder effective care. Option D is incorrect as speaking loudly can be perceived as disrespectful and does not address the core issue of language comprehension. By choosing option B, healthcare providers demonstrate respect for diversity and inclusion, ensuring holistic patient care.

Question 48: Correct Answer: C) Critical thinking includes analyzing information objectively and making informed decisions.

Rationale: Critical thinking for a CMSRN involves the ability to analyze information objectively, consider various perspectives, evaluate evidence, and make informed decisions based on sound reasoning. Option A is incorrect as critical thinking emphasizes considering all available information before making decisions. Option B is inaccurate because critical thinking is a dynamic and iterative process that involves reflection and evaluation. Option D is misleading as critical thinking in nursing requires evidence-based practice rather than relying solely on intuition or personal beliefs.

Question 49: Correct Answer: B) Ensure patient privacy and confidentiality are maintained.

Rationale: During bedside report, it is crucial for the nurse to prioritize patient privacy and confidentiality. Sharing personal information with other healthcare staff (Option A) violates patient confidentiality. Skipping medication reconciliation (Option C) can lead to errors in patient care. Using medical jargon (Option D) can hinder effective communication with the patient. Therefore, ensuring patient privacy and confidentiality (Option B) is the most appropriate and professional approach during bedside report.

Question 50: Correct Answer: B) Ensuring Mrs. Smith has a follow-up appointment with her primary care physician within a week.

Rationale: Effective care coordination and transition management involve ensuring continuity of care for the patient. Providing Mrs. Smith with a follow-up appointment with her primary care physician within a week is crucial for monitoring her recovery progress, addressing any post-operative concerns, and ensuring appropriate follow-up care. Options A, C, and D do not promote comprehensive care coordination as they either lack professional follow-up support, adequate guidance, or may lead to potential complications by not emphasizing the importance of post-operative care under the continuum of care principles.

Question 51: Correct Answer: C) Tailoring the orientation process to the individual's learning needs

Rationale: It is essential to tailor the orientation process to the individual's learning needs to ensure a successful transition into the new role. By customizing the orientation plan, preceptors can address specific learning styles, previous experience, and areas of improvement for each orientee. Providing personalized guidance enhances the orientee's understanding, confidence, and competence in their new role. Options A, B, and D are incorrect as they promote practices that can hinder the orientee's learning experience and potentially compromise patient care.

Question 52: Correct Answer: A) Allow the nursing assistant to remove the dressing under direct supervision.

Rationale: In this scenario, the most appropriate action for the CMSRN to take is to allow the nursing assistant to remove the dressing under direct supervision. Delegation involves entrusting a task to a competent individual while providing guidance and oversight. Allowing the nursing assistant to perform the task under direct supervision ensures patient safety and promotes teamwork. Option B is incorrect as the task should not be delegated independently without supervision. Option C is incorrect as delegating to another nursing assistant without direct supervision may compromise patient care. Option D is incorrect as the CMSRN should focus on supervision and delegation rather than performing tasks that can be safely delegated.

Question 53: Correct Answer: B) Assessing the patient's airway and breathing

Rationale: In the scenario provided, the priority action in managing Mr. Smith's burns is to assess his airway and breathing (Option B). This is crucial in determining if there is any compromise to his respiratory system due to the burns. Administering pain medication (Option A) can come later once the patient's airway and breathing are stabilized. Applying cold compress to the burns (Option C) is contraindicated as it can further damage the skin. Notifying the family (Option D) is important but not the immediate priority compared to ensuring the patient's airway and breathing are intact.

Question 54: Correct Answer: C) Verifying the medication with another nurse before administration.

Rationale: Verifying medications with another nurse before administration is a crucial step in ensuring patient safety and preventing medication errors. This process, known as the "two-check system," helps in confirming the right patient, medication, dose, route, and time. It acts as a double-check mechanism to reduce the risk of errors. Options A and B pose serious risks to patient safety as they can lead to medication errors and adverse effects. Option D is unsafe as using an outdated drug reference guide may result in inaccurate information, potentially compromising patient care. Therefore, option C is the most appropriate and safe practice in medication management.

Question 55: Correct Answer: C) Recording information as soon as possible after providing care

Rationale: Documenting patient care promptly after providing it is essential for accuracy and completeness of medical records. Option A is incorrect as abbreviations can lead to misinterpretation and errors. Option B is incorrect as delaying documentation increases the risk of missing important details. Option D is incorrect as relying on memory compromises the reliability of the documentation. Therefore, the best practice is to record information promptly to ensure the integrity and quality of patient care documentation.

Question 56: Correct Answer: A) Attending a workshop on conflict resolution within healthcare teams.

Rationale: Option A is the correct answer as attending a workshop on conflict resolution within healthcare teams will directly enhance Sarah's nursing teamwork and collaboration skills. This resource will provide her with practical strategies to effectively communicate and work with other healthcare professionals, ultimately improving patient care outcomes. Option B, subscribing to a nursing journal, while informative, may not specifically target nursing teamwork and collaboration. Option C, participating in a social media group, although beneficial for networking, may not offer structured guidance on teamwork skills. Option D, watching online tutorials on basic nursing skills, is important but does not focus on the specific aspect of teamwork and collaboration.

Question 57: Correct Answer: C) Reporting any unsafe conditions or practices promptly

Rationale: Reporting any unsafe conditions or practices promptly is crucial for maintaining workplace safety as a CMSRN. This action helps prevent accidents, injuries, and potential harm to patients, colleagues, and oneself. Option A is incorrect as ignoring safety protocols compromises safety. Option B is incorrect as using PPE inconsistently can lead to exposure risks. Option D is incorrect as disregarding ergonomic principles can result in musculoskeletal injuries. By promptly reporting unsafe conditions or practices, CMSRNs contribute to creating a safe and healthy practice environment, reflecting professional responsibility and commitment to workplace safety.

Question 58: Correct Answer: B) Notify the healthcare provider immediately

Rationale: In this scenario, Mr. Johnson's sudden onset of severe abdominal pain, along with other symptoms, raises concerns for a potentially serious underlying condition such as a perforated viscus or bowel obstruction. As a medical-surgical nurse, critical thinking involves recognizing abnormal findings and taking prompt action to ensure patient safety. Notifying the healthcare provider immediately is crucial to facilitate further evaluation and appropriate interventions. Administering pain medication without further assessment or orders, offering antacids for non-specific symptoms, or solely documenting findings without acting on them could delay necessary medical intervention and jeopardize Mr. Johnson's well-being.

Question 59: Correct Answer: C) Turning and repositioning the patient every two hours

Rationale: Turning and repositioning the patient every two hours is crucial in preventing further skin breakdown and promoting wound healing in pressure ulcers. This intervention helps to relieve pressure on the affected area, improve circulation, and reduce the risk of tissue damage. Applying a hydrocolloid dressing (Option A) is important for wound healing but is not the highest priority in this scenario. Administering oral antibiotics (Option B) is essential for treating infection but does not address the primary prevention of pressure ulcers. Implementing a pressure redistribution mattress (Option D) is beneficial but should be combined with turning and repositioning for optimal pressure ulcer management.

Question 60: Correct Answer: B) Inform the patient that the medication cannot be given without a physician's order.

Rationale: Option A is incorrect because administering medication without a physician's order violates hospital policy and legal requirements, potentially putting the patient at risk. Option C involves unnecessary escalation as the charge nurse may also advise against administering the medication. Option D delays addressing the patient's pain and does not provide a clear explanation. Option B is the correct choice as it upholds legislative and licensure requirements by ensuring medication administration follows proper protocols, protecting both the patient and the nurse legally and ethically.

Question 61: Correct Answer: A) Approach the charge nurse privately to discuss the issue and request a fair redistribution of patients.

Rationale: Option A is the correct answer as it demonstrates staff advocacy by addressing the issue through appropriate channels. The CMSRN should communicate with the charge nurse to ensure fair workload distribution, promoting staff well-being and collaboration. Option B is incorrect as advocating for staff is part of the CMSRN's role in promoting a positive work environment. Option C is incorrect as confronting Sarah directly may not address the root cause of the issue and could lead to conflict. Option D is incorrect as reporting directly to hospital administration without attempting to resolve the issue internally may not promote effective teamwork and collaboration among staff members.

Question 62: Correct Answer: B) Calling for assistance to help reorient and safely transfer the patient back to bed

Rationale: In this scenario, the correct action for the nurse to prioritize during safety rounds is to call for assistance to help reorient and safely transfer the confused patient back to bed. This ensures patient safety by preventing falls or injuries that may occur if the patient attempts to get out of bed unassisted. Administering a sedative (Option A) should not be the first response as it does not address the underlying issue of confusion. Documenting the incident (Option C) is important but should not take precedence over immediate patient safety. Ignoring the behavior (Option D) is not appropriate and could lead to adverse outcomes.

Question 63: Correct Answer: C) Inserted through a peripheral vein with tip placement in the central venous system

Rationale: The correct answer is C) Inserted through a peripheral vein with tip placement in the central venous system. A PICC is a type of central venous access device that is inserted through a peripheral vein, typically in the upper arm, with the tip of the catheter placed in the central venous system. This allows for long-term intravenous therapy while reducing the risk of complications associated with other central venous access devices. Option A, subcutaneous port for medication administration, is incorrect as it describes a subcutaneous port, not a PICC. Option B, external catheter that exits the body, is incorrect as it describes a tunneled central venous catheter, not a PICC. Option D, used for short-term intravenous therapy, is incorrect as PICCs are typically used for long-term intravenous therapy.

Question 64: Correct Answer: A) Provides a fresh perspective and additional expertise.

Rationale: Seeking a second opinion in patient care is a common practice that can enhance the quality of decision-making and patient outcomes. Option A is correct as it highlights the benefits of obtaining a fresh perspective and additional expertise, which can lead to a more comprehensive understanding of the patient's condition and treatment options. In contrast, options B and C are incorrect as they present negative consequences that are not necessarily associated with seeking a second opinion. Option D is also incorrect as seeking a second opinion does not always indicate a lack of trust but rather a proactive approach to ensuring the best possible care for the patient.

Question 65: Correct Answer: B) Encouraging open communication about errors

Rationale: In a "just culture," the emphasis is on promoting open communication about errors without fear of retribution. Option A is incorrect as blaming individuals for errors goes against the principles of a just culture. Option C is incorrect because a just culture focuses on addressing system failures rather than punishing individuals. Option D is also incorrect as ignoring errors does not contribute to a culture of safety and improvement. Encouraging open communication about errors fosters a transparent environment where lessons can be learned and patient safety can be enhanced.

Question 66: Correct Answer: C) Consulting with the healthcare provider to adjust the pain medication due to liver cirrhosis
Rationale: In this scenario, the nurse should prioritize consulting with the healthcare provider to adjust the pain medication due to Mr. Johnson's history of liver cirrhosis. Acetaminophen is metabolized in the liver and can potentially worsen liver function in patients with cirrhosis. Oxycodone, on the other hand, may require dose adjustments or alternative medications due to altered metabolism in liver disease. Option A is incorrect as administering the prescribed medications without considering the patient's liver condition can lead to adverse effects. Option B is a good supportive measure but not the priority in this case. Option D is beneficial for long-term management but does not address the immediate concern of medication adjustment for liver cirrhosis.

Question 67: Correct Answer: C) Coordinate a meeting to discuss and integrate both recommendations.
Rationale: Effective communication and collaboration within the interdisciplinary team are crucial for providing comprehensive care to patients. In this scenario, option C is the correct choice as it demonstrates the nurse's role in facilitating communication between team members to ensure all recommendations are considered and integrated into the patient's care plan. Options A and B are incorrect as they involve favoring one recommendation over the other, which may not be in the patient's best interest. Option D is incorrect as it disregards the expertise of other team members and goes against the principles of interprofessional collaboration.

Question 68: Correct Answer: C) Distraction techniques
Rationale: Distraction techniques, such as guided imagery, music therapy, or deep breathing exercises, have been shown to be effective in managing acute pain in postoperative patients by diverting their attention away from the pain sensation. Heat therapy and cold therapy are more commonly used for musculoskeletal injuries or chronic pain conditions. Massage therapy can be beneficial for relaxation and reducing muscle tension but may not be as effective for acute postoperative pain management. Therefore, distraction techniques are the most suitable non-pharmacological intervention for acute pain in this context.

Question 69: Correct Answer: B) Removing potentially harmful objects from the patient's environment.
Rationale: As a CMSRN, the priority is to ensure patient safety, especially for those at risk for suicide. Removing potentially harmful objects, such as sharp items or medications, from the patient's environment is crucial to prevent self-harm. Allowing the patient to be alone for extended periods (Option A) can increase the risk of suicide. Providing sharp objects (Option C) can be dangerous and goes against safety protocols. Discussing suicide methods in detail (Option D) may trigger or worsen the patient's condition, rather than promoting safety and prevention.

Question 70: Correct Answer: B) Massage therapy
Rationale: Massage therapy is a widely accepted nonpharmacological intervention in chronic pain management due to its ability to promote relaxation, reduce muscle tension, and alleviate stress. Acupuncture (Option A) involves the insertion of thin needles into specific points on the body to help relieve pain, while herbal supplements (Option C) are ingested substances derived from plants that may have medicinal properties but are not typically the primary intervention for chronic pain. Electrotherapy (Option D) uses electrical stimulation for pain relief, but massage therapy is more commonly associated with relaxation and stress

reduction in chronic pain management.

Question 71: Correct Answer: A) Active listening
Rationale: Active listening is a crucial communication skill for a CMSRN when working within an interdisciplinary team. It involves fully concentrating on what is being said, understanding the information, and responding thoughtfully. This skill fosters effective teamwork, enhances collaboration, and promotes a supportive work environment. On the other hand, options B, C, and D are detrimental to effective communication within the team. Interrupting others, avoiding eye contact, and speaking over colleagues can lead to misunderstandings, conflicts, and breakdowns in communication, hindering the quality of patient care and teamwork.

Question 72: Correct Answer: D) Modified Early Warning Score (MEWS)
Rationale: The correct answer is D) Modified Early Warning Score (MEWS). MEWS is a validated tool used to assess and track a patient's physiological parameters over time to detect early signs of clinical deterioration. In this scenario, Mr. Johnson's symptoms of shortness of breath and chest pain indicate a potential deterioration in his condition, making MEWS the most appropriate risk assessment method to monitor his vital signs closely. Comparing the incorrect options: A) Braden Scale: The Braden Scale is used for predicting pressure sore risk in patients, which is not relevant to Mr. Johnson's current symptoms. B) Morse Fall Scale: This scale assesses a patient's risk of falling, which is not the primary concern in Mr. Johnson's case. C) Glasgow Coma Scale: This scale is used to assess a patient's level of consciousness, which is not the immediate priority for Mr. Johnson, given his symptoms of shortness of breath and chest pain.

Question 73: Correct Answer: C) Involving the patient in decision-making and respecting their values.
Rationale: Holistic patient care in end-of-life preferences involves considering the physical, emotional, social, and spiritual aspects of the patient. By involving the patient in decision-making and respecting their values, the nurse acknowledges the importance of the patient's autonomy and individual beliefs. Providing information only on medical interventions (Option A) neglects the emotional and spiritual needs of the patient. Ignoring emotional and spiritual needs (Option B) can lead to inadequate support. Making decisions for the patient (Option D) disregards their autonomy and preferences, contradicting holistic care principles.

Question 74: Correct Answer: C) The physical therapist collaborates with the nurse to develop a mobility plan for Mr. Smith.
Rationale: Interprofessional care involves collaboration among healthcare team members to provide comprehensive and holistic care to patients. In this scenario, option C is the correct answer as it demonstrates collaboration between the physical therapist and nurse to address Mr. Smith's mobility needs, considering his overall health status. Options A and B represent actions taken independently by individual team members, which do not reflect interprofessional care. Option D overlooks the importance of considering the patient's preferences in providing dietary recommendations, which is essential in patient-centered care.

Question 75: Correct Answer: D) Initiating a multidisciplinary team meeting to discuss the patient's discharge plan.
Rationale: Initiating a multidisciplinary team meeting to discuss the patient's discharge plan is the most appropriate action that demonstrates effective nursing teamwork and collaboration in this scenario. This approach involves gathering input from various healthcare professionals, such as physicians, pharmacists, social workers, and physical therapists, to address the patient's complex needs comprehensively. While providing written instructions (Option A) and scheduling a follow-up appointment (Option B) are important aspects of patient care, they do not fully utilize the benefits of teamwork and collaboration. Consulting with the pharmacist (Option C) is valuable but may not address all aspects of the patient's discharge plan. By initiating a multidisciplinary team meeting, the nurse ensures a holistic approach to addressing the

patient's medication management concerns and promotes continuity of care post-discharge.

Question 76: Correct Answer: D) Using alcohol-based hand rub before and after wound care procedures.

Rationale: The correct answer is D) Using alcohol-based hand rub before and after wound care procedures. Current evidence-based practice emphasizes the importance of hand hygiene in infection prevention. Alcohol-based hand rub is preferred over soap and water for routine hand hygiene in healthcare settings as it is more effective in reducing the transmission of microorganisms. Options A, B, and C are incorrect as daily dressing changes with sterile technique, cleaning with hydrogen peroxide, and applying antibiotic ointment are not recommended as routine practices in surgical wound care according to current evidence-based guidelines.

Question 77: Correct Answer: A) Notify the healthcare provider immediately

Rationale: In this scenario, the presence of redness, warmth, tenderness, purulent drainage, and fever at the central line insertion site indicates a potential central line-associated bloodstream infection (CLABSI). The most appropriate initial nursing action is to notify the healthcare provider immediately to ensure timely intervention, such as initiating appropriate antibiotic therapy, obtaining blood cultures, and potentially removing the central line if indicated. Administering antibiotics through the central line without proper evaluation and guidance can lead to further complications. Removing the central line and sending the tip for culture should be done under the healthcare provider's direction to prevent contamination and ensure accurate results. Applying a warm compress is not the priority in this situation and may exacerbate the infection.

Question 78: Correct Answer: B) Telemedicine

Rationale: Telemedicine is a technology trend in health care that enables healthcare professionals to remotely monitor patients' vital signs, provide consultations, and deliver care over a distance. This technology allows for increased access to healthcare services, especially in rural or underserved areas. Electronic Health Records (EHR) focus on digitalizing patient health information for easy access and sharing among healthcare providers. Artificial Intelligence (AI) in Diagnostics involves using algorithms to analyze medical data for diagnostic purposes. Virtual Reality (VR) is utilized for training, pain management, and therapeutic interventions in healthcare settings. However, in the context of remote patient monitoring, telemedicine is the most relevant technology trend.

Question 79: Correct Answer: C) Verifying the patient's identity using two unique identifiers before administering medication.

Rationale: Verifying a patient's identity using two unique identifiers, such as name and date of birth, is a crucial step in medication administration to ensure patient safety and compliance with regulatory requirements and standards of practice. Option A is incorrect as it violates patient safety protocols. Option B is incorrect as documentation should always be based on actual assessments. Option D is incorrect as patient consent is essential for decision-making in healthcare, respecting the patient's autonomy and rights.

Question 80: Correct Answer: B) Providing care outside the scope of practice without proper training

Rationale: Providing care outside the scope of practice without proper training is considered unsafe practice as it can lead to harm or adverse outcomes for the patient. Reporting a medication error, following evidence-based practice guidelines, and collaborating with the healthcare team are all examples of safe and ethical practices that promote patient safety and quality care. It is essential for MSRN to adhere to their scope of practice, seek appropriate resources, and uphold professional standards to ensure safe and effective patient care.

Question 81: Correct Answer: B) Document the time and date of death in the patient's medical record

Rationale: Reporting a patient's death is a critical aspect of nursing practice, especially in Palliative/End-of-Life Care and Holistic Patient Care settings. Option B is the correct choice as it aligns with regulatory requirements to accurately document the time and date of death in the patient's medical record. This documentation is essential for legal and administrative purposes, ensuring proper closure of the patient's medical file and facilitating the necessary procedures following a patient's passing. Options A, C, and D are incorrect as they do not adhere to the standard regulatory protocols for reporting a patient's death, which require timely and accurate documentation to maintain transparency and accountability in healthcare practices.

Question 82: Correct Answer: B) Perform a 12-lead ECG and notify the healthcare provider

Rationale: In this scenario, Mr. Smith is presenting with symptoms suggestive of a possible cardiac event, such as chest pain, diaphoresis, and shortness of breath. His vital signs also indicate potential cardiac compromise. Performing a 12-lead ECG is crucial to assess for any cardiac abnormalities and to determine the appropriate course of action. Notifying the healthcare provider promptly allows for timely intervention and management. Administering oxygen (option A) is important but should not delay the ECG. Offering a warm blanket (option C) is not a priority in this critical situation. Simply documenting the findings (option D) without taking immediate action can compromise patient safety.

Question 83: Correct Answer: A) Implementing a new electronic health record system that leads to increased documentation errors

Rationale: Unintended consequences can arise when changes are made in healthcare settings. In this scenario, option A highlights the unintended consequence of implementing a new electronic health record system, which was intended to streamline documentation but instead led to increased errors. This outcome underscores the importance of carefully evaluating and planning changes to mitigate unintended consequences. Options B, C, and D all describe positive outcomes or intended consequences, which do not align with the concept of unintended consequences in a healthcare setting.

Question 84: Correct Answer: C) Advocating for the patient to receive pain medication based on the patient's self-report

Rationale: Option A is incorrect as administering pain medication without assessing the patient's pain level can lead to inappropriate pain management. Option B is incorrect as it goes against patient advocacy by neglecting the patient's right to pain relief. Option D is incorrect as ignoring the patient's pain complaints contradicts the nurse's role as an advocate. Option C is the correct answer as advocating for pain medication based on the patient's self-report aligns with patient advocacy principles, ensuring the patient's voice is heard and their pain is effectively managed.

Question 85: Correct Answer: A) Evidence-based practice

Rationale: Evidence-based practice is a crucial component of the Nursing professional practice model as it involves integrating the best available evidence with clinical expertise and patient preferences to make informed decisions about patient care. This approach ensures that nurses stay current with the latest research and advancements in healthcare, leading to improved patient outcomes. Cost-effective care focuses on efficient resource utilization, patient-centered care prioritizes individual preferences, and traditional nursing care may not always align with the most current evidence-based practices, making them less ideal choices in the context of quality management and professional concepts.

Question 86: Correct Answer: A) Initiate discussions about hospice care options with Mrs. Smith and her family.

Rationale: Mrs. Smith's expressed wish to discontinue aggressive treatments and focus on comfort care aligns with the principles of palliative and end-of-life care. Initiating discussions about hospice care options respects her preferences for quality of life over aggressive interventions. Increasing pain medication dosage may not address the holistic needs of the patient at this stage. Recommending a new chemotherapy regimen goes against Mrs. Smith's preference for comfort care. Transfer to the intensive care unit would not align with her desire to spend her remaining time at home with family.

Question 87: Correct Answer: C) Notify the healthcare provider about the fluctuating oxygen saturation levels.

Rationale: In this scenario, the most appropriate action for the nursing team is to notify the healthcare provider about the fluctuating oxygen saturation levels in a patient with a history of COPD. Increasing the oxygen flow rate without healthcare provider's order (Option A) can potentially lead to oxygen toxicity. Placing the patient on a non-rebreather mask at a high flow rate (Option B) is not indicated unless there is a medical emergency. Discontinuing oxygen therapy (Option D) without proper assessment and orders can compromise the patient's respiratory status. Therefore, the best course of action is to communicate the concerning findings to the healthcare provider for further evaluation and management.

Question 88: Correct Answer: D) Request a professional medical interpreter fluent in Gujarati to assist with the pain assessment.

Rationale: Option A is incorrect as relying solely on a language translation app may lead to misinterpretation and misunderstanding of critical information due to nuances in language. Option B is not the best choice as family members may not accurately convey medical information, compromising patient care. Option C is inappropriate as using written materials in a language the patient does not understand is ineffective. Option D is the correct answer as it ensures accurate and clear communication by involving a professional medical interpreter who is fluent in Gujarati, aligning with the CMSRN's responsibility to provide holistic patient care and meet cultural and linguistic needs effectively.

Question 89: Correct Answer: C) Compassion fatigue

Rationale: Compassion fatigue is the emotional and physical exhaustion that healthcare professionals may experience when they repeatedly engage in empathetic interactions with patients who are suffering. In this scenario, the nurse's ongoing care for Mr. Smith despite feeling emotionally drained highlights the risk of compassion fatigue. Burnout, although related, is characterized by feelings of exhaustion and detachment from work tasks. Empathy is the ability to understand and share the feelings of another, which the nurse demonstrates towards Mr. Smith. Sympathy involves feelings of pity or sorrow for someone's misfortune, which is not the primary concept depicted in this scenario.

Question 90: Correct Answer: D) Prealbumin level of 10 mg/dL

Rationale: Prealbumin is a sensitive marker for acute changes in nutritional status and reflects protein-energy malnutrition. A prealbumin level of 10 mg/dL indicates severe malnutrition as it falls below the normal range of 15-36 mg/dL. BMI, albumin, and hemoglobin levels can be influenced by factors other than malnutrition, making them less specific indicators. Therefore, a low prealbumin level is a more reliable marker for severe malnutrition in patients.

Question 91: Correct Answer: C) Communication

Rationale: Communication is a fundamental element in interprofessional collaboration for successful problem-solving. Effective communication ensures that all team members understand the patient's needs, treatment plans, and goals, leading to coordinated care delivery. Autonomy, on the other hand, can hinder collaboration by promoting individual decision-making over teamwork. Competition within the team can create conflicts and hinder the sharing of information. Isolation of team members prevents the exchange of ideas and expertise necessary for collaborative problem-solving. Therefore, communication plays a crucial role in fostering teamwork, shared decision-making, and ultimately, improved patient outcomes.

Question 92: Correct Answer: D) Supportive nurse leadership and management

Rationale: A healthy practice environment for CMSRNs is characterized by supportive nurse leadership and management. This includes having leaders who advocate for nurses, provide resources for professional growth, and foster a culture of open communication and teamwork. Option A is incorrect as high nurse-to-patient ratios can lead to burnout and decreased quality of care. Option B is incorrect as interprofessional collaboration is essential for optimal patient outcomes. Option C is incorrect as access to professional development opportunities is crucial for career advancement and maintaining competency.

Question 93: Correct Answer: B) Place a caution sign near the spill and notify the unit manager

Rationale: The correct answer is to place a caution sign near the spill and notify the unit manager. This action ensures that other staff members are aware of the hazard and can avoid the area until it is properly cleaned. Option A is incorrect as the nurse should prioritize alerting others to the spill before attempting to clean it up. Option C is incorrect as the nurse should not delegate the responsibility of cleaning up a hazardous spill to a nursing assistant. Option D is incorrect as ignoring the spill poses a risk to both staff and patients, compromising workplace safety.

Question 94: Correct Answer: A) Provide information on patient assistance programs offered by pharmaceutical companies.

Rationale: It is crucial for CMSRNs to be aware of patient assistance programs provided by pharmaceutical companies to help patients like Ms. Johnson access necessary medications despite financial constraints. Option B is incorrect as skipping doses can lead to ineffective treatment and worsen the patient's condition. Option C is not advisable without consulting the healthcare provider, as over-the-counter alternatives may not be suitable or effective for the patient's specific condition. Option D is unsafe and can have serious consequences on the patient's health. By choosing option A, the CMSRN demonstrates advocacy for the patient's well-being while addressing the financial implications of medication management.

Question 95: Correct Answer: B) Ensuring patient safety

Rationale: Ensuring patient safety is the top priority during a crisis in a medical-surgical unit. This involves assessing the situation, stabilizing the patient, and preventing further harm. Documenting the events, although important for legal and quality improvement purposes, should not take precedence over immediate patient safety. Contacting family members can provide support but is not the primary action during a crisis. Administering medications may be necessary but should come after ensuring the patient's safety and stability. Therefore, the correct answer is to prioritize ensuring patient safety first in a crisis situation.

Question 96: Correct Answer: B) Obtaining informed consent from the patient after explaining the procedure, risks, benefits, and alternatives.

Rationale: In the context of moderate/procedural sedation, obtaining informed consent is a crucial step before any procedure. Option A is incorrect as it violates the ethical principle of autonomy and informed decision-making. Option C is incorrect as patient assessment is essential to ensure safe sedation administration. Option D is incorrect as consent must be obtained directly from the patient unless they are incapacitated, in which case appropriate legal steps should be followed. Therefore, option B is the correct choice as it aligns with ethical and legal standards in patient care management.

Question 97: Correct Answer: B) Organize a team meeting to discuss the importance of teamwork in patient care.

Rationale: Option B is the correct answer as it promotes open communication and collaboration among team members, fostering a supportive environment essential for effective patient care. This approach encourages team members to understand the significance of teamwork in achieving positive patient outcomes. Options A, C, and D are incorrect as they do not address the root cause of the issue and may lead to further disengagement and conflict within the team. Effective leadership in promoting awareness of teamwork and collaboration is crucial in enhancing patient care quality and outcomes.

Question 98: Correct Answer: B) Attending interdisciplinary team meetings regularly

Rationale: Attending interdisciplinary team meetings regularly is crucial for effective collaboration in healthcare settings. It allows nurses to discuss patient care plans, share insights, and receive feedback from other team members, fostering a collaborative approach to decision-making. Options A, C, and D promote individualistic behaviors that hinder teamwork and collaboration, emphasizing the importance of teamwork and communication in providing optimal patient care.

Question 99: Correct Answer: B) To provide timely alerts and notifications for potential crises

Rationale: Early warning systems in healthcare are designed to provide timely alerts and notifications for potential crises, allowing healthcare professionals to take proactive measures to prevent or mitigate adverse events. Option A is incorrect as the purpose is not to create panic but to ensure preparedness. Option C is incorrect as the goal is to streamline response efforts, not increase workload. Option D is incorrect as the aim is to reduce response time and improve outcomes in emergency situations. Therefore, the correct answer is B as it aligns with the primary objective of early warning systems in healthcare settings.

Question 100: Correct Answer: C) Encouraging the preceptor to provide constructive feedback and support

Rationale: Providing constructive feedback and support is essential in preceptor best practices as it fosters a positive learning environment, enhances the orientee's skills, and promotes professional growth. Assigning multiple preceptors may lead to confusion and inconsistency in training. Focusing solely on clinical skills neglects the importance of holistic nursing practice. Minimizing communication hinders the development of a strong preceptor-orientee relationship, which is crucial for successful orientation and integration into the nursing team.

Question 101: Correct Answer: B) Notifying the healthcare provider immediately

Rationale: In this scenario, the nurse should prioritize notifying the healthcare provider immediately. The patient's symptoms indicate a potential respiratory distress or hypoxemia, which requires prompt medical attention to prevent further complications. Administering pain medication (Option A) may mask the symptoms and delay appropriate interventions. Documenting findings (Option C) is important but not the priority in an acute situation. Providing a warm blanket (Option D) is not the appropriate intervention for addressing respiratory distress. Timely communication with the healthcare provider is crucial for ensuring patient safety and prompt management of potential complications.

Question 102: Correct Answer: A) Providing the patient with a detailed explanation of the treatment plan.

Rationale: Providing the patient with a detailed explanation of the treatment plan reflects patient-centered care by involving the patient in decision-making and promoting shared decision-making. This approach respects the patient's autonomy, preferences, and values, which are essential components of patient-centered care. Options B, C, and D are incorrect as they do not prioritize the patient's active involvement in the care process, which is crucial for effective patient-centered care. Making decisions for the patient, disregarding their preferences, or neglecting their cultural beliefs can lead to decreased patient satisfaction, non-adherence to treatment, and compromised health outcomes.

Question 103: Correct Answer: C) N95 respirator

Rationale: When caring for a patient on airborne precautions, healthcare workers must wear an N95 respirator to protect themselves from inhaling infectious airborne particles. A surgical mask (option B) does not provide adequate protection against airborne pathogens. Gown and gloves (option A) are typically used for contact precautions, while a face shield (option D) is not specifically required for airborne precautions. The N95 respirator is designed to filter out at least 95% of airborne particles, making it

the most appropriate choice for healthcare workers in this scenario.

Question 104: Correct Answer: C) Respiratory rate

Rationale: Monitoring respiratory rate is essential in the PACU as it provides immediate insight into the patient's oxygenation status and respiratory function post-surgery. Changes in respiratory rate can indicate respiratory distress, airway obstruction, or inadequate oxygenation, requiring prompt intervention. While blood pressure, temperature, and capillary refill time are also important parameters to monitor, respiratory rate takes precedence due to its direct correlation with oxygen exchange and early detection of respiratory complications, making it the most critical vital sign to assess frequently in the postoperative period.

Question 105: Correct Answer: C) Noise in the environment

Rationale: Physical communication barriers refer to obstacles that hinder the effective exchange of information due to environmental factors. In this case, noise in the environment can disrupt the message being conveyed, leading to miscommunication or misunderstanding. Options A and B pertain to semantic and cultural barriers, respectively, which are different from physical barriers. Option D relates to psychological barriers such as emotional blockages, contrasting with the physical barrier of noise. Therefore, the correct answer is C as it directly impacts the transmission of the message.

Question 106: Correct Answer: C) To assess the risk of infection associated with the patient's comorbidities

Rationale: In this scenario, the purpose of conducting an FMEA is to assess the risk of infection associated with the patient's comorbidities. FMEA is a proactive risk assessment method used to identify potential failure modes in a process, system, or service to prevent adverse events. Option A is incorrect as FMEA focuses on processes rather than patients. Option B is not directly related to the purpose of FMEA in this context. Option D is incorrect as FMEA is not used to review medical history but to analyze potential failure modes and their effects. Conducting an FMEA in this scenario will help the healthcare team mitigate the risk of infection and enhance patient safety during the surgical process.

Question 107: Correct Answer: A) Administering medications on time

Rationale: Care bundles in medical-surgical settings are structured interventions that, when implemented together, have been shown to improve patient outcomes. Administering medications on time is a crucial aspect of patient care as it ensures therapeutic effectiveness and prevents complications. Options B, C, and D, although important for patient comfort and satisfaction, do not directly impact patient safety or clinical outcomes as significantly as timely medication administration. Therefore, the correct answer is A.

Question 108: Correct Answer: A) The ability to understand and use healthcare information to make informed decisions.

Rationale: Health literacy refers to an individual's capacity to obtain, process, and understand basic health information and services needed to make appropriate health decisions. Option A is correct as it aligns with the definition of health literacy, emphasizing the importance of comprehending healthcare information to empower patients in decision-making. Options B, C, and D are incorrect as they do not capture the essence of health literacy, which is not solely about memorization, reading speed, or formal medical training, but rather about the practical application of health information in decision-making for improved health outcomes.

Question 109: Correct Answer: B) Speaking in a calm and empathetic tone

Rationale: Patient-centered care emphasizes the importance of effective communication that is empathetic, respectful, and tailored to the individual patient's needs. Speaking in a calm and empathetic tone fosters trust, promotes understanding, and enhances the patient's overall experience. Using medical jargon (option A) can lead to confusion and hinder effective communication. Providing minimal information (option C) may leave the patient feeling uninformed and anxious. Rushing through explanations (option D) can make the patient feel neglected and impact their perception of the quality of care received.

Question 110: Correct Answer: D) Providing timely pain medication as prescribed by the healthcare provider

Rationale: It is crucial for the CMSRN to prioritize providing timely pain medication as prescribed by the healthcare provider for a patient experiencing moderate pain post-abdominal surgery. This approach ensures effective pain management, promotes quicker recovery, and enhances patient comfort. Options A, B, and C are not ideal as administering pain medication only upon request may lead to inadequate pain relief, relying solely on non-pharmacological techniques may not address moderate post-operative pain adequately, and delaying medication until pain is severe can compromise patient comfort and recovery. Therefore, the correct option is to adhere to the prescribed pain management plan for optimal patient care.

Question 111: Correct Answer: C) Incorporating the best available evidence with clinical expertise and patient preferences

Rationale: Evidence-based practice in nursing involves integrating the most current and relevant research evidence with clinical expertise and considering individual patient preferences and values. This approach ensures that patient care is based on the best available evidence, leading to improved outcomes. Options A and D are incorrect as they go against the principles of evidence-based practice by either relying on outdated methods or disregarding patient-centered care. Option B is incorrect as evidence-based practice emphasizes using the most up-to-date research findings to guide clinical decision-making.

Question 112: Correct Answer: A) Notify the healthcare provider immediately

Rationale: In this scenario, the nurse should prioritize notifying the healthcare provider immediately as Mr. Smith is displaying signs of deterioration. Early warning systems emphasize prompt communication with the healthcare team when a patient shows signs of clinical deterioration. Increasing intravenous fluids or administering oxygen therapy may be necessary interventions but should not delay the urgent communication with the healthcare provider. Performing a thorough head-to-toe assessment is important but should not take precedence over timely notification of the healthcare provider in a critical situation like this.

Question 113: Correct Answer: B) Ensuring timely and accurate entry of vital signs

Rationale: In the scenario provided, the correct answer is B) Ensuring timely and accurate entry of vital signs. Vital signs are essential indicators of a patient's health status and can provide crucial information for the interprofessional team to make informed decisions regarding the patient's care. Timely and accurate documentation of vital signs in the EHR ensures that all team members have access to real-time data, facilitating effective communication and coordination of care. Options A, C, and D, although important aspects of patient care, do not directly impact interprofessional care coordination as significantly as the timely and accurate recording of vital signs.

Question 114: Correct Answer: C) Allocating resources based on acuity and need

Rationale: Resource allocation in a medical-surgical setting should prioritize patients based on acuity and need to ensure that those who require immediate attention receive timely care. Option A, equal distribution of resources to all patients, may not address the urgency of certain cases. Option B, prioritizing based on insurance coverage, goes against ethical principles and may compromise patient care. Option D, providing resources first come, first served, does not consider the severity of conditions. Therefore, the most appropriate approach is to allocate resources based on acuity and need to optimize patient outcomes and ensure efficient resource utilization.

Question 115: Correct Answer: B) Respect Ms. Patel's wishes and work with the healthcare team to integrate Ayurvedic treatments into her care plan.

Rationale: It is essential to respect and honor the cultural beliefs and preferences of patients, such as Ms. Patel's interest in Ayurvedic treatments. Integrating traditional practices with conventional medical care can enhance patient satisfaction, comfort, and overall well-being. Option A is incorrect as it dismisses Ms. Patel's cultural background. Option C is inappropriate as it neglects the importance of cultural competence in healthcare. Option D fails to acknowledge the significance of incorporating patient-centered care that respects individual beliefs and values.

Question 116: Correct Answer: A) Phlebitis

Rationale: Phlebitis is a common complication associated with central lines, characterized by inflammation of the vein where the catheter is inserted. It can lead to pain, redness, and swelling at the insertion site. Hypertension (option B) is not directly related to central lines but may be managed in patients with central lines. Hyperglycemia (option C) can occur due to stress or medications but is not a direct complication of central lines. Bradycardia (option D) is a condition of slow heart rate and is not typically associated with central line complications. Therefore, option A is the correct answer as phlebitis is a significant concern in patients with central lines.

Question 117: Correct Answer: C) Returning them to a pharmacy or authorized collection site

Rationale: Returning unused or expired medications to a pharmacy or authorized collection site is the safest and most environmentally friendly method of disposal. Flushing medications down the toilet can lead to water contamination, while throwing them in the trash risks accidental ingestion by children or pets. Burying medications in the backyard can also lead to environmental harm. Returning medications to a pharmacy ensures proper disposal by trained professionals, preventing misuse and protecting the environment. It is crucial for nurses to educate patients on the importance of safe drug disposal to prevent harm and promote public health.

Question 118: Correct Answer: C) Moral distress

Rationale: Moral distress occurs when a healthcare provider knows the ethically appropriate action to take but is unable to do so due to various constraints. In this scenario, Sarah is facing moral distress as she is aware of the right course of action but feels powerless to implement it due to external factors like staffing shortages. Burnout (Option A) is characterized by emotional exhaustion and reduced personal accomplishment, often caused by prolonged stress. Compassion fatigue (Option B) is the emotional and physical burden felt by healthcare providers due to caring for patients in distress. Moral resilience (Option D) refers to the ability to maintain moral standards despite facing moral adversity, which is not the case for Sarah in this scenario.

Question 119: Correct Answer: C) Control Chart

Rationale: Control charts are essential tools in Continuous Quality and Process Improvement as they help in monitoring process performance over time by displaying data points in relation to control limits. Control charts provide a visual representation of trends, variations, and patterns in a process, enabling healthcare professionals to identify when a process is out of control or experiencing unusual variation. In contrast, Pareto charts are used to prioritize issues, Scatter diagrams show relationships between variables, and Fishbone diagrams help in identifying root causes of problems, but they do not specifically display trends and variations over time like Control charts do.

Question 120: Correct Answer: C) Collecting patient data

Rationale: During the assessment phase of the nursing process, the priority action is to collect comprehensive and accurate patient data. This step involves gathering information about the patient's health status, medical history, current symptoms, and any other relevant data. By collecting thorough data, the nurse can establish a baseline for the patient's care and identify any potential health issues or risks. Administering medications (option A) occurs during the implementation phase, developing a care plan (option B) is part of the planning phase, and evaluating patient outcomes (option D) is done during the evaluation phase. Therefore, the correct answer is to collect patient data during the assessment phase to ensure effective patient care management and safety.

Question 121: Correct Answer: A) Patient falls

Rationale: Nursing sensitive indicators are specific to nursing care and reflect the structure, process, and outcomes of nursing care. Patient falls are a well-established nursing sensitive indicator as they are directly related to the quality of nursing care provided. Hospital readmission rates, physician satisfaction scores, and hospital revenue generation, although important in healthcare, are not specific to nursing care quality and do not fall under nursing sensitive indicators as per evidence-based guidelines. Therefore, the correct option is A) Patient falls.

Question 122: Correct Answer: C) Placing a hand on Mr. Johnson's shoulder and saying, "I can see you're feeling worried. Can you tell me more about your chest pain?"

Rationale: Option A is incorrect as interrupting the patient can hinder effective communication and does not demonstrate active listening. Option B is also incorrect as nodding while focusing on documentation shows a lack of engagement with the patient. Option D is incorrect as focusing on the IV infusion rate instead of the patient's concerns is not an example of active listening. Option C is the correct answer as it involves showing empathy by acknowledging the patient's emotions, using non-verbal cues, and encouraging further expression of symptoms, which are key components of active listening in healthcare settings.

Question 123: Correct Answer: A) Apologize to Mr. Johnson and explain the reasons for the delay in pain medication administration.

Rationale: Option A is the correct answer as it demonstrates empathy, accountability, and transparency in addressing Mr. Johnson's concerns. By apologizing and providing an explanation for the delay, the nurse acknowledges the issue and shows a commitment to resolving it. This approach aligns with service recovery principles by focusing on patient satisfaction and communication. Options B, C, and D are incorrect as they do not address the patient's concerns effectively. Dismissing or ignoring complaints can escalate the situation and lead to further dissatisfaction. Offering a discount may not be appropriate in this scenario and does not address the root cause of the issue, which is the delay in pain medication administration.

Question 124: Correct Answer: C) Investigating, identifying, and rectifying the medication error promptly.

Rationale: In this scenario, the correct answer is C) Investigating, identifying, and rectifying the medication error promptly. This action aligns with the principles of a high accountable organization focused on patient safety culture and effective patient management. Option A is incorrect as ignoring the error would compromise patient safety. Option B is also incorrect as reporting the error at the end of the shift delays necessary actions. Option D is incorrect as seeking assistance without addressing the error directly does not ensure immediate patient safety. The nurse's prompt investigation, identification, and correction of the medication error demonstrate a proactive approach to ensuring patient safety and quality care.

Question 125: Correct Answer: B) Use simple language and visual aids to explain hypertension management.

Rationale: Option B is the correct choice as it aligns with the principles of health promotion and holistic patient care. Using simple language and visual aids helps enhance patient understanding and engagement in managing their health. Options A, C, and D are incorrect as they do not prioritize effective communication or patient-centered education. Providing written materials in medical jargon may confuse the patient,

recommending online resources without explanation lacks personalized guidance, and discussing advanced treatment options without assessing readiness can overwhelm the patient. Effective health information delivery involves clear communication tailored to the patient's needs, which option B fulfills.

Question 126: Correct Answer: B) Communicating clearly and regularly with team members

Rationale: Effective communication is crucial in disaster planning and management to ensure coordination, timely response, and optimal patient outcomes. Clear and regular communication among team members helps in sharing vital information, coordinating efforts, and addressing challenges promptly. Assigning tasks based on individual preferences may not always align with the needs of the situation and can lead to inefficiencies. Working independently can hinder teamwork and collaboration, impacting the overall response effectiveness. Ignoring input from other healthcare professionals can result in missed opportunities for valuable insights and contributions, undermining the collaborative effort essential in managing disasters successfully.

Question 127: Correct Answer: C) Shared decision-making is a collaborative process between healthcare providers and patients to make healthcare decisions together.

Rationale: Shared decision-making is a patient-centered approach that involves active participation of both healthcare providers and patients in making healthcare decisions. Option A is incorrect as it goes against the essence of shared decision-making, which emphasizes patient involvement. Option B is incorrect as shared decision-making involves collaboration among all team members, not just the most senior provider. Option D is incorrect as shared decision-making requires patients to be well-informed about their treatment options to actively participate in the decision-making process.

Question 128: Correct Answer: C) Attending interprofessional team meetings to discuss patient care

Rationale: Effective interprofessional collaboration involves active participation in team meetings where healthcare professionals from various disciplines come together to discuss and plan patient care. Option A is incorrect as providing care without consulting other team members goes against the principles of interprofessional collaboration. Option B is limited in scope as effective communication should extend beyond the nursing team. Option D is not aligned with interprofessional collaboration, as decisions should be made collectively, considering input from all disciplines involved in patient care. Therefore, option C is the most appropriate choice as it promotes teamwork, communication, and shared decision-making, essential elements of successful interprofessional care coordination.

Question 129: Correct Answer: B) Approach Mr. Johnson calmly and maintain a non-threatening posture.

Rationale: In this scenario, the most effective de-escalation technique is to approach Mr. Johnson calmly and maintain a non-threatening posture. This approach helps to prevent escalating the situation further and promotes a sense of safety and trust. Option A is incorrect as matching his intensity can escalate the situation. Option C is incorrect as ignoring the behavior can lead to increased agitation. Option D is incorrect as threatening to withhold medication can worsen the patient's behavior and compromise care. Effective verbal intervention involves staying calm, using a soothing tone, and actively listening to the patient's concerns to address them appropriately.

Question 130: Correct Answer: C) Implementing early ambulation with assistive devices

Rationale: Implementing early ambulation with assistive devices is crucial in promoting mobility for Mr. Johnson post hip replacement surgery. This intervention helps prevent complications such as deep vein thrombosis and muscle atrophy. Encouraging passive range of motion exercises (Option A) is important but not as effective as early ambulation. Limiting weight-bearing activities on the affected hip (Option B) may hinder recovery and delay mobility progress. Keeping the patient on strict bed rest for 48 hours (Option D) can increase the risk of postoperative complications and slow down the rehabilitation process. Early ambulation with assistive devices is the most evidence-based and beneficial intervention for enhancing mobility and preventing complications in postoperative patients like Mr. Johnson.

Question 131: Correct Answer: C) Collaborating and sharing information openly

Rationale: Collaboration and open information sharing are fundamental for an effective interprofessional care team. Working in silos (option A) hinders communication and coordination, leading to fragmented care. Delaying sharing patient information (option B) can result in treatment delays and errors. Ignoring input from other team members (option D) undermines the value of a multidisciplinary approach. Therefore, option C is the correct choice as it promotes teamwork, enhances patient outcomes, and ensures comprehensive care delivery.

Question 132: Correct Answer: C) Diabetes mellitus

Rationale: Diabetes mellitus is a metabolic disorder where the body either does not produce enough insulin or cannot effectively use the insulin it produces. This results in high blood sugar levels, leading to various complications. Hypothyroidism (Option A) is a condition where the thyroid gland does not produce enough thyroid hormone. Celiac disease (Option B) is an autoimmune disorder triggered by gluten consumption. Chronic obstructive pulmonary disease (Option D) is a lung disease characterized by chronic bronchitis and emphysema. Comparatively, only diabetes mellitus aligns with the description provided in the question.

Question 133: Correct Answer: C) Regular follow-up appointments with healthcare provider

Rationale: Regular follow-up appointments with healthcare provider are essential in preventing readmissions and ensuring continuity of care. Patients with scheduled follow-ups are more likely to receive timely interventions and support. On the other hand, factors such as lack of social support, history of non-compliance with medications, and limited health literacy are known to increase the risk of readmissions. Patients lacking social support may struggle with self-care post-discharge, non-compliance with medications can lead to exacerbation of conditions, and limited health literacy may hinder understanding of discharge instructions, all contributing to higher readmission rates.

Question 134: Correct Answer: B) Pause the procedure, conduct a thorough search for the missing instrument

Rationale: The correct action for the circulating nurse in this scenario is to pause the procedure and conduct a thorough search for the missing instrument. Patient safety is paramount in the operating room, and any discrepancies or missing equipment must be addressed immediately to prevent harm to the patient. Option A is incorrect as proceeding with the surgery without the necessary instrument can compromise patient safety. Option C is not the best course of action as the circulating nurse should take the lead in resolving the issue. Option D is also incorrect as it disregards the importance of having all required instruments available before proceeding with the surgery. Conducting a thorough search ensures that the surgical team can proceed safely and effectively.

Question 135: Correct Answer: B) Offer small, frequent meals with foods he enjoys within his dietary restrictions

Rationale: Option B is the most appropriate intervention as it addresses Mr. Smith's poor appetite and nausea by offering small, frequent meals with foods he enjoys within his dietary restrictions. This approach promotes individualized nutritional care, ensuring that Mr. Smith receives adequate nutrition while considering his preferences and medical conditions. Options A and C are more invasive measures that are not indicated at this stage. Option D disregards Mr. Smith's dietary restrictions and preferences, which can negatively impact his compliance and nutritional status. Therefore, option B is the best choice to meet Mr. Smith's

individualized nutritional needs effectively.

Question 136: Correct Answer: B) Promoting evidence-based practice

Rationale: In the context of a nursing professional practice model, promoting evidence-based practice is crucial for delivering high-quality patient care. Evidence-based practice involves integrating the best available evidence with clinical expertise and patient preferences to make informed healthcare decisions. While ensuring adequate staffing levels is important for patient safety, it is not the primary focus of a nursing professional practice model. Providing patient education on heart failure and administering medications are essential nursing interventions but do not encompass the comprehensive approach of a nursing professional practice model, which emphasizes evidence-based care delivery to improve patient outcomes.

Question 137: Correct Answer: C) Demonstrating empathy and understanding

Rationale: Active listening is a crucial skill in patient-centered care, emphasizing the importance of demonstrating empathy and understanding towards the patient. Options A and B are incorrect as they disrupt the flow of communication and do not prioritize the patient's perspective. Option D is also incorrect as it shifts the focus away from the patient's needs. By choosing option C, nurses can establish a therapeutic relationship, gain valuable insights into the patient's concerns, and promote a holistic approach to care.

Question 138: Correct Answer: A) Dysphagia

Rationale: Dysphagia, or difficulty swallowing, is a common indication for alternate nutrition administration in patients. Patients with dysphagia may have difficulty ingesting food orally, leading to the need for alternate methods such as enteral or parenteral nutrition. Hypertension, urinary tract infection, and skin rash are not direct indications for alternate nutrition administration. While these conditions may impact a patient's overall health, they do not specifically necessitate the use of alternate nutrition methods. Therefore, option A is the correct choice as it aligns with the indication for alternate nutrition administration in patients with dysphagia.

Question 139: Correct Answer: C) Using a warm blanket on a patient with peripheral vascular disease

Rationale: Heat therapy is contraindicated for acute inflammation as it can exacerbate swelling and pain. Applying heat to a fresh post-operative incision can increase the risk of bleeding and delay healing. Administering heat to an open wound can lead to infection. In contrast, using a warm blanket on a patient with peripheral vascular disease can help improve circulation and provide comfort without causing harm. Heat therapy in the form of a warm blanket is a safe and effective non-pharmacological intervention for patients with peripheral vascular disease, making option C the correct choice.

Question 140: Correct Answer: C) Mr. Johnson is exhibiting signs of acute pancreatitis.

Rationale: The correct interpretation based on Mr. Johnson's clinical presentation is acute pancreatitis. The symptoms of severe abdominal pain, nausea, vomiting, fever, tachycardia, elevated white blood cell count, and abdominal tenderness are indicative of acute pancreatitis. Option A is incorrect as the symptoms are not consistent with an acute myocardial infarction. Option B is incorrect as the symptoms are not specific to a urinary tract infection. Option D is incorrect as the symptoms do not suggest deep vein thrombosis. By carefully analyzing the patient's symptoms and vital signs, the nurse can accurately interpret Mr. Johnson's condition as acute pancreatitis.

Question 141: Correct Answer: D) Continuous quality improvement

Rationale: Continuous quality improvement is a fundamental principle in healthcare quality management that focuses on ongoing assessment, evaluation, and enhancement of processes to ensure optimal patient outcomes. This approach involves identifying areas for improvement, implementing changes, and monitoring the results to make further refinements. Options A, B, and C are incorrect as they do not align with the core principles of quality management. Cost reduction at the expense of quality compromises patient care, a reactive approach is not proactive, and emphasizing individual blame hinders a culture of teamwork and learning.

Question 142: Correct Answer: B) To assess Mrs. Smith's swallowing function and recommend appropriate diet modifications.
Rationale: Speech consultation in this scenario aims to evaluate Mrs. Smith's swallowing ability through clinical assessments such as bedside swallow evaluation or modified barium swallow study. The goal is to recommend specific diet modifications, such as texture modifications or positional strategies, to ensure safe oral intake and prevent complications like aspiration pneumonia. Option A is incorrect as strict oral intake restriction may not be necessary if appropriate modifications can enable safe swallowing. Option C is incorrect as tube feeding is typically considered if oral intake is unsafe. Option D is incorrect as resuming a regular diet without modifications can pose a risk of aspiration for Mrs. Smith.

Question 143: Correct Answer: B) Encouraging regular exercise and physical activity
Rationale: Health promotion in holistic patient care involves empowering individuals to take control of their health. Encouraging regular exercise and physical activity aligns with this principle by promoting overall well-being, reducing the risk of chronic diseases, and enhancing mental health. Administering medications, monitoring vital signs, and providing wound care are essential nursing interventions but do not directly address the holistic aspect of health promotion. By choosing option B, nurses can actively engage patients in self-care practices that contribute to their physical, emotional, and mental health, reflecting a comprehensive approach to holistic patient care.

Question 144: Correct Answer: C) Advocating for the prompt initiation of oxygen therapy for Mr. Johnson.
Rationale: In this scenario, the most appropriate action that aligns with patient safety culture is option C, advocating for the prompt initiation of oxygen therapy for Mr. Johnson. Patient safety culture emphasizes the importance of advocating for the well-being of patients and taking proactive measures to ensure their safety. While notifying the charge nurse (option A) and documenting vital signs accurately (option B) are essential aspects of nursing practice, the immediate priority in this situation is to address the patient's declining oxygen saturation levels. Administering pain medication (option D) is not the most critical intervention at this time, as ensuring adequate oxygenation takes precedence in promoting patient safety and preventing further complications.

Question 145: Correct Answer: A) Effective Communication and Collaboration
Rationale: In this scenario, the nurse demonstrates the professional behavior of effective communication and collaboration by promptly informing the nursing team about the deteriorating patient condition and working together efficiently to provide necessary care. While time management and prioritization are essential skills, they are not the primary focus in this situation. Patient advocacy and empowerment, although important, do not directly address the teamwork and collaboration aspect highlighted in the scenario. Clinical judgment and decision-making are crucial but are secondary to the immediate need for teamwork and communication in this critical situation.

Question 146: Correct Answer: C) To improve communication among healthcare team members
Rationale: Checklists play a crucial role in enhancing communication among healthcare team members by ensuring that all necessary steps in patient care are systematically followed. By utilizing checklists within care bundles, healthcare professionals can effectively coordinate tasks, reduce errors, and enhance patient safety. Options A, B, and D are incorrect as they do not

align with the primary purpose of checklists in care bundles. Increasing costs, decreasing adherence to evidence-based practices, and reducing patient engagement are not the intended outcomes of utilizing checklists in patient care.

Question 147: Correct Answer: B) Report the error to the charge nurse or supervisor privately.
Rationale: Speaking up for patient safety is a crucial aspect of a nurse's role in ensuring quality care. In this scenario, option B is the correct course of action as it aligns with the principles of patient safety culture. Reporting the error to the charge nurse or supervisor privately allows for a timely and appropriate resolution of the issue without causing embarrassment to the colleague involved. Options A, C, and D are incorrect as confronting the colleague publicly may lead to conflict and hinder effective resolution, ignoring the error compromises patient safety, and involving the patient's family without proper protocol breaches confidentiality and may not lead to the desired outcome.

Question 148: Correct Answer: A) Hospice care services
Rationale: Hospice care services focus on providing comprehensive support to patients with life-limiting illnesses, such as advanced cancer, by addressing their physical, emotional, and spiritual needs. These services offer symptom management, pain control, emotional support, and assistance with end-of-life decision-making. In contrast, options B, C, and D are not suitable for a patient like Ms. Thompson who requires palliative and end-of-life care. Chemotherapy treatment centers focus on active cancer treatment, weight loss clinics on weight management, and cosmetic surgery facilities on elective procedures, none of which address the holistic needs of a patient in palliative care. Therefore, recommending hospice care services aligns with the principles of holistic patient care and support for Ms. Thompson and her family during this challenging time.

Question 149: Correct Answer: B) Smoking status
Rationale: Smoking status is the most significant demographic factor that poses a high risk to Mrs. Smith's health status. Smoking is a well-known risk factor for various health conditions such as cardiovascular diseases, respiratory disorders, and cancer. While age, living alone, and medical history are important demographic factors to consider, smoking has a direct and immediate impact on Mrs. Smith's current and future health outcomes. Encouraging smoking cessation and providing support for this behavior change is crucial in improving Mrs. Smith's overall health and reducing the risk of complications associated with her existing medical conditions.

Question 150: Correct Answer: C) Using bed and chair alarms for high-risk patients
Rationale: Using bed and chair alarms for high-risk patients is an evidence-based practice to prevent falls in healthcare settings. These alarms alert healthcare providers when a patient attempts to get out of bed or a chair without assistance, allowing for timely intervention. Placing the call bell within reach is important but may not prevent falls directly. Keeping the room well-lit is beneficial but may not address the immediate risk of falls. Administering sedatives can increase the risk of falls by causing drowsiness and confusion, thus contradicting fall prevention efforts. Therefore, using bed and chair alarms is the most effective option for preventing falls in high-risk patients.

CMSRN Exam Practice Questions [SET 4]

Question 1: Scenario: Mr. Smith, a 65-year-old patient, is admitted to the medical-surgical unit with a diagnosis of pneumonia. The healthcare team has initiated a care bundle to improve patient outcomes and reduce the risk of healthcare-associated infections. As part of the care bundle, which intervention should the nurse prioritize to prevent ventilator-associated pneumonia (VAP)?

A) Administering prophylactic antibiotics
B) Elevating the head of the bed to 30-45 degrees
C) Providing oral care with chlorhexidine solution
D) Changing the ventilator circuit every 48 hours

Question 2: Which action by a nurse demonstrates an appropriate response to moral distress related to unintended consequences in a healthcare setting?

A) Ignoring the situation and continuing with routine tasks
B) Seeking guidance from a supervisor to address the issue
C) Blaming colleagues for the situation
D) Avoiding the patient involved in the distressing situation

Question 3: In a healthcare setting, which type of survey is commonly used to assess patient customer experience based on data results?

A) Randomized controlled trial
B) Case-control study
C) Cross-sectional survey
D) Patient satisfaction survey

Question 4: Scenario: Mr. Patel, a 65-year-old patient, is admitted to the medical-surgical unit with a complex medical history. He speaks limited English and appears confused during the assessment. The healthcare team needs to communicate important information regarding his treatment plan. Which action is most appropriate to ensure effective communication with Mr. Patel?

A) Utilize a family member who speaks the same language to interpret.
B) Use a bilingual staff member from a different department to interpret.
C) Employ a professional medical interpreter service.
D) Communicate through gestures and basic English words.

Question 5: Ms. Johnson, a 65-year-old postoperative patient, is recovering in the medical-surgical unit. The nurse notices that the room temperature is too cold for the patient's comfort. Which action by the nurse best promotes a healthy practice environment for Ms. Johnson?

A) Providing an extra blanket for the patient
B) Adjusting the thermostat to a warmer setting
C) Offering the patient a hot beverage
D) Closing the window to block the draft

Question 6: In the context of nursing teamwork and collaboration, what is the primary purpose of establishing a professional network?

A) To compete with other healthcare professionals
B) To gain recognition and awards
C) To enhance patient care and outcomes
D) To socialize with colleagues

Question 7: Scenario: Mr. Johnson, a 68-year-old patient, is admitted to the medical-surgical unit with a diagnosis of congestive heart failure. As the CMSRN on duty, you are responsible for ensuring regulatory and compliance standards are met. Which action demonstrates adherence to regulatory standards in this scenario?

A) Administering medications without verifying the patient's identity
B) Documenting vital signs every 4 hours instead of every 2 hours as ordered
C) Allowing family members to stay overnight in the patient's room
D) Using two patient identifiers before administering medications

Question 8: In the context of Care Coordination and Transition Management, which community resource plays a vital role in providing support and assistance to individuals with chronic illnesses?

A) Local Gyms offering discounted memberships
B) Public Libraries providing free internet access
C) Food Banks offering emergency food supplies
D) Retail Stores with seasonal discounts

Question 9: When documenting in a patient's medical record, which of the following is the most crucial element for ensuring effective interprofessional care coordination?

A) Using abbreviations to save time
B) Providing detailed and accurate information
C) Delaying documentation until the end of the shift
D) Including personal opinions about the patient

Question 10: When implementing restraints as a safety measure for a patient, which action by the nurse is essential to ensure patient safety and compliance with protocols?

A) Secure the restraint straps tightly to limit movement
B) Check the patient's circulation and skin integrity regularly
C) Leave the patient unattended while restrained to respect their privacy
D) Apply restraints without obtaining consent from the patient or family

Question 11: Which of the following is a key benefit of using electronic health records (EHRs) in medical-surgical nursing practice?

A) Increased risk of data breaches
B) Limited accessibility to patient information
C) Improved coordination of care among healthcare team members
D) Higher likelihood of medication errors

Question 12: Which of the following diseases is characterized by chronic inflammation of the airways, airflow obstruction, and bronchospasm?

A) Pneumonia
B) Asthma
C) Tuberculosis
D) Emphysema

Question 13: Which action by the nurse best demonstrates effective patient-centered care in the context of Patient/Care Management?

A) Providing the patient with a detailed explanation of their diagnosis and treatment plan.
B) Involving the patient in shared decision-making regarding their care.
C) Administering medications without discussing potential side effects with the patient.
D) Following the care plan without considering the patient's preferences or values.

Question 14: Scenario: Mr. Johnson, a 65-year-old patient, is admitted to the medical-surgical unit with a history of hypertension and anxiety. He becomes agitated and starts yelling at the nursing staff due to a misunderstanding about his medication schedule. As a Certified Medical Surgical Registered Nurse (CMSRN), which communication technique would be most appropriate to de-escalate the situation with Mr. Johnson?
A) Raising your voice to match his level of agitation
B) Maintaining a calm tone and using therapeutic communication
C) Ignoring his outburst and walking away
D) Threatening to restrain him if he does not calm down

Question 15: Scenario: Mr. Johnson, a 45-year-old patient admitted for a surgical procedure, has a history of depression and suicidal ideation. He has been expressing feelings of hopelessness and isolation since his admission. During a routine check, the nurse finds Mr. Johnson sitting alone in his room, staring blankly out of the window. He appears withdrawn and tearful. What should be the nurse's immediate action based on patient safety protocols?
A) Leave Mr. Johnson alone to have some privacy.
B) Engage Mr. Johnson in a conversation about his favorite hobbies.
C) Notify the healthcare team about Mr. Johnson's behavior and concerns.
D) Provide Mr. Johnson with a sharp object to help him cope with his emotions.

Question 16: During a morning huddle on a medical-surgical unit, the charge nurse discusses a patient, Mr. Johnson, who is scheduled for discharge today. The nurse mentions that Mr. Johnson has a history of falls and requires assistance with ambulation. The team decides to ensure that a walker is readily available for him post-discharge. What is the primary purpose of this huddle discussion?
A) To share important patient information and ensure a safe discharge process.
B) To discuss the latest medical research on fall prevention in elderly patients.
C) To plan a surprise farewell party for Mr. Johnson.
D) To review the hospital's financial goals for the quarter.

Question 17: In a hospital setting, the rapid response team is activated when:
A) A patient is experiencing a sudden change in condition
B) A routine medication administration is due
C) A family member requests additional blankets for the patient
D) A physician is conducting rounds

Question 18: In a healthcare setting, what is the primary purpose of a huddle?
A) To discuss patient care plans and updates
B) To schedule staff vacations
C) To organize office supplies
D) To plan social events for the team

Question 19: When educating patients and families as part of holistic patient care, which approach is most effective in promoting understanding and compliance?
A) Providing information only when asked by the patient or family.
B) Using medical jargon to ensure accuracy and precision.
C) Tailoring education to the individual's learning style and preferences.
D) Presenting all information at once to avoid confusion.

Question 20: Scenario: Mr. Johnson, a 65-year-old male patient, is admitted to the medical-surgical unit with a history of hypertension, diabetes, and recent myocardial infarction. During the initial assessment, the nurse notes that Mr. Johnson is experiencing shortness of breath and has crackles in his lung bases. His vital signs are as follows: temperature 99.2 ℉, heart rate 110 bpm, respiratory rate 24/min, blood pressure 160/90 mmHg. Mr. Johnson mentions feeling fatigued and having difficulty sleeping due to his breathing. Which of the following conditions is most likely contributing to Mr. Johnson's current symptoms?
A) Pulmonary embolism
B) Pneumonia
C) Chronic obstructive pulmonary disease (COPD)
D) Heart failure

Question 21: Scenario: Mr. Smith, a 65-year-old patient with a history of hypertension and diabetes, is admitted to the medical-surgical unit for the treatment of pneumonia. The physician orders the administration of a new medication to manage his pneumonia. As the nurse caring for Mr. Smith, you understand the importance of pharmacological interventions in his care. Which of the following factors should the nurse consider when administering medications to Mr. Smith to ensure patient safety and optimal outcomes?
A) Assessing the patient's vital signs before medication administration
B) Administering the medication at the same time every day
C) Encouraging the patient to self-administer the medication
D) Mixing the medication with food to enhance absorption

Question 22: Scenario: Mrs. Smith, a 65-year-old patient, is scheduled for a cardiac catheterization procedure. As a CMSRN, which of the following actions is within your scope of practice related to procedures for this patient?
A) Administering conscious sedation during the procedure
B) Interpreting the results of the cardiac catheterization
C) Performing the actual cardiac catheterization procedure
D) Monitoring vital signs and assessing for complications post-procedure

Question 23: Which of the following is NOT a key factor in promoting employee engagement in the context of Leadership, Nursing Teamwork, and Collaboration?
A) Providing opportunities for professional development
B) Recognizing and rewarding employees' contributions
C) Implementing strict hierarchical structures
D) Encouraging open communication and feedback

Question 24: Scenario: During a busy shift on a medical-surgical unit, a patient named Mr. Smith, who underwent a major surgery, starts experiencing sudden shortness of breath and chest pain. The nurse in charge notices the situation and immediately informs the healthcare team. The team members gather around to assess the patient's condition and decide on the next steps to provide prompt and effective care. Which action by the nurse in charge demonstrates effective leadership in this scenario?
A) Delegating the tasks to other team members without actively participating in the patient assessment.
B) Taking charge of the situation, coordinating the team's efforts, and ensuring timely interventions for the patient.
C) Ignoring the patient's symptoms and continuing with routine tasks.
D) Leaving the patient's room to seek assistance from a more experienced nurse.

Question 25: Scenario: Mr. Johnson, a 65-year-old patient, is admitted to the medical-surgical unit with a diagnosis of

pneumonia. During the morning rounds, the nurse notices that Mr. Johnson appears anxious and is having difficulty breathing. The nurse asks Mr. Johnson how he is feeling, and he responds, "I can't catch my breath, and I'm scared." Which response by the nurse demonstrates effective verbal communication skills in this situation?
A) "Don't worry, everything will be fine."
B) "Let me get you some water to help you relax."
C) "I understand you're feeling scared. I will stay with you and help you breathe easier."
D) "Try to calm down and take deep breaths."

Question 26: In the context of patient advocacy, which action best demonstrates a nurse's commitment to holistic patient care?
A) Administering medications strictly based on the physician's orders.
B) Engaging in open communication with the patient to understand their cultural beliefs and preferences.
C) Following hospital protocols without considering the patient's individual needs.
D) Prioritizing tasks efficiently to ensure timely completion of nursing duties.

Question 27: What is the primary purpose of safety huddles in a medical-surgical setting?
A) To discuss staff scheduling issues
B) To review patient satisfaction surveys
C) To identify and address potential safety risks
D) To plan social events for the healthcare team

Question 28: Which of the following is a crucial step in medication reconciliation during the discharge process for a patient being transitioned to home care?
A) Contacting the primary care physician for medication list verification
B) Providing the patient with a new set of medications without reviewing the current list
C) Disregarding the patient's self-reported medication history
D) Failing to communicate medication changes to the patient

Question 29: Scenario: Mr. Johnson, a 65-year-old postoperative patient, suddenly develops shortness of breath, tachycardia, and confusion. The nurse suspects a possible pulmonary embolism. The nurse initiates the rapid response team (RRT) to assess the patient's condition promptly. Which action is the priority for the nurse to take while waiting for the RRT to arrive?
A) Administer oxygen at 2 liters per minute via nasal cannula.
B) Prepare to assist with intubation if needed.
C) Administer a dose of intravenous pain medication.
D) Obtain a set of vital signs and prepare to report to the RRT.

Question 30: Which social determinant of health plays a significant role in patient safety assessments and reporting for Certified Medical Surgical Registered Nurses (CMSRNs)?
A) Education level
B) Blood type
C) Favorite color
D) Shoe size

Question 31: Scenario: Mr. Smith, a 65-year-old postoperative patient, is being transferred from the recovery room to the surgical unit. The nurse provides a detailed report to the receiving nurse about the patient's condition, medications, and any specific instructions. The receiving nurse acknowledges the report, repeats back the key points, and clarifies any uncertainties. This process is an example of:

A) Open-loop communication
B) Closed-loop communication
C) One-way communication
D) Non-verbal communication

Question 32: In the context of conflict management within nursing teamwork and collaboration, which approach is most effective for resolving conflicts between healthcare team members?
A) Avoidance and ignoring the conflict
B) Confrontation and aggressive behavior
C) Collaboration and open communication
D) Compromise and giving in to demands

Question 33: Which statement best reflects the nursing philosophy related to Leadership, Nursing Teamwork, and Collaboration?
A) Nursing leadership is solely about making decisions without involving the team.
B) Effective nursing teamwork is not essential for providing quality patient care.
C) Collaboration among healthcare professionals is unnecessary in the nursing field.
D) Nursing leadership involves guiding and supporting the team to achieve optimal patient outcomes.

Question 34: In a decentralized nursing care delivery system, which characteristic best describes the decision-making process?
A) Centralized decision-making by a single authority
B) Decision-making shared among all team members
C) Decision-making solely by the nurse manager
D) Decision-making based on patient preferences

Question 35: Which factor plays a crucial role in successful change management within a medical-surgical nursing team?
A) Resistance to change
B) Lack of communication
C) Strong leadership
D) Individualistic approach

Question 36: Scenario: Mr. Patel, a 65-year-old patient from India, is admitted to the medical-surgical unit. During the initial assessment, the nurse notices that Mr. Patel avoids making direct eye contact and frequently nods his head in agreement. He prefers to communicate with family members present in the room rather than directly with the healthcare team. Which cultural sign should the nurse recognize and respect when providing care for Mr. Patel?
A) Avoiding eye contact and nodding head in agreement
B) Preferring to communicate through family members
C) Speaking softly and using gentle gestures
D) Maintaining a close physical distance during interactions

Question 37: In the context of delegation and supervision, which action by the registered nurse demonstrates appropriate scope of practice?
A) Administering a medication without verifying the patient's identity
B) Delegating wound care to a nursing assistant without providing proper training
C) Supervising a licensed practical nurse (LPN) in administering intravenous (IV) medications
D) Performing a complex procedure without consulting the healthcare provider

Question 38: Which of the following best describes critical thinking in the context of a Certified Medical Surgical Registered Nurse (CMSRN)?

A) Accepting information at face value without questioning
B) Relying solely on intuition and personal beliefs
C) Evaluating evidence, considering implications, and making informed decisions
D) Following protocols and guidelines without deviation

Question 39: Scenario: Mr. Johnson, a 65-year-old patient, is admitted to the medical-surgical unit with a history of heart failure. He is prescribed multiple medications, including a new anticoagulant. The nurse notices that the anticoagulant dosage seems higher than usual. What action should the nurse take first?
A) Administer the medication as prescribed
B) Consult with the healthcare provider regarding the dosage
C) Discuss the dosage concern with the patient's family
D) Wait and monitor the patient for any adverse effects

Question 40: During interprofessional rounding, the medical surgical registered nurse is discussing a patient's care plan with the healthcare team. The patient, Mr. Smith, has a complex medical history and is scheduled for surgery tomorrow. The nurse notices a discrepancy in the medication orders provided by the physician and the pharmacist. What is the most appropriate action for the nurse to take in this situation?
A) Proceed with the surgery as scheduled and inform the patient post-operation.
B) Discuss the discrepancy with the pharmacist only.
C) Raise the concern immediately with the healthcare team during rounding.
D) Wait until after the surgery to address the medication discrepancy.

Question 41: Scenario: Mr. Smith, a 65-year-old male, is admitted to the medical-surgical unit with a suspected bacterial infection. The healthcare team has initiated antibiotic therapy. As the CMSRN overseeing his care, you are responsible for ensuring appropriate antimicrobial stewardship. Which action best demonstrates adherence to antimicrobial stewardship principles in this scenario?
A) Continuing the current broad-spectrum antibiotic therapy without reassessment.
B) Ordering additional antibiotics to cover a wider range of potential pathogens.
C) Performing a thorough clinical reassessment to narrow the antibiotic spectrum based on culture results.
D) Discontinuing all antibiotics immediately to prevent resistance development.

Question 42: Scenario: Mr. Johnson, a 65-year-old patient, is admitted to the medical-surgical unit with a complex medical history including diabetes, hypertension, and recent myocardial infarction. He is experiencing difficulty managing his medications and monitoring his blood glucose levels due to vision impairment. The healthcare team consisting of nurses, physicians, and pharmacists collaborates to develop a comprehensive care plan for Mr. Johnson. Which action best demonstrates interprofessional collaboration in managing Mr. Johnson's care?
A) The nurse independently adjusts Mr. Johnson's insulin dosage based on blood glucose readings.
B) The physician prescribes new medications without consulting the patient's primary care provider.
C) The pharmacist provides education on proper medication administration and side effects to Mr. Johnson.
D) The nurse refers Mr. Johnson to an ophthalmologist without informing the rest of the healthcare team.

Question 43: In the context of human trafficking, which action is essential for Certified Medical Surgical Registered Nurses (CMSRNs) to prioritize in patient care management?
A) Identifying potential signs of human trafficking in patients
B) Administering medications as prescribed
C) Ensuring patients have clean linens
D) Providing extra snacks to patients upon request

Question 44: Scenario: Mrs. Smith, a 65-year-old postoperative patient, has been experiencing increased restlessness, confusion, and tachycardia since the past hour. Her blood pressure is slightly elevated, and she is complaining of sudden onset chest pain. The nurse notes decreased urine output and cool, clammy skin. Mrs. Smith underwent abdominal surgery two days ago and has a history of hypertension and diabetes. Which action should the nurse prioritize based on clinical judgment?
A) Administer pain medication for chest pain.
B) Notify the healthcare provider immediately.
C) Increase the IV fluid rate.
D) Reassure the patient and continue monitoring.

Question 45: Which of the following is a key aspect of maintaining a healthy practice environment for Certified Medical Surgical Registered Nurses (CMSRNs) in terms of physical well-being?
A) Ensuring proper ventilation in the workplace
B) Using personal protective equipment only during emergencies
C) Ignoring ergonomic principles when lifting patients
D) Disregarding safety protocols when handling hazardous materials

Question 46: Which nutrition administration modality is suitable for a patient with dysphagia who is unable to swallow safely?
A) Total Parenteral Nutrition (TPN)
B) Enteral Nutrition via Nasogastric Tube
C) Oral Nutrition Supplements
D) Intravenous Fluids

Question 47: Scenario: Mr. Johnson, a 65-year-old patient, is admitted to the medical-surgical unit with a history of heart failure and diabetes. He is experiencing shortness of breath and edema in his lower extremities. The healthcare team has initiated diuretic therapy to manage his symptoms. As the CMSRN caring for Mr. Johnson, which action demonstrates an effective strategy to individualize his care?
A) Implementing a standardized care plan for all patients with heart failure
B) Collaborating with the dietitian to provide a generic heart-healthy diet
C) Adjusting the diuretic dosage based on Mr. Johnson's response and renal function
D) Scheduling routine nursing assessments at fixed intervals for all patients

Question 48: Which action is an essential component of antimicrobial stewardship in the context of infection prevention and patient/care management?
A) Prescribing broad-spectrum antibiotics for all suspected infections
B) Administering antibiotics for the shortest effective duration
C) Encouraging self-medication with antibiotics for minor illnesses
D) Using antibiotics without considering microbial susceptibility testing

Question 49: Scenario: Ms. Johnson, a 78-year-old patient, is admitted to the medical-surgical unit following a hip

replacement surgery. She is at risk for falls due to postoperative weakness and dizziness. As the CMSRN on duty, which intervention is the most appropriate to prevent falls in this patient?
A) Placing the call bell within the patient's reach
B) Administering sedative medication to promote rest
C) Encouraging the patient to walk unassisted for exercise
D) Keeping the patient's room dimly lit to promote sleep

Question 50: Mr. Johnson, a 65-year-old patient, is admitted to the medical-surgical unit with a diagnosis of heart failure. He is receiving intravenous diuretics to manage his fluid overload. The nurse notes that Mr. Johnson has developed hypokalemia. Which intervention is most appropriate for the nurse to implement?
A) Administer potassium supplements orally with a glass of water.
B) Increase the rate of intravenous diuretics to enhance diuresis.
C) Encourage the patient to consume a banana with breakfast daily.
D) Notify the healthcare provider to adjust the diuretic regimen.

Question 51: What is a crucial aspect of post-mortem care in the context of Palliative/End-of-Life Care and Holistic Patient Care?
A) Providing emotional support to the family members
B) Administering pain medication to the deceased
C) Performing a full physical assessment on the deceased
D) Initiating resuscitation efforts on the deceased

Question 52: Which of the following interventions is essential for preventing pressure ulcers in bedridden patients?
A) Massaging bony prominences every hour
B) Keeping the skin moist with powders
C) Repositioning the patient every 2 hours
D) Using donut-shaped cushions under bony areas

Question 53: Ms. Johnson, a 65-year-old patient, was admitted for a total knee replacement surgery. The surgical team ensured proper pre-operative education, pain management, and post-operative rehabilitation. Ms. Johnson's surgery was successful, and she is now ready for discharge. Which of the following quality patient outcome measures is most appropriate to evaluate the effectiveness of care coordination and transition management in this scenario?
A) Patient satisfaction with the hospital food
B) Timeliness of medication administration during the hospital stay
C) Rate of hospital-acquired infections post-surgery
D) Patient adherence to the prescribed home exercise program after discharge

Question 54: Scenario: Mr. Johnson, a 65-year-old patient, is admitted to the medical-surgical unit with a history of hypertension and diabetes. While in the hospital, he suddenly develops chest pain, shortness of breath, and diaphoresis. His blood pressure drops, and he becomes tachycardic. The nurse notes that he is pale and anxious. What should be the nurse's immediate action in this crisis situation?
A) Administer pain medication
B) Call a code blue
C) Offer the patient a glass of water
D) Document the findings in the patient's chart

Question 55: Scenario: Sarah, a 45-year-old patient recovering from abdominal surgery, is experiencing severe pain. She has a history of opioid misuse. As a CMSRN, what is the most appropriate action to take in this situation to ensure self-regulation?
A) Administer the prescribed opioid pain medication as ordered.

B) Assess the patient's pain level using a pain scale and explore non-pharmacological pain management techniques.
C) Withhold all pain medications due to the patient's history of opioid misuse.
D) Consult with the healthcare team to consider alternative pain management strategies.

Question 56: In the context of staffing for Certified Medical Surgical Registered Nurses (CMSRN), which factor is crucial for ensuring a healthy practice environment?
A) Assigning nurses to units based solely on their availability
B) Providing adequate orientation and training for new staff
C) Implementing mandatory overtime for all nursing staff
D) Ignoring nurse-to-patient ratios to cut costs

Question 57: Which of the following is a primary health promotion goal for a Certified Medical Surgical Registered Nurse (CMSRN) in the context of holistic patient care?
A) Encouraging smoking cessation programs
B) Promoting regular physical activity
C) Advocating for excessive alcohol consumption
D) Suggesting high intake of saturated fats

Question 58: Scenario: Sarah, a 35-year-old Medical Surgical Registered Nurse, has been experiencing increased fatigue, irritability, and a lack of motivation at work. She finds it challenging to concentrate during her shifts and has been feeling emotionally drained. Despite her passion for nursing, Sarah is beginning to feel overwhelmed and exhausted. Which of the following actions is most appropriate for Sarah to address her symptoms of burnout?
A) Increasing her work hours to stay on top of her responsibilities.
B) Ignoring her feelings and continuing to work without seeking help.
C) Engaging in regular exercise, mindfulness practices, and seeking support from colleagues.
D) Taking on additional tasks to distract herself from her burnout symptoms.

Question 59: Scenario: Mr. Johnson, a 65-year-old postoperative patient, experiences a sudden onset of shortness of breath, chest pain, and confusion. The nurse suspects a potential adverse event related to his recent surgery. What is the most appropriate action for the nurse to take first?
A) Notify the physician immediately
B) Administer oxygen therapy
C) Document the findings in the patient's chart
D) Conduct a thorough assessment of the patient's vital signs

Question 60: In the context of service recovery in healthcare, which action best demonstrates a patient-centered approach to resolving a complaint?
A) Ignoring the patient's complaint and moving on to the next task.
B) Acknowledging the patient's concern, apologizing, and actively listening to understand the issue.
C) Blaming the patient for the issue and providing no further assistance.
D) Offering a generic solution without addressing the specific complaint.

Question 61: Scenario: Mrs. Smith, a 65-year-old patient, was admitted for a surgical procedure. Due to a mix-up in scheduling, her surgery was delayed by several hours, causing her significant distress and anxiety. As a CMSRN, how should you handle this situation to ensure effective service recovery and patient satisfaction?
A) Apologize to Mrs. Smith and explain the situation, offering her a

complimentary meal.

B) Ignore the delay and proceed with the surgery without addressing the issue.

C) Blame the delay on the operating room staff to alleviate Mrs. Smith's concerns.

D) Communicate with Mrs. Smith, express empathy for the inconvenience, and involve her in the revised plan.

Question 62: Which of the following actions by a Certified Medical Surgical Registered Nurse (CMSRN) demonstrates a commitment to promoting a healthy practice environment in terms of environmental safety?

A) Reusing disposable gloves to reduce waste

B) Proper disposal of hazardous materials in designated bins

C) Ignoring spills on the floor during rounds

D) Leaving medication cart unlocked for easier access

Question 63: In the healthcare setting, the chain of command refers to:

A) A hierarchical structure that outlines the order of authority and communication within an organization.

B) A group of nurses working together in a team.

C) A system of random communication flow among healthcare providers.

D) A structure that allows patients to make decisions regarding their care.

Question 64: In the context of financial stewardship within nursing leadership, which action best demonstrates effective management of resources?

A) Implementing cost-cutting measures that compromise patient care

B) Allocating funds for staff education and training programs

C) Ignoring budget constraints to meet patient demands

D) Overlooking financial reports and expenditures

Question 65: Which of the following is a crucial step in the organ donation process for a patient in palliative/end-of-life care?

A) Initiating the organ donation process without consent

B) Ensuring the patient's comfort and dignity are maintained

C) Withholding pain management to preserve organ function

D) Disregarding the patient's wishes regarding organ donation

Question 66: Scenario: Mrs. Smith, a 65-year-old patient, is admitted to the medical-surgical unit with chronic lower back pain. As part of her pain management plan, which nonpharmacological intervention would be most appropriate for the nurse to recommend to help alleviate Mrs. Smith's pain?

A) Transcutaneous Electrical Nerve Stimulation (TENS) therapy

B) Intravenous opioid administration

C) Continuous passive motion (CPM) machine

D) Heat application using a heating pad

Question 67: Scenario: Mr. Smith, a 65-year-old patient with multiple comorbidities, is admitted to the medical-surgical unit. The healthcare team is discussing the allocation of resources for his care. The team is considering various interventions to manage his complex health needs. Which intervention demonstrates effective resource allocation for Mr. Smith?

A) Ordering unnecessary daily laboratory tests to monitor all possible parameters

B) Implementing a multidisciplinary team approach to coordinate his care efficiently

C) Providing excessive medications to cover all potential symptoms

D) Keeping Mr. Smith isolated in his room to prevent any potential

infections

Question 68: Ms. Johnson, a 58-year-old patient recovering from abdominal surgery, expresses a strong desire to actively participate in her care plan and rehabilitation process. She frequently asks questions, seeks clarification, and engages with the healthcare team. Which leadership style would be most effective in supporting Ms. Johnson's desire for involvement and collaboration in her care?

A) Authoritative leadership

B) Democratic leadership

C) Laissez-faire leadership

D) Transactional leadership

Question 69: Scenario: Mrs. Smith, a 65-year-old patient, has been admitted for a surgical procedure. As part of her care plan, the nurse needs to educate her on post-operative exercises. Mrs. Smith is a visual learner and prefers hands-on demonstrations. Which teaching method would be most effective for educating Mrs. Smith on post-operative exercises?

A) Providing her with written instructions

B) Verbally explaining the exercises

C) Demonstrating the exercises using visual aids

D) Discussing the exercises in a group setting

Question 70: Ms. Smith, a CMSRN, is reflecting on a recent incident where a medication error occurred in her unit. She is contemplating how to approach this situation and learn from it. Which action best demonstrates reflective practice in this scenario?

A) Ignoring the incident and hoping it does not happen again.

B) Discussing the error openly with colleagues to understand what went wrong.

C) Blaming a coworker for the error to shift responsibility.

D) Avoiding any discussion about the incident to prevent conflict.

Question 71: Scenario: Mr. Smith, a 55-year-old patient, is admitted to the medical-surgical unit with a diagnosis of pneumonia. While providing care to Mr. Smith, the nurse notices that the room temperature is unusually high, causing discomfort to the patient. Which action by the nurse is most appropriate to ensure a healthy practice environment for Mr. Smith?

A) Provide extra blankets to Mr. Smith to keep him warm.

B) Adjust the thermostat to a comfortable temperature for Mr. Smith.

C) Open the windows to allow fresh air circulation in the room.

D) Offer Mr. Smith a warm beverage to regulate his body temperature.

Question 72: Scenario: Ms. Rodriguez, a 65-year-old Hispanic female, is admitted to the medical-surgical unit with a diagnosis of heart failure exacerbation. During the assessment, the nurse notes that Ms. Rodriguez lives alone in a low-income neighborhood with limited access to fresh produce and healthcare facilities. She expresses concerns about affording her medications. Which social determinant of health is most likely impacting Ms. Rodriguez's current health status?

A) Education level

B) Socioeconomic status

C) Occupation

D) Marital status

Question 73: Which action by a nurse best demonstrates stewardship in safe drug management and disposal?

A) Flushing expired medications down the toilet

B) Donating unused medications to a local pharmacy
C) Discarding medications in the household trash
D) Returning unused medications to a designated take-back program

Question 74: Scenario: Mr. Smith, a 65-year-old patient, is scheduled for a surgical procedure requiring the use of a hemostat. Which instrument would be most appropriate for the nurse to select to assist the surgeon during the procedure?
A) Scalpel
B) Forceps
C) Retractor
D) Hemostat

Question 75: Which action by the nurse best demonstrates a commitment to patient safety in the context of Patient/Care Management?
A) Administering medications without checking the patient's identification
B) Double-checking the patient's identification before administering medications
C) Ignoring a patient's call light while attending to paperwork
D) Leaving a patient unattended during a procedure to answer a personal phone call

Question 76: Ms. Johnson, a 65-year-old patient recovering from abdominal surgery, is prescribed a clear liquid diet. Which of the following food items would be appropriate for Ms. Johnson's diet?
A) Chicken broth
B) Vanilla pudding
C) Mashed potatoes
D) Oatmeal

Question 77: Scenario: Mr. Smith, a 65-year-old patient recovering from a total knee replacement surgery, is scheduled for physical therapy sessions to aid in his rehabilitation process. As a CMSRN, you are responsible for coordinating his care and ensuring optimal outcomes. During the initial assessment, Mr. Smith expresses concerns about his mobility and pain levels, seeking guidance on the appropriate exercises to improve his strength and flexibility. Which of the following physical therapy interventions would be most beneficial for Mr. Smith at this stage of his recovery?
A) Passive Range of Motion (PROM) exercises
B) High-impact aerobic exercises
C) Isometric strengthening exercises
D) Resistance band exercises

Question 78: Scenario: Mr. Smith, a 65-year-old patient with a history of heart failure, diabetes, and hypertension, is admitted to the medical-surgical unit for exacerbation of heart failure. The healthcare team consists of a medical doctor, nurse practitioner, registered nurse, physical therapist, and dietitian. The team meets to discuss Mr. Smith's care plan, including medication adjustments, dietary modifications, and physical therapy goals. Which team member is primarily responsible for coordinating the interprofessional care plan for Mr. Smith?
A) Registered Nurse
B) Medical Doctor
C) Nurse Practitioner
D) Physical Therapist

Question 79: Scenario: Ms. Patel, a 65-year-old South Asian woman, has been admitted to the medical-surgical unit for post-operative care following a cholecystectomy. The healthcare team is discussing her nutritional needs, taking into consideration her cultural background. Ms. Patel's family has brought her traditional South Asian dishes to eat during her hospital stay. Which action by the nurse best demonstrates culturally sensitive care for Ms. Patel's nutritional needs?
A) Encouraging Ms. Patel to eat only hospital-provided meals for standardized nutrition.
B) Allowing Ms. Patel to eat only the traditional South Asian dishes brought by her family.
C) Providing a menu that includes a mix of hospital meals and traditional South Asian options.
D) Advising Ms. Patel to avoid her cultural foods for better post-operative recovery.

Question 80: Which action is the priority when managing a deteriorating patient in a crisis situation?
A) Administering medication without consulting the healthcare team
B) Notifying the healthcare provider immediately
C) Waiting for the next vital sign assessment
D) Documenting the changes in the patient's condition for the next shift

Question 81: Scenario: Mr. Johnson, a 65-year-old patient, has been admitted to the medical-surgical unit with a diagnosis of pneumonia. During the morning rounds, the nurse notices that Mr. Johnson is experiencing increased shortness of breath and restlessness. On further assessment, the nurse observes that Mr. Johnson's oxygen saturation has dropped to 88%. The nurse decides to inform the healthcare provider immediately. What is the most appropriate action for the nurse to take next?
A) Wait for the next scheduled provider visit to discuss Mr. Johnson's condition.
B) Document the findings in the patient's chart and continue routine care.
C) Call the healthcare provider immediately to report Mr. Johnson's change in condition.
D) Administer supplemental oxygen without consulting the healthcare provider.

Question 82: Scenario: Mr. Johnson, a 65-year-old patient, is admitted to the medical-surgical unit with complaints of severe post-operative pain following a knee replacement surgery. The healthcare team has prescribed pain management interventions to address his discomfort. As the CMSRN, you assess Mr. Johnson's pain level using a pain scale and note his vital signs. Which intervention should you prioritize to manage Mr. Johnson's pain effectively?
A) Administering a non-opioid analgesic such as acetaminophen
B) Initiating patient-controlled analgesia (PCA) with morphine
C) Applying heat therapy to the surgical site
D) Suggesting relaxation techniques and guided imagery

Question 83: Which action by a Certified Medical Surgical Registered Nurse (CMSRN) best demonstrates patient/family-centered care in the context of Care Coordination and Transition Management?
A) Providing discharge instructions only to the patient
B) Involving the patient's family in care planning and decision-making
C) Making decisions without considering the patient's preferences
D) Disregarding the patient's cultural beliefs and practices

Question 84: Scenario: A nurse working in a local hospital encounters a situation where a patient's family member requests confidential information about the patient's condition over the phone. The nurse is aware of the importance of patient confidentiality and privacy. What action should the

nurse take based on the scope of practice and code of ethics for nurses per local and regional nursing bodies?
A) Provide the requested information to the family member to maintain good relations.
B) Politely decline to provide the information and offer to discuss it in person at the hospital.
C) Ask the family member to confirm their identity and then share the information.
D) Transfer the call to the patient's primary physician for disclosure of information.

Question 85: Which of the following actions by a Certified Medical Surgical Registered Nurse (CMSRN) ensures patient safety regarding equipment use?
A) Placing a malfunctioning equipment back in the storage room.
B) Using equipment without checking the expiration date.
C) Following manufacturer's guidelines for equipment maintenance.
D) Sharing equipment without proper disinfection.

Question 86: When delegating tasks to unlicensed assistive personnel (UAP), the Certified Medical Surgical Registered Nurse (CMSRN) should prioritize which of the following actions?
A) Providing clear instructions and expectations
B) Allowing the UAP to choose the method of task completion
C) Avoiding supervision once the task is delegated
D) Not providing feedback on task performance

Question 87: Scenario: Sarah, a 25-year-old female, presents to the emergency department with multiple unexplained injuries and appears fearful when questioned about how she sustained them. She avoids making eye contact and seems hesitant to provide personal information. The nurse notices that Sarah's companion is overly controlling and answers most questions on her behalf. Sarah's medical history shows frequent visits to different healthcare facilities with inconsistent complaints. Which action should the nurse prioritize when suspecting human trafficking in this scenario?
A) Discharge Sarah with instructions to follow up with a primary care provider.
B) Notify the hospital social worker about the suspicions of human trafficking.
C) Document the injuries and history in the medical record without further investigation.
D) Confront Sarah's companion directly to inquire about the injuries.

Question 88: When documenting patient care, which action by the Certified Medical Surgical Registered Nurse (CMSRN) demonstrates adherence to professional reporting standards?
A) Using abbreviations and acronyms to save time
B) Including subjective opinions in the documentation
C) Documenting care provided by another healthcare provider as their own
D) Recording information accurately and objectively

Question 89: Scenario: Mr. Johnson, a 65-year-old patient, is admitted to the medical-surgical unit with a stage IV pressure ulcer on his sacrum. The wound is showing signs of infection, with surrounding erythema and purulent drainage. The healthcare team has initiated wound care management, including appropriate dressing changes and antibiotic therapy. As the CMSRN overseeing Mr. Johnson's care, what is the most crucial aspect to prioritize in the management of his infected pressure ulcer?
A) Ensuring adequate nutrition and hydration for the patient
B) Administering pain medication to alleviate discomfort

C) Implementing strict isolation precautions to prevent the spread of infection
D) Monitoring and documenting the wound characteristics and response to treatment

Question 90: Which of the following is a potential benefit of probiotics in the context of Certified Medical Surgical Registered Nurse(CMSRN) practice?
A) Prevention of antibiotic-associated diarrhea
B) Treatment of hypertension
C) Management of type 2 diabetes
D) Improvement of vision

Question 91: When resolving conflicts in a medical-surgical setting, which communication approach is most effective in promoting a positive outcome?
A) Avoiding the conflict altogether
B) Using aggressive communication to assert dominance
C) Employing active listening and empathy
D) Blaming others for the conflict

Question 92: Scenario: Ms. Rodriguez, a 45-year-old Hispanic female, presents to the clinic with uncontrolled hypertension. During the assessment, it is revealed that she works two jobs to support her family, has limited access to fresh produce in her neighborhood, and experiences high levels of stress due to financial constraints. Which social determinant of health is most likely contributing to Ms. Rodriguez's uncontrolled hypertension?
A) Limited access to healthcare facilities
B) High levels of stress
C) Lack of physical exercise
D) Inadequate health literacy

Question 93: Scenario: Mr. Johnson, a 65-year-old patient, is admitted to the medical-surgical unit with complaints of chest pain and shortness of breath. As the nurse, you approach Mr. Johnson to assess his condition. He appears anxious and is having difficulty expressing himself clearly due to his distress. How should you demonstrate active listening in this situation?
A) Interrupt him to gather information quickly.
B) Maintain eye contact and nod periodically.
C) Check your watch frequently to manage time efficiently.
D) Provide solutions before he finishes speaking.

Question 94: In the context of human trafficking, what is a crucial aspect of patient safety assessments and reporting for Certified Medical Surgical Registered Nurses (CMSRNs)?
A) Recognizing signs of physical abuse only
B) Identifying potential victims and reporting suspicions
C) Focusing solely on medical treatment without involvement in social issues
D) Disregarding patient history related to social determinants

Question 95: Which of the following is a key step in the research process for evidence-based practice in nursing?
A) Conducting a literature review
B) Administering medications to patients
C) Documenting vital signs
D) Answering phone calls at the nursing station

Question 96: Which of the following interventions is essential for preventing pressure ulcers in bedridden patients?
A) Massaging bony prominences every hour
B) Keeping the skin clean and dry
C) Applying direct pressure to reddened areas
D) Using donut-shaped cushions for prolonged sitting

Question 97: Scenario: Mr. Johnson, a 65-year-old patient, is admitted to the medical-surgical unit for post-operative care following a hip replacement surgery. The nurse observes that the patient is experiencing increased pain and requests pain medication. The nurse notices that the medication prescribed is incorrect but the physician is unavailable at the moment. What should the nurse do first to ensure patient safety culture?
A) Administer the incorrect medication to relieve the patient's pain.
B) Consult with the pharmacist to verify the medication order.
C) Wait for the physician to become available before taking any action.
D) Inform the patient that the medication will be delayed.

Question 98: Scenario: During hourly rounding, the nurse finds a patient, Mr. Johnson, complaining of severe abdominal pain. The patient rates the pain as 8/10 on the pain scale. He appears restless and diaphoretic. On assessment, the nurse notes tachycardia and increased blood pressure. What should be the nurse's immediate action based on the situation described?
A) Administer pain medication as ordered
B) Notify the healthcare provider immediately
C) Reassure the patient and continue with the rounding
D) Document the findings in the patient's chart

Question 99: In the context of 'check-back' communication technique, what is the primary purpose of this strategy?
A) To confirm that the message sent by the sender is correctly received by the receiver.
B) To interrupt the flow of communication for clarification.
C) To assert dominance in the conversation.
D) To ignore the information shared by the sender.

Question 100: Scenario: Mr. Smith, a 65-year-old patient, has been discharged from the hospital with multiple medications. As part of safe drug management and disposal, which action by the nurse is most appropriate to ensure proper medication disposal?
A) Flush the medications down the toilet
B) Throw the medications in the household trash
C) Mix the medications with coffee grounds or kitty litter before disposal
D) Return the medications to a pharmacy or participate in a drug take-back program

Question 101: Scenario: During the handover report, the nurse mentions to the oncoming nurse that the patient in room 302 is allergic to penicillin. The oncoming nurse repeats back, "Patient in room 302 is allergic to penicillin." This communication technique is known as:
A) Paraphrasing
B) Reflecting
C) Read-back
D) Summarizing

Question 102: Which intervention is crucial in preventing patient falls in a medical-surgical setting?
A) Encouraging patients to walk unassisted
B) Keeping call bells within reach of patients
C) Restraining agitated patients to prevent wandering
D) Minimizing staff presence on the unit

Question 103: Scenario: Mr. Johnson, a 65-year-old patient, is admitted to the medical-surgical unit with a diagnosis of congestive heart failure. The healthcare team includes a medical doctor, a nurse practitioner, a physical therapist, and a social worker. The team meets regularly to discuss Mr. Johnson's care plan and progress. What is the role of the Certified Medical Surgical Registered Nurse (CMSRN) within the interdisciplinary team caring for Mr. Johnson?
A) Coordinate care and communicate with all team members
B) Prescribe medications and treatments for the patient
C) Perform physical therapy sessions with the patient
D) Assist the social worker in completing paperwork for the patient

Question 104: Which of the following best describes moral injury in the context of a Healthy Practice Environment for Certified Medical Surgical Registered Nurses (CMSRNs)?
A) Moral injury is solely caused by intentional harm or wrongdoing.
B) Moral injury results from a discrepancy between what one believes to be right and the actions taken in a high-stress work environment.
C) Moral injury is a term used interchangeably with burnout.
D) Moral injury is a rare occurrence and does not significantly impact healthcare professionals.

Question 105: Which of the following is an example of an adverse reaction to medication?
A) Increased heart rate after taking a beta-blocker
B) Decreased blood pressure after taking an ACE inhibitor
C) Improved blood sugar levels after taking insulin
D) Reduced pain after taking an analgesic

Question 106: Scenario: Ms. Johnson, a 68-year-old postoperative patient, requires frequent wound dressing changes and vital sign monitoring. As the charge nurse, you need to delegate these tasks to the nursing team. Which task can be appropriately delegated to the nursing assistant?
A) Assessing the wound for signs of infection
B) Changing the wound dressing using sterile technique
C) Monitoring vital signs every 4 hours
D) Providing patient education on wound care

Question 107: Scenario: Mr. Johnson, a 65-year-old patient, is admitted to the medical-surgical unit for post-operative care following a knee replacement surgery. The healthcare team plans to utilize technology to enhance interprofessional care for Mr. Johnson. Which technological tool would be most beneficial in facilitating communication and collaboration among the healthcare team members involved in Mr. Johnson's care?
A) Electronic Health Record (EHR) system
B) Social media platforms
C) Personal email communication
D) Fax machine

Question 108: In Failure Mode and Effects Analysis (FMEA), which step involves assigning a numerical value to the frequency of occurrence, likelihood of detection, and severity of the potential failure mode?
A) Step 1: Define the scope and boundaries of the analysis
B) Step 2: Assemble a multidisciplinary team
C) Step 3: Identify potential failure modes
D) Step 4: Assign a Risk Priority Number (RPN) to each potential failure mode

Question 109: Which leadership model emphasizes the leader's ability to inspire and motivate team members through a compelling vision and strong personal values?
A) Transactional Leadership
B) Servant Leadership
C) Transformational Leadership
D) Laissez-Faire Leadership

Question 110: Scenario: Ms. Johnson, a 68-year-old patient, is admitted to the medical-surgical unit with a diagnosis of heart failure. The healthcare team is discussing the implementation of a new nursing care delivery system to improve patient outcomes and satisfaction. As the CMSRN, which nursing care delivery system focuses on providing individualized care by assigning one nurse to oversee all aspects of a patient's care during a 12-hour shift?
A) Team Nursing
B) Total Patient Care
C) Primary Nursing
D) Case Management

Question 111: Ms. Johnson, a 65-year-old patient, is being discharged from the hospital after undergoing a surgical procedure. As the Certified Medical Surgical Registered Nurse (CMSRN) responsible for her care coordination and transition management, which action is most crucial to ensure a smooth transition and continuity of care for Ms. Johnson?
A) Providing her with a list of community resources for post-operative care.
B) Ensuring she has a follow-up appointment scheduled with her primary care physician.
C) Sending her home with detailed written instructions about her medications.
D) Recommending a new diet plan for her recovery period.

Question 112: Scenario: Mrs. Smith, a 68-year-old patient with advanced cancer, is admitted to the palliative care unit. She is experiencing severe pain that is impacting her quality of life. As a CMSRN, which intervention is most appropriate for managing Mrs. Smith's pain effectively?
A) Administering non-opioid analgesics such as acetaminophen
B) Scheduling regular pain assessments every 12 hours
C) Initiating opioid therapy with morphine as per the WHO analgesic ladder
D) Using distraction techniques to divert Mrs. Smith's attention from pain

Question 113: Which social determinant of health plays a significant role in patient safety assessments and reporting for Certified Medical Surgical Registered Nurses (CMSRNs)?
A) Education level
B) Blood type
C) Favorite color
D) Shoe size

Question 114: Which of the following is a key aspect of Career Development Relationships in nursing education?
A) Building strong communication skills with patients
B) Establishing mentorship with experienced nurses
C) Attending regular educational seminars
D) Participating in physical fitness programs

Question 115: Which of the following statements regarding acupuncture is true?
A) Acupuncture is a form of massage therapy.
B) Acupuncture involves the use of herbal remedies.
C) Acupuncture is based on the concept of meridians and energy flow.
D) Acupuncture is primarily used for surgical procedures.

Question 116: Scenario: During hourly rounding, the Certified Medical Surgical Registered Nurse (CMSRN) finds a patient, Mr. Smith, complaining of severe abdominal pain. The nurse assesses the patient and notes that the pain is localized to the right lower quadrant. Mr. Smith rates the pain as 8/10 on the pain scale. Vital signs are stable, and there are no signs of peritonitis. What action should the nurse take next?
A) Administer pain medication as ordered
B) Notify the healthcare provider immediately
C) Reassess the patient's pain level in 30 minutes
D) Document the findings in the patient's chart

Question 117: Which of the following is a key component of patient-centered care in setting health goals?
A) Dictating goals to the patient
B) Ignoring patient preferences
C) Collaborating with the patient
D) Excluding the patient from decision-making

Question 118: During a disaster situation, which action by the medical surgical registered nurse demonstrates effective teamwork and collaboration in emergency procedures?
A) Taking charge of the situation without consulting other team members
B) Following individual protocols without coordinating with other healthcare providers
C) Communicating effectively with the interdisciplinary team to prioritize patient care
D) Ignoring the input of other team members and making decisions independently

Question 119: In the context of patient-centered care, which action best demonstrates the importance of family involvement in the care of a patient?
A) Allowing family members to visit only during restricted visiting hours.
B) Providing family members with limited information about the patient's condition.
C) Involving family members in care decisions and treatment planning.
D) Restricting family involvement to avoid interference in medical care.

Question 120: Scenario: Mrs. Smith, a 65-year-old patient, was admitted to a high accountable organization for a surgical procedure. During her stay, the nursing staff consistently followed the hospital's protocols, engaged in effective communication, and ensured Mrs. Smith's safety and well-being at all times. The organization emphasized a culture of patient safety and prioritized patient-centered care management. Which characteristic best describes a high accountable organization in the context of patient safety culture and patient/care management?
A) Prioritizing cost-cutting measures over patient safety
B) Focusing on individual performance rather than teamwork
C) Emphasizing open communication and collaboration among healthcare team members
D) Neglecting patient preferences and feedback

Question 121: Scenario: Mr. Johnson, a 65-year-old male patient, is admitted to the medical-surgical unit with a diagnosis of heart failure. The healthcare team is discussing the implementation of a new evidence-based practice related to heart failure management. As a CMSRN, which action demonstrates the nurse's commitment to evidence-based practice?
A) Following the traditional heart failure management protocol
B) Consulting the latest clinical practice guidelines for heart failure
C) Implementing a practice based on personal experience
D) Disregarding research findings and relying on intuition

Question 122: Scenario: Mr. Johnson, a 65-year-old patient admitted for pneumonia, suddenly becomes unresponsive, with shallow breathing and a weak pulse. The nurse notes

cyanosis around his lips. His oxygen saturation is 82%. What should the nurse do first?
A) Administer a dose of pain medication
B) Call a code blue and initiate CPR
C) Increase the rate of the IV fluids
D) Re-position the patient in bed

Question 123: Scenario: Mr. Smith, a 65-year-old patient, was admitted to the medical-surgical unit for post-operative care following a hip replacement surgery. He appears frustrated and agitated, frequently asking questions about his treatment plan and expressing concerns about his recovery. Despite the nurse's attempts to provide explanations, Mr. Smith continues to appear distressed and uncooperative. Which of the following communication barriers is most likely affecting the interaction between Mr. Smith and the nurse?
A) Language barriers
B) Emotional barriers
C) Physical barriers
D) Cultural barriers

Question 124: When receiving a verbal order from a physician, the nurse should:
A) Immediately implement the order without questioning
B) Write down the order and then inform the physician
C) Ignore the order and wait for a written confirmation
D) Disregard the order as verbal orders are not valid

Question 125: Scenario: Mr. Smith, a 65-year-old patient, is admitted to the medical-surgical unit with a diagnosis of pneumonia. The nurse is preparing to perform a tracheostomy care procedure for Mr. Smith. Which of the following actions by the nurse demonstrates current evidence-based practice for infection control and prevention procedures?
A) Wearing gloves only during tracheostomy care.
B) Using alcohol-based hand sanitizer before and after tracheostomy care.
C) Cleaning the inner cannula with tap water and soap.
D) Reusing the same tracheostomy tube inner cannula for multiple care sessions.

Question 126: During the assessment phase of the nursing process, the nurse should prioritize which action?
A) Implementing interventions without further evaluation
B) Formulating a nursing diagnosis based on assumptions
C) Collecting comprehensive and accurate patient data
D) Skipping the assessment phase and proceeding directly to planning

Question 127: Scenario: Mr. Smith, a 65-year-old patient, is admitted to the medical-surgical unit with a history of heart failure. He is anxious about his condition and frequently expresses his concerns to the nursing staff. As a Certified Medical Surgical Registered Nurse (CMSRN), which communication technique would be most appropriate to use when mediating Mr. Smith's anxiety?
A) Offering reassurance and empathy while actively listening to Mr. Smith's concerns.
B) Providing quick solutions to alleviate Mr. Smith's anxiety and move on to other tasks.
C) Ignoring Mr. Smith's expressions of anxiety to avoid escalating the situation.
D) Interrupting Mr. Smith to redirect the conversation towards medical interventions.

Question 128: Ms. Johnson, a 65-year-old patient, is admitted with a diagnosis of chronic kidney disease (CKD) stage 3. Which dietary modification is most appropriate for Ms.

Johnson's condition?
A) Increase protein intake
B) Limit phosphorus-rich foods
C) Encourage high potassium foods
D) Promote fluid intake as desired

Question 129: Which resource is commonly used for alternate nutrition administration in patients unable to tolerate oral intake?
A) Percutaneous endoscopic gastrostomy (PEG) tube
B) Intravenous (IV) fluids
C) Nasogastric (NG) tube
D) Rectal suppositories

Question 130: In the context of Leadership, Nursing Teamwork, and Collaboration, which strategy is most effective for improving recruitment and retention of medical-surgical nurses?
A) Offering competitive salary and benefits packages
B) Implementing mandatory overtime shifts
C) Providing limited opportunities for professional growth
D) Ignoring staff feedback and suggestions

Question 131: In the context of 'read-back' as a communication strategy in healthcare, what is the primary purpose of this practice?
A) To confirm and verify information exchanged during verbal communication.
B) To speed up the communication process and save time.
C) To avoid documentation of important details.
D) To rely solely on memory for retaining information.

Question 132: Scenario: Mr. Smith, a 65-year-old postoperative patient, is experiencing respiratory distress. The nurse suspects a possible malfunction with the oxygen delivery system. Which action should the nurse prioritize in troubleshooting the equipment?
A) Check the oxygen flow meter for proper settings.
B) Increase the oxygen flow rate immediately.
C) Disconnect the oxygen tubing and reconnect it.
D) Switch the patient to a different oxygen delivery device.

Question 133: In the context of 'Role within the interdisciplinary team' in Interprofessional Collaboration and Elements of Interprofessional Care, which action by a Certified Medical Surgical Registered Nurse (CMSRN) best demonstrates effective teamwork?
A) Providing patient care independently without consulting other team members
B) Attending team meetings regularly and actively participating in discussions
C) Ignoring input from other healthcare professionals during patient care planning
D) Refusing to collaborate with allied health professionals in the care of a patient

Question 134: In an interdisciplinary healthcare team, what is the primary purpose of information sharing?
A) To create barriers between team members
B) To enhance collaboration and patient care
C) To promote individualistic decision-making
D) To limit communication channels

Question 135: Scenario: Mr. Smith, a 65-year-old male, is admitted to the medical-surgical unit with a diagnosis of pneumonia. He has been started on empirical broad-spectrum antibiotics. After 48 hours, the culture results indicate that the causative organism is sensitive to a narrower spectrum antibiotic. The healthcare team decides to de-escalate the antibiotic therapy. Which action best demonstrates antimicrobial stewardship in this scenario?

A) Continuing the broad-spectrum antibiotics to cover for potential resistant organisms.

B) Stopping all antibiotics to prevent antibiotic resistance.

C) De-escalating the antibiotic therapy to a narrower spectrum based on culture results.

D) Rotating through different classes of antibiotics to prevent resistance.

Question 136: Which of the following is an example of primary prevention in health maintenance and disease prevention for patients and families?

A) Administering antibiotics for an active infection

B) Providing smoking cessation counseling to prevent lung cancer

C) Monitoring blood glucose levels in diabetic patients

D) Performing physical therapy after a hip replacement surgery

Question 137: Which of the following is a potential complication associated with epidural analgesia?

A) Hypertension

B) Hypoglycemia

C) Bradycardia

D) Hyperkalemia

Question 138: Which resource is most appropriate for a patient/family seeking information on managing a chronic condition at home?

A) Social media platforms

B) Online support groups

C) Hospital library

D) Certified patient education materials

Question 139: Which of the following best defines a positive patient safety culture in a healthcare setting?

A) Blaming individuals for errors

B) Prioritizing speed over accuracy in patient care

C) Open communication about errors and near misses

D) Ignoring staff concerns about patient safety

Question 140: When prioritizing tasks as a Certified Medical Surgical Registered Nurse (CMSRN), which action demonstrates effective delegation and supervision?

A) Completing all tasks independently to ensure accuracy

B) Delegating tasks based on personal preference

C) Assigning tasks according to each team member's scope of practice

D) Ignoring tasks that are time-consuming

Question 141: Which of the following is a key pre-procedural unit standard that should be adhered to in surgical/procedural nursing management?

A) Ensuring the patient has signed the consent form

B) Administering post-operative medications

C) Documenting vital signs post-procedure

D) Allowing the patient to eat immediately before the procedure

Question 142: Ms. Johnson, a 65-year-old patient, is admitted to the medical-surgical unit with a diagnosis of heart failure. During the initial assessment, the nurse discusses health goals with Ms. Johnson. Which of the following goals reflects the principles of patient-centered care for Ms. Johnson?

A) Decrease sodium intake to 2,000 mg per day.

B) Increase daily water intake to 3 liters.

C) Walk for 30 minutes every day.

D) Reduce stress through meditation techniques.

Question 143: Scenario: Mrs. Smith, a 65-year-old patient, was admitted to the medical-surgical unit with a diagnosis of congestive heart failure. She is experiencing shortness of breath, fatigue, and pedal edema. During the assessment, the nurse notes crackles in Mrs. Smith's lungs, elevated blood pressure, and decreased urine output. Mrs. Smith expresses fear and anxiety about her condition and upcoming treatments. Which intervention by the nurse best demonstrates holistic patient care for Mrs. Smith?

A) Administering diuretics to reduce pedal edema

B) Providing emotional support and reassurance to address Mrs. Smith's fear and anxiety

C) Monitoring blood pressure and urine output closely

D) Educating Mrs. Smith on dietary restrictions for managing congestive heart failure

Question 144: Ms. Johnson, a 65-year-old patient, is scheduled for an exploratory laparotomy tomorrow. As the nurse preparing Ms. Johnson for surgery, which action is the highest priority in the preoperative phase?

A) Administering preoperative antibiotics

B) Ensuring the patient has signed the informed consent form

C) Verifying the patient's identification using two unique identifiers

D) Confirming that the surgical site is correctly marked

Question 145: Which of the following best defines the scope of practice for a Certified Medical Surgical Registered Nurse (CMSRN)?

A) Performing surgical procedures independently

B) Prescribing medications without physician oversight

C) Providing post-operative care and education to patients

D) Making final decisions on patient diagnoses

Question 146: In the context of fiscal efficiency in nursing, which action by the Registered Nurse demonstrates effective budgetary considerations?

A) Ordering excessive supplies to ensure availability

B) Implementing evidence-based practice to reduce unnecessary costs

C) Ignoring cost-saving suggestions from the nursing team

D) Overstaffing shifts to prevent shortages

Question 147: Which medication is commonly used for moderate/procedural sedation in a medical-surgical setting?

A) Furosemide

B) Midazolam

C) Metoprolol

D) Omeprazole

Question 148: Which of the following is a modifiable risk factor for patient safety in the context of Patient/Care Management?

A) Age

B) Gender

C) Smoking

D) Genetic predisposition

Question 149: Scenario: Mrs. Smith, a 78-year-old patient, is admitted to the medical-surgical unit following a hip replacement surgery. She is at risk for falls due to post-operative weakness and dizziness. While assessing Mrs. Smith, the nurse notes that she is attempting to get out of bed without calling for assistance. Which intervention should the nurse prioritize to prevent falls in this patient?

A) Place a bed alarm on Mrs. Smith's bed.

B) Instruct Mrs. Smith to call for help before getting out of bed.

C) Apply physical restraints to Mrs. Smith's wrists.

D) Encourage Mrs. Smith to walk to the bathroom independently.

Question 150: Which strategy is essential when individualizing care for a patient in the context of the Nursing Process/Clinical Judgement Measurement Model and Elements of Interprofessional Care?

A) Implementing standardized care plans for all patients

B) Ignoring patient preferences to maintain consistency in care delivery

C) Tailoring care based on the patient's unique needs and preferences

D) Following a one-size-fits-all approach to care provision

ANSWER WITH DETAILED EXPLANATION SET [4]

Question 1: Correct Answer: B) Elevating the head of the bed to 30-45 degrees

Rationale: Elevating the head of the bed to 30-45 degrees is a crucial intervention in preventing ventilator-associated pneumonia (VAP) by reducing the risk of aspiration. This position helps to prevent the pooling of secretions in the lungs, thus decreasing the chances of developing VAP. Administering prophylactic antibiotics may contribute to antibiotic resistance and is not a standard preventive measure for VAP. Providing oral care with chlorhexidine solution is essential for oral hygiene but is not directly related to preventing VAP. Changing the ventilator circuit every 48 hours is important for infection control but does not specifically target VAP prevention.

Question 2: Correct Answer: B) Seeking guidance from a supervisor to address the issue

Rationale: Seeking guidance from a supervisor to address the issue is the most appropriate response to moral distress related to unintended consequences. This action demonstrates a proactive approach to resolving the ethical dilemma and seeking support from a higher authority to address the situation effectively. Options A, C, and D are not appropriate responses as they involve either ignoring the issue, blaming others, or avoiding the patient, which do not address the root cause of moral distress and may lead to further ethical challenges in the healthcare environment.

Question 3: Correct Answer: D) Patient satisfaction survey

Rationale: Patient satisfaction surveys are specifically designed to gather feedback from patients regarding their experiences with healthcare services. These surveys focus on aspects such as quality of care, communication with healthcare providers, wait times, and overall satisfaction. In contrast, randomized controlled trials and case-control studies are research study designs used to investigate treatment outcomes and associations between variables, while cross-sectional surveys provide a snapshot of a population at a specific point in time. Therefore, the correct option for assessing patient customer experience based on data results in a healthcare setting is the patient satisfaction survey.

Question 4: Correct Answer: C) Employ a professional medical interpreter service.

Rationale: Utilizing a professional medical interpreter service (Option C) is the most appropriate choice when communicating with a patient who has limited English proficiency. This ensures accurate and confidential communication, preventing misunderstandings that could impact patient care. Options A and B may lead to breaches in patient confidentiality and potential misinterpretation of medical information. Option D is not a reliable method for conveying complex medical information and may result in errors or miscommunication, compromising the quality of care provided to the patient.

Question 5: Correct Answer: B) Adjusting the thermostat to a warmer setting

Rationale: Adjusting the thermostat to a warmer setting is the best action to promote a healthy practice environment for the patient. Maintaining a comfortable room temperature is essential for patient well-being and aids in the recovery process. Providing an extra blanket (option A) or offering a hot beverage (option C) may provide temporary relief but does not address the root cause of the issue. Closing the window (option D) may help block the draft but may not effectively regulate the room temperature. By adjusting the thermostat, the nurse ensures a consistent and comfortable environment for the patient, promoting optimal healing and recovery.

Question 6: Correct Answer: C) To enhance patient care and outcomes

Rationale: Establishing a professional network in nursing is crucial for enhancing patient care and outcomes. While options A and B focus on personal gains and competition, option D emphasizes social aspects. However, the primary purpose of a professional network in nursing is to collaborate, share knowledge, seek advice, and support each other to provide the best possible care for patients. By connecting with other healthcare professionals, nurses can access resources, stay updated on best practices, and ultimately improve the quality of patient care through effective teamwork and collaboration.

Question 7: Correct Answer: D) Using two patient identifiers before administering medications

Rationale: Option D is the correct answer as using two patient identifiers, such as asking for the patient's name and date of birth, is a standard practice to ensure the right patient receives the right medication. This process aligns with regulatory standards to prevent medication errors. Options A, B, and C are incorrect as they do not directly relate to regulatory and compliance standards. Administering medications without proper identification, deviating from ordered documentation frequency, and allowing family members to stay overnight, though important for patient care, do not specifically address regulatory and compliance standards in this scenario.

Question 8: Correct Answer: C) Food Banks offering emergency food supplies

Rationale: Food banks are essential community resources that provide emergency food supplies to individuals and families in need, including those with chronic illnesses who may struggle with food insecurity. While local gyms, public libraries, and retail stores offer valuable services, they do not directly address the immediate nutritional needs of individuals dealing with chronic illnesses. Food banks play a crucial role in supporting the overall well-being and health management of individuals by ensuring access to nutritious food, making them a key resource in the realm of Care Coordination and Transition Management.

Question 9: Correct Answer: B) Providing detailed and accurate information

Rationale: Documenting detailed and accurate information in a patient's medical record is essential for effective interprofessional care coordination. This ensures that all healthcare team members have access to the most up-to-date and relevant information about the patient's condition, treatment plan, and progress. Using abbreviations can lead to misinterpretation and errors in communication. Delaying documentation can result in crucial information being missed or forgotten. Including personal opinions about the patient is subjective and may not contribute to the overall care coordination process. Therefore, option B is the correct choice as it promotes clear communication and continuity of care among healthcare providers.

Question 10: Correct Answer: B) Check the patient's circulation and skin integrity regularly

Rationale: It is crucial for the nurse to regularly assess the patient's circulation and skin integrity when using restraints to prevent complications such as impaired circulation, skin breakdown, or nerve damage. Option A is incorrect as securing restraints too tightly can lead to circulation issues and injury. Option C is incorrect as the patient should never be left unattended while restrained for safety reasons. Option D is incorrect as obtaining consent is a necessary ethical and legal requirement when using restraints to ensure patient autonomy and rights are respected. Regular monitoring of circulation and skin integrity is vital to prevent harm and ensure patient safety.

Question 11: Correct Answer: C) Improved coordination of care among healthcare team members

Rationale: Electronic health records (EHRs) play a crucial role in enhancing communication and collaboration among healthcare team members, leading to improved coordination of care for patients. Option A is incorrect as EHRs, when implemented securely, actually reduce the risk of data breaches compared to paper records. Option B is inaccurate as EHRs provide quick and easy access to patient information for authorized personnel. Option D is false as EHRs help in reducing medication errors through features like alerts and medication reconciliation, thus decreasing the likelihood of such errors.

Question 12: Correct Answer: B) Asthma

Rationale: Asthma is a chronic respiratory condition involving inflammation of the airways, leading to bronchospasm and airflow obstruction. Pneumonia is an acute infection of the lung tissue, not primarily associated with chronic inflammation. Tuberculosis is a bacterial infection affecting the lungs with specific symptoms different from asthma. Emphysema is a type of chronic obstructive pulmonary disease (COPD) characterized by damage to the air sacs in the lungs, distinct from the pathophysiology of asthma. Therefore, the correct answer is B) Asthma, as it aligns with the described disease process of chronic airway inflammation and bronchospasm.

Question 13: Correct Answer: B) Involving the patient in shared decision-making regarding their care.

Rationale: In patient-centered care, involving the patient in shared decision-making is crucial as it respects the patient's autonomy, preferences, and values. This approach promotes better adherence to treatment plans, improves patient satisfaction, and enhances overall health outcomes. Options A, C, and D do not prioritize the patient's active involvement in their care, which may lead to decreased patient satisfaction, non-compliance, and potential adverse outcomes. Effective patient-centered care focuses on collaboration between healthcare providers and patients, ensuring that care plans align with the patient's goals and preferences.

Question 14: Correct Answer: B) Maintaining a calm tone and using therapeutic communication

Rationale: Option B is the correct answer as maintaining a calm tone and using therapeutic communication is essential in de-escalating situations involving agitated patients. By staying calm, the nurse can help Mr. Johnson feel heard and understood, which can help diffuse the situation. Option A is incorrect as matching the patient's agitation level can escalate the situation further. Option C is incorrect as ignoring the outburst can make the patient feel neglected and escalate the situation. Option D is incorrect as threatening to restrain the patient can lead to increased agitation and is not in line with de-escalation techniques.

Question 15: Correct Answer: C) Notify the healthcare team about Mr. Johnson's behavior and concerns.

Rationale: The correct answer is to notify the healthcare team about Mr. Johnson's behavior and concerns. This action aligns with patient safety protocols as it ensures that appropriate measures are taken to address the patient's risk of self-harm. Option A is incorrect as leaving a patient with suicidal ideation alone can increase the risk of harm. Option B is incorrect as engaging in a conversation about hobbies may not address the immediate safety concern. Option D is incorrect as providing a sharp object can pose a significant risk to the patient's safety. In such cases, timely communication with the healthcare team is crucial to ensure the patient receives the necessary support and interventions.

Question 16: Correct Answer: A) To share important patient information and ensure a safe discharge process.

Rationale: The correct answer is A) To share important patient information and ensure a safe discharge process. During huddles, healthcare teams come together to communicate essential patient details, coordinate care plans, and address any potential risks or concerns. In this scenario, the focus is on Mr. Johnson's safety

during discharge, considering his history of falls and mobility needs. Options B, C, and D are incorrect as they do not align with the primary purpose of a huddle, which is to facilitate effective communication and collaboration among healthcare providers to deliver safe and quality patient care.

Question 17: Correct Answer: A) A patient is experiencing a sudden change in condition

Rationale: The correct answer is A) A patient is experiencing a sudden change in condition. The rapid response team is summoned when a patient's condition deteriorates unexpectedly, requiring immediate intervention to prevent further decline or potential cardiac or respiratory arrest. This team is composed of healthcare professionals trained to assess, stabilize, and manage critical situations promptly. Options B, C, and D are incorrect as they do not warrant the activation of the rapid response team. Option B refers to routine care, Option C is a non-urgent request, and Option D involves regular physician activities unrelated to acute patient deterioration.

Question 18: Correct Answer: A) To discuss patient care plans and updates

Rationale: A huddle in a healthcare setting serves as a brief and focused meeting where team members come together to share important information, discuss patient care plans, and provide updates on current cases. It is a crucial communication tool that enhances teamwork, promotes efficiency, and ensures that all team members are informed and aligned regarding patient care. Options B, C, and D are incorrect as they do not align with the primary purpose of a huddle in a medical context, which is centered around patient care and professional communication.

Question 19: Correct Answer: C) Tailoring education to the individual's learning style and preferences.

Rationale: Tailoring education to the individual's learning style and preferences is the most effective approach in promoting understanding and compliance among patients and families. This method acknowledges that each person learns differently, whether visually, auditory, kinesthetically, or through reading/writing. By customizing the education to suit the individual's preferred learning style, the information is more likely to be absorbed and retained, leading to better comprehension and adherence to the healthcare plan. Options A, B, and D are not ideal as they do not consider the diverse learning needs of patients and families, which are crucial in achieving successful patient education outcomes.

Question 20: Correct Answer: D) Heart failure

Rationale: Mr. Johnson's symptoms of shortness of breath, crackles in the lung bases, fatigue, and difficulty sleeping are indicative of heart failure. In heart failure, the heart is unable to pump blood effectively, leading to fluid accumulation in the lungs (crackles) and other parts of the body. While pulmonary embolism and pneumonia can also present with shortness of breath, they are less likely given Mr. Johnson's medical history and symptoms. COPD typically presents with a chronic cough and wheezing, which are not prominent in this scenario. Therefore, the most likely cause of Mr. Johnson's symptoms is heart failure.

Question 21: Correct Answer: A) Assessing the patient's vital signs before medication administration

Rationale: Assessing the patient's vital signs before medication administration is crucial to ensure patient safety and monitor for any potential adverse reactions or interactions. Vital signs provide valuable information about the patient's current physiological status, helping the nurse make informed decisions regarding medication administration. Administering the medication at the same time every day (option B) is important for medication adherence but does not directly impact patient safety. Encouraging self-administration (option C) can be risky, especially for elderly patients with comorbidities. Mixing medication with food (option D) may alter absorption rates and effectiveness, leading to suboptimal outcomes.

Question 22: Correct Answer: D) Monitoring vital signs and assessing for complications post-procedure

Rationale: As a CMSRN, it is within your scope of practice to monitor vital signs and assess for complications post-procedure. This includes observing for signs of bleeding, infection, or other adverse reactions. Administering conscious sedation (Option A) is typically done by a provider trained in sedation administration. Interpreting results of the procedure (Option B) is usually the responsibility of the healthcare provider who ordered the test. Performing the actual cardiac catheterization procedure (Option C) is performed by an interventional cardiologist or a specially trained healthcare provider, not within the CMSRN scope of practice. Monitoring vital signs and assessing for complications post-procedure is crucial in ensuring the patient's safety and recovery, making it the correct answer in this scenario.

Question 23: Correct Answer: C) Implementing strict hierarchical structures

Rationale: Employee engagement thrives in environments that foster open communication, collaboration, and empowerment. Implementing strict hierarchical structures can hinder engagement by creating barriers to communication, stifling creativity, and limiting employee autonomy. In contrast, options A, B, and D are essential strategies for promoting employee engagement. Providing opportunities for professional development shows investment in employees' growth, recognizing and rewarding contributions boosts morale and motivation, and encouraging open communication and feedback enhances teamwork and trust within the organization.

Question 24: Correct Answer: B) Taking charge of the situation, coordinating the team's efforts, and ensuring timely interventions for the patient.

Rationale: In this scenario, the most effective leadership action is demonstrated by option B. Effective leadership in nursing teamwork and collaboration involves taking charge during critical situations, coordinating team efforts, and ensuring timely and appropriate interventions for the patient. This approach ensures that the patient receives prompt and efficient care, leading to better outcomes. Options A, C, and D are incorrect as they do not prioritize the patient's urgent needs or demonstrate effective leadership qualities in a healthcare setting.

Question 25: Correct Answer: C) "I understand you're feeling scared. I will stay with you and help you breathe easier."

Rationale: Option A is dismissive and does not address Mr. Johnson's concerns, which can further escalate his anxiety. Option B focuses on providing water, but it does not directly address Mr. Johnson's emotional state. Option D instructs Mr. Johnson to calm down without acknowledging his feelings of fear. Option C is the correct answer as it demonstrates empathy, active listening, and a commitment to providing support to the patient. By acknowledging Mr. Johnson's fear and offering assistance, the nurse establishes trust and shows a patient-centered approach to care.

Question 26: Correct Answer: B) Engaging in open communication with the patient to understand their cultural beliefs and preferences.

Rationale: Patient advocacy involves advocating for the patient's best interests, which includes understanding their unique cultural background, beliefs, and preferences. By engaging in open communication and actively listening to the patient, nurses can provide care that is tailored to the individual's holistic needs. This approach fosters a patient-centered care environment where the patient feels respected, valued, and actively involved in their own care. Administering medications solely based on orders, following rigid protocols, or focusing solely on task completion may overlook the patient's holistic needs and preferences, thus not fully embodying the essence of patient advocacy in holistic patient care.

Question 27: Correct Answer: C) To identify and address potential safety risks

Rationale: Safety huddles in a medical-surgical setting are structured brief meetings where healthcare team members come together to proactively identify and address potential safety risks that could impact patient care. Option A is incorrect as safety huddles focus on patient safety, not staff scheduling. Option B is incorrect as patient satisfaction surveys are not the primary focus of safety huddles. Option D is incorrect as safety huddles are not intended for planning social events but rather for enhancing patient safety and care quality through risk assessment and management discussions.

Question 28: Correct Answer: A) Contacting the primary care physician for medication list verification

Rationale: Contacting the primary care physician for medication list verification is essential during medication reconciliation to ensure accuracy and prevent medication errors. This step helps in cross-referencing the patient's current medications with the prescribed list, reducing the risk of adverse drug events. Providing the patient with a new set of medications without reviewing the current list (Option B) can lead to duplication or omission of medications. Disregarding the patient's self-reported medication history (Option C) can result in overlooking important medications. Failing to communicate medication changes to the patient (Option D) can lead to confusion and non-adherence. Therefore, option A is the correct choice for effective medication reconciliation and patient safety.

Question 29: Correct Answer: D) Obtain a set of vital signs and prepare to report to the RRT.

Rationale: In a rapid response situation, the priority action for the nurse is to assess the patient's condition by obtaining vital signs and preparing to report to the RRT. This step ensures that the RRT has accurate and up-to-date information upon arrival, facilitating prompt and effective intervention. Administering oxygen (option A) is important but should be based on the patient's oxygen saturation levels. Intubation (option B) and pain medication (option C) may be necessary interventions but are not the immediate priority in this scenario.

Question 30: Correct Answer: A) Education level

Rationale: Education level is a crucial social determinant of health that impacts patient safety assessments and reporting. Patients with lower education levels may have challenges understanding medical instructions, leading to errors in self-care management and medication adherence. This can result in adverse outcomes and affect patient safety. Blood type, favorite color, and shoe size are not social determinants of health that directly influence patient safety assessments and reporting in the medical-surgical nursing context. It is essential for CMSRNs to consider social determinants like education level to provide holistic and effective patient care.

Question 31: Correct Answer: B) Closed-loop communication

Rationale: Closed-loop communication is a structured form of information sharing where the sender initiates a message, the receiver acknowledges the message, repeats back the key points, and seeks clarification if needed. In this scenario, the nurse providing the report and the receiving nurse engage in closed-loop communication by ensuring that the information is accurately transmitted and understood. Option A, open-loop communication, lacks the feedback component essential for clarity and confirmation. Option C, one-way communication, does not involve active participation from both parties. Option D, non-verbal communication, focuses on gestures and body language rather than verbal interaction, which is not the primary mode of communication in this scenario.

Question 32: Correct Answer: C) Collaboration and open communication

Rationale: Collaboration and open communication are essential in conflict resolution among healthcare team members. This approach encourages active listening, sharing perspectives, and working together to find mutually beneficial solutions. Avoidance (Option A) can lead to unresolved issues, affecting team dynamics. Confrontation (Option B) and aggressive behavior often escalate conflicts, creating a hostile environment. Compromise (Option D) may not address the root cause of the conflict. In contrast, collaboration fosters trust, respect, and understanding, promoting a positive work environment and effective teamwork.

Question 33: Correct Answer: D) Nursing leadership involves guiding and supporting the team to achieve optimal patient outcomes.

Rationale: Nursing philosophy emphasizes the crucial role of leadership in guiding and supporting the healthcare team to deliver high-quality patient care. Effective leadership involves fostering teamwork, communication, and collaboration among team members to ensure positive patient outcomes. Option A is incorrect as nursing leadership involves active team involvement. Option B is incorrect as teamwork is fundamental in providing holistic patient care. Option C is incorrect as collaboration among healthcare professionals, including nurses, is vital for comprehensive patient care and positive health outcomes.

Question 34: Correct Answer: B) Decision-making shared among all team members

Rationale: In a decentralized nursing care delivery system, decision-making is shared among all team members, promoting teamwork and collaboration. This approach empowers nurses to contribute their expertise, insights, and perspectives to enhance patient care outcomes. Centralized decision-making (Option A) by a single authority limits input from other team members. Decision-making solely by the nurse manager (Option C) may overlook valuable input from frontline staff. Decision-making based on patient preferences (Option D) is important but does not specifically address the organizational structure of decision-making within the nursing care delivery system.

Question 35: Correct Answer: C) Strong leadership

Rationale: Strong leadership is essential for successful change management within a medical-surgical nursing team. A strong leader can effectively communicate the need for change, motivate team members, and provide guidance throughout the transition process. Resistance to change (Option A) and lack of communication (Option B) are common barriers that strong leadership can help overcome. An individualistic approach (Option D) may hinder teamwork and collaboration, which are vital for implementing changes effectively in a medical-surgical setting. Therefore, the correct option is C) Strong leadership.

Question 36: Correct Answer: B) Preferring to communicate through family members

Rationale: In this scenario, the correct cultural sign that the nurse should recognize and respect when providing care for Mr. Patel is his preference to communicate through family members. This cultural practice is common in many cultures, including Indian culture, where family members often play a significant role in healthcare decision-making and communication. Options A, C, and D are common misconceptions and may not necessarily align with Mr. Patel's cultural background. It is essential for the nurse to be culturally sensitive and respectful of diverse communication preferences to ensure holistic patient care.

Question 37: Correct Answer: C) Supervising a licensed practical nurse (LPN) in administering intravenous (IV) medications

Rationale: Delegation and supervision are crucial aspects of nursing teamwork and collaboration. Option C is the correct choice as it aligns with the registered nurse's scope of practice to supervise and delegate tasks to other healthcare team members, such as LPNs. Supervising an LPN in administering IV medications ensures patient safety and quality care delivery. Options A, B, and D involve actions that exceed the registered nurse's scope of practice, risking patient safety and violating professional standards. It is essential for registered nurses to delegate tasks appropriately, provide supervision, and collaborate effectively within the healthcare team to optimize patient outcomes.

Question 38: Correct Answer: C) Evaluating evidence, considering implications, and making informed decisions

Rationale: Critical thinking is a crucial skill for CMSRNs as it involves analyzing information, recognizing biases, evaluating evidence, and making informed decisions. Option A is incorrect as critical thinking involves questioning and analyzing information rather than accepting it blindly. Option B is incorrect as critical thinking requires a balance of intuition and evidence-based practice, not solely relying on intuition. Option D is incorrect as critical thinking involves using guidelines as a foundation but also considering individual patient needs and circumstances to make the best decisions. Therefore, option C is the correct choice as it encompasses the essence of critical thinking in nursing practice.

Question 39: Correct Answer: B) Consult with the healthcare provider regarding the dosage

Rationale: In this scenario, the nurse's first action should be to consult with the healthcare provider regarding the dosage concern. This aligns with the nurse's scope of practice to advocate for the patient's safety and ensure appropriate medication administration. Option A is incorrect as administering a potentially incorrect dosage without clarification can jeopardize the patient's well-being. Option C is incorrect as discussing the concern with the family does not address the immediate need to verify the dosage. Option D is incorrect as waiting and monitoring without clarification can lead to adverse outcomes. Consulting with the healthcare provider is crucial to uphold ethical standards and provide safe patient care.

Question 40: Correct Answer: C) Raise the concern immediately with the healthcare team during rounding.

Rationale: In the scenario described, the most appropriate action for the medical surgical registered nurse during interprofessional rounding is to address the medication discrepancy with the healthcare team immediately. This ensures timely resolution of the issue before the surgery, promoting patient safety and quality care. Option A is incorrect as proceeding with the surgery without addressing the discrepancy can lead to potential harm to the patient. Option B is not sufficient as the nurse should involve the entire healthcare team in decision-making. Option D is also incorrect as delaying the resolution of the discrepancy can compromise patient safety. Therefore, option C is the best course of action to promote effective interprofessional collaboration and patient-centered care.

Question 41: Correct Answer: C) Performing a thorough clinical reassessment to narrow the antibiotic spectrum based on culture results.

Rationale: Option C is the correct answer as it aligns with antimicrobial stewardship principles by emphasizing the importance of reassessment and tailoring antibiotic therapy based on culture results. This approach helps optimize treatment efficacy, minimize side effects, and prevent the development of antibiotic resistance. Options A and B promote overuse of broad-spectrum antibiotics, which can contribute to resistance and adverse effects. Option D is not recommended as abrupt discontinuation of antibiotics can lead to treatment failure and potential harm to the patient.

Question 42: Correct Answer: C) The pharmacist provides education on proper medication administration and side effects to Mr. Johnson.

Rationale: In the scenario provided, the pharmacist's action of educating Mr. Johnson on medication administration and side effects exemplifies interprofessional collaboration. This approach involves the pharmacist working in conjunction with other healthcare team members to ensure comprehensive care for the patient. Option A is incorrect as adjusting medication dosage without interprofessional consultation can lead to adverse effects. Option B is incorrect as prescribing new medications without consulting the primary care provider disregards the importance of collaborative decision-making. Option D is incorrect as referring the patient to an ophthalmologist without informing the team disrupts the collaborative effort in Mr. Johnson's care.

Question 43: Correct Answer: A) Identifying potential signs of human trafficking in patients

Rationale: Certified Medical Surgical Registered Nurses (CMSRNs) play a crucial role in patient safety assessments and reporting, including recognizing signs of human trafficking. By identifying indicators such as unexplained injuries, inconsistencies in the patient's story, or a controlling companion, nurses can intervene and report suspected cases to appropriate authorities. Administering medications, ensuring clean linens, and providing snacks, while important, do not directly address the critical issue of patient safety in the context of human trafficking. Therefore, option A is the correct choice as it aligns with the CMSRN's responsibility to advocate for patient well-being and safety.

Question 44: Correct Answer: B) Notify the healthcare provider immediately.

Rationale: In this scenario, Mrs. Smith is displaying signs of potential complications such as restlessness, confusion, tachycardia, chest pain, decreased urine output, and cool, clammy skin, which could indicate a cardiac event or hypovolemic shock. The nurse should prioritize notifying the healthcare provider immediately to ensure prompt assessment and intervention. Administering pain medication without further assessment could mask symptoms and delay appropriate treatment. Increasing IV fluids may not address the underlying issue, and reassurance alone is insufficient in this critical situation. Therefore, prompt communication with the healthcare provider is crucial for Mrs. Smith's safety and well-being.

Question 45: Correct Answer: A) Ensuring proper ventilation in the workplace

Rationale: Proper ventilation in the workplace is crucial for maintaining a healthy practice environment for CMSRNs. It helps in reducing the risk of exposure to airborne contaminants, ensuring a safe and comfortable atmosphere for both patients and healthcare providers. Options B, C, and D are incorrect as they promote unsafe practices that can jeopardize the physical well-being of nurses. Using personal protective equipment only during emergencies, ignoring ergonomic principles when lifting patients, and disregarding safety protocols when handling hazardous materials can lead to increased risks of injuries, infections, and occupational hazards.

Question 46: Correct Answer: B) Enteral Nutrition via Nasogastric Tube

Rationale: Enteral nutrition via nasogastric tube is the appropriate modality for patients with dysphagia as it provides necessary nutrition directly to the gastrointestinal tract. TPN is used when the GI tract is non-functional, not for dysphagia. Oral nutrition supplements are not suitable for patients who cannot swallow safely. Intravenous fluids do not provide adequate nutrition for patients with dysphagia. Therefore, enteral nutrition via nasogastric tube is the most suitable option in this scenario, ensuring the patient receives essential nutrients while bypassing the swallowing difficulties.

Question 47: Correct Answer: C) Adjusting the diuretic dosage based on Mr. Johnson's response and renal function

Rationale: Individualizing care involves tailoring interventions to meet the specific needs of each patient. In Mr. Johnson's case, adjusting the diuretic dosage based on his response and renal function is crucial to optimize therapeutic outcomes and prevent complications. Options A and B suggest standardized and generic approaches, which do not address Mr. Johnson's unique needs. Option D of fixed nursing assessments does not account for the dynamic nature of Mr. Johnson's condition and the need for personalized adjustments. Therefore, option C is the most appropriate choice for individualizing Mr. Johnson's care.

Question 48: Correct Answer: B) Administering antibiotics for the shortest effective duration

Rationale: Antimicrobial stewardship aims to optimize antibiotic use to improve patient outcomes while minimizing resistance and other adverse effects. Administering antibiotics for the shortest effective duration is a key strategy in antimicrobial stewardship to reduce the development of resistance, decrease healthcare costs, and prevent unnecessary exposure to antibiotics. Options A, C, and D are incorrect as they promote practices that can contribute to antibiotic resistance, inappropriate antibiotic use, and adverse effects on patients. Therefore, the correct answer is B as it aligns with the principles of antimicrobial stewardship.

Question 49: Correct Answer: A) Placing the call bell within the patient's reach

Rationale: Placing the call bell within the patient's reach is the most appropriate intervention to prevent falls in a high-risk patient like Ms. Johnson. This enables her to call for assistance promptly if needed, reducing the likelihood of attempting to move independently and risking a fall. Administering sedatives (option B) can increase the risk of falls by causing drowsiness and impairing balance. Encouraging unassisted walking (option C) may be unsafe for a postoperative patient with weakness. Keeping the room dimly lit (option D) can further increase the risk of falls by reducing visibility.

Question 50: Correct Answer: D) Notify the healthcare provider to adjust the diuretic regimen.

Rationale: In the scenario provided, Mr. Johnson is experiencing hypokalemia, which can be exacerbated by diuretic therapy. Administering potassium supplements orally without adjusting the diuretic regimen can lead to further electrolyte imbalances. Increasing the diuretic rate may worsen the hypokalemia. While consuming potassium-rich foods like bananas is beneficial, it may not provide an adequate and timely correction for Mr. Johnson's low potassium levels. Therefore, the most appropriate action is for the nurse to notify the healthcare provider to adjust the diuretic regimen to prevent complications associated with hypokalemia.

Question 51: Correct Answer: A) Providing emotional support to the family members

Rationale: Providing emotional support to the family members is a critical component of post-mortem care in the context of Palliative/End-of-Life Care and Holistic Patient Care. This support helps the family members cope with their loss, understand the situation, and begin the grieving process. Administering pain medication to the deceased (option B) is not necessary as the patient is no longer experiencing pain. Performing a full physical assessment on the deceased (option C) is not a priority after death. Initiating resuscitation efforts on the deceased (option D) is not appropriate as the patient has already passed away. Emotional support plays a key role in ensuring a compassionate and holistic approach to post-mortem care.

Question 52: Correct Answer: C) Repositioning the patient every 2 hours

Rationale: Repositioning the patient every 2 hours is a crucial patient safety protocol to prevent pressure ulcers by relieving pressure on bony prominences. Massaging bony areas can actually increase the risk of pressure ulcers by causing friction and shearing forces on the skin. Keeping the skin moist with powders can lead to maceration and skin breakdown. Donut-shaped cushions can also contribute to pressure ulcers by concentrating pressure on specific areas rather than distributing it evenly. Therefore, regular repositioning is the most effective strategy for preventing pressure ulcers in bedridden patients.

Question 53: Correct Answer: D) Patient adherence to the prescribed home exercise program after discharge

Rationale: In this scenario, evaluating patient adherence to the prescribed home exercise program after discharge is crucial in assessing the effectiveness of care coordination and transition management. This measure reflects the continuity of care beyond the hospital setting, ensuring that the patient is actively participating in their recovery process. Options A and B focus on aspects within the hospital stay and do not directly assess post-discharge care. Option C, while important, pertains more to infection control practices rather than care coordination and transition management. Therefore, monitoring patient adherence to the home exercise program provides valuable insights into the continuity of care and patient outcomes.

Question 54: Correct Answer: B) Call a code blue

Rationale: In this scenario, Mr. Johnson is displaying signs and symptoms of a potential myocardial infarction (heart attack) such as chest pain, shortness of breath, diaphoresis, hypotension, tachycardia, pallor, and anxiety. These are critical indicators of a medical emergency requiring immediate intervention. Calling a code blue will activate the hospital's emergency response team to provide prompt assessment and treatment to address the cardiac event. Administering pain medication or offering water would delay necessary interventions, and documenting findings, although important, is not the priority in this acute crisis situation.

Question 55: Correct Answer: B) Assess the patient's pain level using a pain scale and explore non-pharmacological pain management techniques.

Rationale: In this scenario, the most appropriate action for self-regulation as a CMSRN is to assess the patient's pain level using a pain scale and explore non-pharmacological pain management techniques. This approach aligns with critical thinking skills by ensuring a comprehensive assessment of the patient's needs and considering the individual's history of opioid misuse. Option A is incorrect as administering opioid pain medication without proper assessment may not be safe. Option C is incorrect as withholding all pain medications can compromise the patient's comfort and recovery. Option D is incorrect as consulting with the healthcare team should follow the initial assessment and exploration of non-pharmacological options.

Question 56: Correct Answer: B) Providing adequate orientation and training for new staff

Rationale: Providing adequate orientation and training for new staff is essential for ensuring a healthy practice environment. This approach helps in acclimating new nurses to the unit's workflow, policies, and procedures, ultimately enhancing patient care quality and safety. Options A, C, and D are incorrect as they promote practices that can lead to burnout, compromised patient care, and increased risks. Assigning nurses based solely on availability may result in mismatches between skills and unit needs. Implementing mandatory overtime can lead to fatigue and decreased job satisfaction. Ignoring nurse-to-patient ratios compromises patient safety and quality of care. Thus, option B stands out as the most appropriate choice for promoting a healthy practice environment.

Question 57: Correct Answer: B) Promoting regular physical activity

Rationale: Promoting regular physical activity is a primary health promotion goal for CMSRNs as it contributes to overall well-being, reduces the risk of chronic diseases, and enhances mental health. Encouraging smoking cessation programs (Option A) is important but not the primary goal. Advocating for excessive alcohol consumption (Option C) and suggesting high intake of saturated fats (Option D) are contrary to health promotion goals as they can lead to various health issues. By promoting regular physical activity, CMSRNs support patients in maintaining a healthy lifestyle and preventing illness, aligning with the holistic approach to patient care.

Question 58: Correct Answer: C) Engaging in regular exercise, mindfulness practices, and seeking support from colleagues.

Rationale: Engaging in regular exercise, mindfulness practices, and seeking support from colleagues is the most appropriate action for Sarah to address her symptoms of burnout. These strategies can help her manage stress, improve her mental well-being, and prevent further emotional exhaustion. Option A would only exacerbate her burnout symptoms by increasing her workload. Option B is not advisable as ignoring her feelings can lead to worsening burnout. Option D would not address the root cause of her burnout and may increase her stress levels. By choosing option C, Sarah can take proactive steps towards self-care and emotional recovery, promoting a healthy practice environment for herself and

enhancing her professional concepts.

Question 59: Correct Answer: A) Notify the physician immediately

Rationale: In the scenario described, the nurse's priority should be to notify the physician immediately when a patient experiences sudden onset symptoms that could indicate a serious adverse event. Prompt communication with the physician is crucial to ensure timely intervention and appropriate management of the patient's condition. Administering oxygen therapy or conducting a thorough assessment are important actions but notifying the physician takes precedence in situations where patient safety may be compromised. Documenting the findings is essential but should follow immediate notification and intervention to address the potential adverse event effectively.

Question 60: Correct Answer: B) Acknowledging the patient's concern, apologizing, and actively listening to understand the issue.

Rationale: In service recovery, a patient-centered approach involves empathetically acknowledging the patient's concern, apologizing for any inconvenience caused, and actively listening to fully understand the issue. This approach shows respect for the patient's perspective and helps build trust. Options A, C, and D do not prioritize the patient's needs or address the complaint effectively, which can lead to dissatisfaction and hinder the service recovery process. Active listening and genuine empathy are key components of patient-centered care and contribute to holistic patient satisfaction management.

Question 61: Correct Answer: D) Communicate with Mrs. Smith, express empathy for the inconvenience, and involve her in the revised plan.

Rationale: Option D is the correct answer as effective service recovery in this scenario involves open communication, empathy, and involving the patient in the revised plan. By acknowledging the delay, expressing empathy, and including Mrs. Smith in the decision-making process, the nurse demonstrates patient-centered care and holistic patient management. Options A, B, and C are incorrect as they do not address the patient's emotional needs, fail to provide a solution, and may further escalate the situation. Effective service recovery focuses on addressing the issue, showing empathy, and involving the patient in the resolution process to enhance patient satisfaction and overall care quality.

Question 62: Correct Answer: B) Proper disposal of hazardous materials in designated bins

Rationale: Proper disposal of hazardous materials in designated bins is crucial for maintaining a safe and healthy practice environment. By following correct disposal procedures, the nurse helps prevent accidents, contamination, and environmental harm. Options A, C, and D are incorrect as they pose risks to both the nurse and the environment. Reusing disposable gloves can lead to cross-contamination, ignoring spills compromises safety, and leaving medication carts unlocked violates security protocols. Therefore, option B is the most appropriate choice for ensuring workplace safety and promoting a healthy practice environment.

Question 63: Correct Answer: A) A hierarchical structure that outlines the order of authority and communication within an organization.

Rationale: The correct answer is A) because the chain of command in healthcare establishes a clear line of authority and communication flow, ensuring that decisions are made efficiently and effectively. It helps in maintaining order, promoting accountability, and enhancing patient safety. Option B is incorrect as it does not define the chain of command. Option C is incorrect as random communication flow can lead to confusion and errors. Option D is incorrect as patients are not part of the chain of command in healthcare settings. It is essential for nurses to understand and follow the chain of command to promote effective communication and collaboration in patient care.

Question 64: Correct Answer: B) Allocating funds for staff education and training programs

Rationale: Allocating funds for staff education and training programs is a key aspect of financial stewardship in nursing leadership. This action not only enhances the skills and knowledge of the nursing team but also contributes to improved patient outcomes and overall quality of care. In contrast, options A, C, and D are not aligned with effective financial stewardship practices. Implementing cost-cutting measures that compromise patient care can lead to adverse effects on patient safety and satisfaction. Ignoring budget constraints may result in financial instability, while overlooking financial reports and expenditures can hinder informed decision-making and resource utilization. Therefore, option B stands out as the most appropriate choice for demonstrating financial stewardship in nursing leadership.

Question 65: Correct Answer: B) Ensuring the patient's comfort and dignity are maintained

Rationale: In palliative/end-of-life care, the primary focus is on providing comfort and dignity to the patient. It is essential to respect the patient's wishes regarding organ donation while ensuring their physical and emotional well-being. Initiating the organ donation process without consent (Option A) violates ethical principles and patient autonomy. Withholding pain management (Option C) goes against the principles of holistic patient care. Disregarding the patient's wishes (Option D) is unethical and does not align with patient-centered care in the organ donation process. Therefore, option B is the correct choice as it emphasizes the importance of holistic patient care in the organ donation process.

Question 66: Correct Answer: A) Transcutaneous Electrical Nerve Stimulation (TENS) therapy

Rationale: Transcutaneous Electrical Nerve Stimulation (TENS) therapy is a nonpharmacological intervention commonly used in pain management. It works by delivering small electrical impulses through electrodes placed on the skin, which can help reduce pain perception. In Mrs. Smith's case, TENS therapy can be beneficial for managing her chronic lower back pain without the need for medications. Comparing the incorrect options: - Option B, Intravenous opioid administration, involves pharmacological intervention and is not a nonpharmacological approach. - Option C, Continuous passive motion (CPM) machine, is typically used for joint rehabilitation and not specifically indicated for chronic lower back pain. - Option D, Heat application using a heating pad, is a nonpharmacological intervention but may not be as effective as TENS therapy for chronic pain management.

Question 67: Correct Answer: B) Implementing a multidisciplinary team approach to coordinate his care efficiently

Rationale: Effective resource allocation in the context of a healthy practice environment involves optimizing the use of available resources to provide high-quality patient care. In this scenario, implementing a multidisciplinary team approach (Option B) is the most appropriate intervention for Mr. Smith. This approach ensures that healthcare professionals from different disciplines collaborate to address his complex health needs efficiently, leading to better outcomes. Options A, C, and D involve unnecessary or excessive use of resources, which may not align with the principles of efficient resource allocation and patient-centered care.

Question 68: Correct Answer: B) Democratic leadership

Rationale: Democratic leadership style encourages active participation, open communication, and shared decision-making among team members and patients. In Ms. Johnson's case, involving her in the care plan aligns with this approach, fostering a sense of empowerment and collaboration. Authoritative leadership, although effective in certain situations, may not fully support Ms. Johnson's desire for involvement. Laissez-faire leadership, characterized by minimal guidance, could lead to confusion for Ms. Johnson, impacting her engagement. Transactional leadership, based on rewards and punishments, may not resonate well with Ms. Johnson's proactive approach to her care.

Question 69: Correct Answer: C) Demonstrating the exercises using visual aids

Rationale: Visual learners, like Mrs. Smith, comprehend information best through visual aids and hands-on demonstrations. Providing written instructions (Option A) may not be as effective for her learning style. Verbally explaining the exercises (Option B) might not fully engage her visual learning preference. Discussing the exercises in a group setting (Option D) may not cater to Mrs. Smith's individualized learning needs. Therefore, demonstrating the exercises using visual aids (Option C) is the most suitable teaching method for Mrs. Smith to grasp the post-operative exercises effectively.

Question 70: Correct Answer: B) Discussing the error openly with colleagues to understand what went wrong.

Rationale: Reflective practice involves critically analyzing situations to improve future practice. Option B is the correct choice as it shows Ms. Smith's willingness to engage in open dialogue with her colleagues, fostering a culture of learning and collaboration. Options A, C, and D are incorrect as they do not promote self-reflection, teamwork, or professional growth. By discussing the error openly, Ms. Smith can identify root causes, implement preventive measures, and enhance patient safety through shared learning experiences.

Question 71: Correct Answer: B) Adjust the thermostat to a comfortable temperature for Mr. Smith.

Rationale: In this scenario, the most appropriate action to ensure a healthy practice environment for Mr. Smith is to adjust the thermostat to a comfortable temperature. This action promotes workplace safety by preventing patient discomfort due to extreme room temperatures. Providing extra blankets (Option A) may exacerbate the issue of high room temperature, while opening the windows (Option C) may not be feasible in all healthcare settings. Offering a warm beverage (Option D) does not address the root cause of the discomfort. Adjusting the thermostat ensures a conducive environment for patient recovery, aligning with professional concepts of patient-centered care.

Question 72: Correct Answer: B) Socioeconomic status

Rationale: Socioeconomic status (SES) plays a significant role in determining an individual's access to resources such as healthcare, healthy food options, and medication affordability. In this scenario, Ms. Rodriguez's living situation in a low-income neighborhood directly affects her ability to access essential resources for managing her heart failure. While education level, occupation, and marital status can also influence health outcomes, socioeconomic status encompasses a broader range of factors that impact overall well-being, making it the most relevant social determinant in this case.

Question 73: Correct Answer: D) Returning unused medications to a designated take-back program

Rationale: Stewardship in safe drug management and disposal involves responsible practices to prevent environmental harm and misuse of medications. Returning unused medications to a designated take-back program ensures proper disposal, reducing the risk of contamination of water sources or accidental ingestion. Flushing medications (Option A) can lead to water pollution. Donating medications (Option B) may pose risks of improper use. Discarding in household trash (Option C) can result in accidental ingestion by children or pets. Therefore, the best practice aligning with stewardship principles is returning medications to authorized take-back programs.

Question 74: Correct Answer: D) Hemostat

Rationale: A hemostat is a surgical tool used to control bleeding by clamping blood vessels. In this scenario, for a surgical procedure requiring hemostasis, the most appropriate instrument for the nurse to select would be a hemostat. A scalpel (Option A) is used for making incisions, forceps (Option B) are used for grasping tissues, and retractors (Option C) are used to hold back tissues or organs during surgery. These options are not suitable for achieving hemostasis, making them incorrect choices in this scenario.

Question 75: Correct Answer: B) Double-checking the patient's identification before administering medications

Rationale: Patient safety is a critical aspect of nursing care, and one key element is medication administration. Double-checking the patient's identification before administering medications helps prevent medication errors and ensures that the right medication is given to the right patient. Options A, C, and D all pose risks to patient safety by either skipping essential steps in care (A, C) or leaving a patient unattended (D), which can lead to adverse events. Double-checking patient identification is a standard safety practice that helps prevent medication errors and ensures patient well-being.

Question 76: Correct Answer: A) Chicken broth

Rationale: Clear liquid diets are often prescribed post-surgery to provide hydration and some nutrients without taxing the digestive system. Chicken broth is a suitable option as it is clear, easily digestible, and provides essential fluids and electrolytes. Vanilla pudding, mashed potatoes, and oatmeal are not appropriate for a clear liquid diet as they contain solid particles or fiber that may be difficult for the patient to digest at this stage of recovery. It is crucial to follow the prescribed diet plan to support the patient's healing process and prevent complications.

Question 77: Correct Answer: A) Passive Range of Motion (PROM) exercises

Rationale: In the scenario provided, Mr. Smith is in the early stages of recovery post total knee replacement surgery, making Passive Range of Motion (PROM) exercises the most suitable intervention. PROM exercises involve gentle movements of the joint by an external force, helping prevent stiffness and maintain joint flexibility without causing strain or stress on the healing tissues. High-impact aerobic exercises (Option B) would be contraindicated due to the potential impact on the surgical site. Isometric strengthening exercises (Option C) and resistance band exercises (Option D) may be introduced in later stages of rehabilitation once Mr. Smith's knee has healed sufficiently.

Question 78: Correct Answer: C) Nurse Practitioner

Rationale: In this scenario, the nurse practitioner is primarily responsible for coordinating the interprofessional care plan for Mr. Smith. Nurse practitioners are advanced practice nurses who are trained to assess, diagnose, and manage patients with complex health conditions. They work closely with the healthcare team to develop and implement comprehensive care plans that address the physical, emotional, and social needs of the patient. While all team members play important roles in Mr. Smith's care, the nurse practitioner is best positioned to coordinate the interprofessional collaboration and ensure continuity of care across disciplines. The registered nurse provides direct patient care, the medical doctor oversees medical management, and the physical therapist focuses on rehabilitation goals, but the nurse practitioner serves as the central coordinator of care in this scenario.

Question 79: Correct Answer: C) Providing a menu that includes a mix of hospital meals and traditional South Asian options.

Rationale: Option A is incorrect as it disregards Ms. Patel's cultural preferences, which are essential for her well-being and recovery. Option B, while well-intentioned, may not provide a balanced nutritional intake necessary for post-operative care. Option D is incorrect as it goes against the principles of culturally competent care, which emphasizes respecting and incorporating patients' cultural beliefs and practices. Option C is the most appropriate choice as it acknowledges and respects Ms. Patel's cultural background while ensuring she receives a well-rounded and suitable diet for her recovery.

Question 80: Correct Answer: B) Notifying the healthcare provider immediately

Rationale: In a crisis situation with a deteriorating patient, the priority action is to notify the healthcare provider immediately. This ensures timely intervention and appropriate management of the patient's condition. Administering medication without consulting the healthcare team can be dangerous as it may not address the underlying cause of deterioration. Waiting for the next vital sign assessment or documenting changes for the next shift can lead to delays in providing necessary care, potentially compromising patient safety. Effective communication and prompt action are crucial in managing deteriorating patients.

Question 81: Correct Answer: C) Call the healthcare provider immediately to report Mr. Johnson's change in condition.

Rationale: In this scenario, the nurse should prioritize patient safety and communication by promptly notifying the healthcare provider about the significant change in Mr. Johnson's condition. Option A is incorrect as it delays necessary intervention, risking Mr. Johnson's health. Option B is inappropriate as it disregards the urgency of the situation. Option D is unsafe without provider guidance and assessment. Effective communication with the healthcare provider is crucial in ensuring timely and appropriate interventions for patients experiencing acute changes in their condition.

Question 82: Correct Answer: B) Initiating patient-controlled analgesia (PCA) with morphine

Rationale: Initiating patient-controlled analgesia (PCA) with morphine is the most appropriate intervention for managing severe post-operative pain in Mr. Johnson. PCA allows the patient to self-administer small doses of pain medication within safe limits, providing better pain control while minimizing the risk of overmedication. Option A, administering acetaminophen, may not be sufficient for severe pain management post-surgery. Option C, applying heat therapy, may offer some comfort but is not the primary intervention for severe pain. Option D, relaxation techniques, can be beneficial but may not provide adequate pain relief for Mr. Johnson's current level of discomfort.

Question 83: Correct Answer: B) Involving the patient's family in care planning and decision-making

Rationale: Patient/family-centered care emphasizes the importance of involving the patient's family in care planning and decision-making processes. This approach recognizes the integral role that family members play in the patient's well-being and recovery. By actively engaging the patient's family, the nurse promotes a collaborative and supportive environment that enhances the overall quality of care. Options A, C, and D are incorrect as they do not align with the principles of patient/family-centered care, which prioritize inclusive decision-making, respect for patient preferences, and cultural sensitivity.

Question 84: Correct Answer: B) Politely decline to provide the information and offer to discuss it in person at the hospital.

Rationale: Option B is the correct answer as per the scope of practice and code of ethics for nurses. Nurses are bound by confidentiality requirements and should not disclose patient information over the phone to protect patient privacy. By declining to provide the information and suggesting an in-person discussion, the nurse upholds ethical standards and ensures that patient confidentiality is maintained. Options A, C, and D are incorrect as they all involve sharing patient information over the phone, which goes against the principles of patient confidentiality and privacy.

Question 85: Correct Answer: C) Following manufacturer's guidelines for equipment maintenance.

Rationale: Following the manufacturer's guidelines for equipment maintenance is crucial for ensuring patient safety. By adhering to these guidelines, the nurse can prevent equipment malfunctions, reduce the risk of harm to patients, and maintain the equipment's effectiveness. Options A, B, and D pose significant risks to patient safety as they involve using malfunctioning equipment, neglecting expiration dates, and compromising infection control practices, respectively. Therefore, option C is the correct choice as it aligns with best practices for equipment management in a medical-surgical setting.

Question 86: Correct Answer: A) Providing clear instructions and expectations

Rationale: Providing clear instructions and expectations is crucial when delegating tasks to UAP as it ensures that the UAP understands what is required, leading to safe and effective task completion. Option B is incorrect as the method of task completion should be specified by the nurse to maintain consistency and quality of care. Option C is incorrect as ongoing supervision is necessary to monitor progress and address any issues promptly. Option D is incorrect as feedback is essential for continuous improvement and learning. Therefore, option A is the most appropriate action for the CMSRN to prioritize when delegating tasks to UAP.

Question 87: Correct Answer: B) Notify the hospital social worker about the suspicions of human trafficking.

Rationale: In cases of suspected human trafficking, healthcare providers play a crucial role in identifying and reporting such instances to the appropriate authorities. By notifying the hospital social worker, the nurse can ensure that Sarah receives the necessary support and intervention from trained professionals who can handle human trafficking cases sensitively. Discharging Sarah without further assessment, documenting without action, or confronting the companion directly may escalate the risk to Sarah's safety and well-being. Reporting suspicions to the social worker allows for a comprehensive and coordinated response to protect the patient from potential harm.

Question 88: Correct Answer: D) Recording information accurately and objectively

Rationale: Accurate and objective documentation is a crucial aspect of professional reporting for CMSRNs. Using abbreviations and acronyms (option A) can lead to misinterpretation and errors in communication. Including subjective opinions (option B) can bias the documentation and affect patient care. Documenting care provided by another healthcare provider as their own (option C) is unethical and violates professional standards. Therefore, the correct choice is option D as it ensures clear, precise, and unbiased documentation, reflecting the highest standards of professional reporting and resources in nursing practice.

Question 89: Correct Answer: D) Monitoring and documenting the wound characteristics and response to treatment

Rationale: In the management of an infected pressure ulcer, the most critical aspect is to monitor and document the wound characteristics and the response to treatment. This includes assessing the size, depth, drainage, odor, and surrounding tissue condition of the wound regularly. By closely monitoring these parameters, the healthcare team can evaluate the effectiveness of the current treatment plan, make necessary adjustments, and prevent further complications. Options A, B, and C are important aspects of patient care but do not take precedence over the continuous assessment and documentation of the wound status in the context of infected pressure ulcers.

Question 90: Correct Answer: A) Prevention of antibiotic-associated diarrhea

Rationale: Probiotics have been shown to be beneficial in preventing antibiotic-associated diarrhea by restoring the balance of gut microbiota disrupted by antibiotics. While probiotics have shown promise in various health aspects, such as immune function and digestive health, there is limited evidence to support their role in treating hypertension, managing type 2 diabetes, or improving vision. Therefore, the correct option is A as it aligns with the antimicrobial stewardship and infection prevention aspects relevant to CMSRN practice.

Question 91: Correct Answer: C) Employing active listening and empathy

Rationale: In conflict resolution within a medical-surgical environment, employing active listening and empathy is crucial for fostering a positive outcome. This approach allows nurses to understand the perspectives of all parties involved, leading to effective communication and mutual respect. Avoiding the conflict (Option A) can escalate the issue, while using aggressive communication (Option B) may lead to further tension and hinder

resolution. Blaming others (Option D) is counterproductive and can damage professional relationships. Therefore, active listening and empathy stand out as the most effective strategies for conflict resolution in healthcare settings.

Question 92: Correct Answer: B) High levels of stress

Rationale: In this scenario, the most significant social determinant impacting Ms. Rodriguez's uncontrolled hypertension is high levels of stress. While limited access to healthcare facilities, lack of physical exercise, and inadequate health literacy are important factors in overall health, chronic stress can directly contribute to hypertension by elevating blood pressure levels. Ms. Rodriguez's multiple jobs, financial strain, and lack of access to healthy food options are likely sources of stress that need to be addressed to effectively manage her hypertension.

Question 93: Correct Answer: B) Maintain eye contact and nod periodically.

Rationale: Active listening is a crucial component of patient-centered care, emphasizing empathy and understanding. In this scenario, maintaining eye contact and nodding periodically demonstrates attentiveness and encourages Mr. Johnson to continue expressing his concerns. Option A is incorrect as interrupting can hinder effective communication. Option C shows a lack of focus on the patient's needs. Option D jumps to conclusions without fully understanding the patient's situation, which can lead to misinterpretation. Therefore, option B is the most appropriate response to facilitate effective active listening and holistic patient care.

Question 94: Correct Answer: B) Identifying potential victims and reporting suspicions

Rationale: Recognizing signs of physical abuse is important, but human trafficking involves various forms of exploitation beyond just physical harm. CMSRNs play a vital role in identifying potential victims by being attentive to behavioral cues, unexplained injuries, inconsistencies in patient stories, and signs of control by others. Reporting suspicions to appropriate authorities is crucial for ensuring the safety and well-being of potential victims. Focusing solely on medical treatment neglects the holistic care approach required in such cases, and disregarding patient history related to social determinants can lead to overlooking crucial information that may indicate human trafficking involvement.

Question 95: Correct Answer: A) Conducting a literature review

Rationale: Conducting a literature review is a crucial step in the research process for evidence-based practice in nursing. It involves reviewing existing research studies, articles, and evidence to gather information on the topic of interest. This step helps nurses stay informed about the latest findings, best practices, and interventions in healthcare. Administering medications to patients, documenting vital signs, and answering phone calls at the nursing station are important nursing responsibilities but are not directly related to the research process for evidence-based practice. Conducting a literature review is essential for nurses to base their practice on the best available evidence and improve patient outcomes.

Question 96: Correct Answer: B) Keeping the skin clean and dry

Rationale: Keeping the skin clean and dry is crucial in preventing pressure ulcers as moisture can increase the risk of skin breakdown. Massaging bony prominences can actually cause more harm by increasing friction and pressure on the skin. Applying direct pressure to reddened areas can further damage the skin and worsen the condition. Donut-shaped cushions, although commonly used, can lead to uneven pressure distribution and exacerbate pressure ulcer formation. Therefore, the best practice to prevent pressure ulcers is to maintain skin integrity by keeping it clean and dry.

Question 97: Correct Answer: B) Consult with the pharmacist to verify the medication order.

Rationale: Option B is the correct answer as consulting with the pharmacist to verify the medication order ensures patient safety by confirming the correct medication before administration. Administering the incorrect medication (Option A) can lead to adverse effects on the patient's health. Waiting for the physician (Option C) may cause unnecessary delays in addressing the issue. Informing the patient about the delay (Option D) is important but ensuring medication safety takes precedence in this scenario. Consulting with the pharmacist promotes a culture of double-checking and verifying orders to prevent medication errors, aligning with patient safety culture principles.

Question 98: Correct Answer: B) Notify the healthcare provider immediately

Rationale: In this scenario, the patient's presentation with severe abdominal pain, restlessness, diaphoresis, tachycardia, and increased blood pressure indicates a potentially serious condition that requires prompt attention. The correct action for the nurse in this situation is to notify the healthcare provider immediately to ensure timely assessment and intervention. Administering pain medication without further evaluation could mask underlying issues. Reassuring the patient is important but not the priority in this critical situation. Documenting findings is essential but should follow after the patient's immediate needs are addressed.

Question 99: Correct Answer: A) To confirm that the message sent by the sender is correctly received by the receiver.

Rationale: The 'check-back' communication technique is utilized in healthcare settings to ensure accurate information transfer between healthcare providers. Option A is correct as it aligns with the primary purpose of 'check-back,' which is to confirm that the message sent is accurately understood by the receiver. Options B, C, and D are incorrect as they do not reflect the essence of 'check-back.' Interrupting the flow, asserting dominance, or ignoring information goes against the collaborative and patient-centered approach that 'check-back' aims to promote.

Question 100: Correct Answer: D) Return the medications to a pharmacy or participate in a drug take-back program

Rationale: The correct answer is to return the medications to a pharmacy or participate in a drug take-back program. This ensures safe and environmentally friendly disposal of medications, preventing misuse or harm. Flushing medications can contaminate water sources, throwing them in the trash can lead to accidental ingestion, and mixing with coffee grounds or kitty litter may not fully deactivate the drugs. Returning medications to a pharmacy or using drug take-back programs is the recommended method for proper disposal, promoting community safety and reducing environmental impact.

Question 101: Correct Answer: C) Read-back

Rationale: The correct answer is C) Read-back. Read-back is a communication technique where the receiver repeats back or reads back the information received to confirm understanding and ensure accuracy. In this scenario, the oncoming nurse repeated the information about the patient's penicillin allergy to confirm that the message was accurately received. Paraphrasing involves restating information in one's own words, reflecting involves mirroring the speaker's emotions, and summarizing involves providing a concise overview of information, which are not the techniques demonstrated in the scenario.

Question 102: Correct Answer: B) Keeping call bells within reach of patients

Rationale: Patient falls are a significant concern in healthcare settings, and keeping call bells within reach of patients is a crucial intervention to prevent falls. Option A is incorrect as encouraging unassisted walking can increase fall risk. Option C is incorrect as restraining patients can lead to agitation and increase fall risk. Option D is incorrect as staff presence is essential for patient safety and fall prevention. By ensuring call bells are easily accessible, patients can promptly request assistance, reducing the likelihood of falls and promoting patient safety.

Question 103: Correct Answer: A) Coordinate care and communicate with all team members

Rationale: Option A is the correct answer as the role of a CMSRN within the interdisciplinary team involves coordinating care and facilitating communication among all team members. This includes ensuring that the patient's care plan is implemented effectively, advocating for the patient's needs, and promoting collaboration among healthcare professionals. Options B, C, and D are incorrect as prescribing medications and treatments, performing physical therapy, and assisting with paperwork are not within the scope of practice for a CMSRN. It is essential for CMSRNs to work collaboratively with other healthcare professionals to provide holistic and patient-centered care.

Question 104: Correct Answer: B) Moral injury results from a discrepancy between what one believes to be right and the actions taken in a high-stress work environment.

Rationale: Moral injury in healthcare settings often arises when healthcare professionals face situations where their ethical beliefs or values are compromised due to system failures, resource constraints, or conflicting responsibilities. It differs from burnout, which is primarily characterized by emotional exhaustion and depersonalization. Moral injury can lead to profound psychological distress, impacting job satisfaction and overall well-being. Recognizing and addressing moral injury is crucial in fostering a Healthy Practice Environment and supporting the mental health of CMSRNs.

Question 105: Correct Answer: A) Increased heart rate after taking a beta-blocker

Rationale: Adverse drug reactions refer to harmful or unintended responses to medications. In this case, an increased heart rate after taking a beta-blocker is an adverse reaction as beta-blockers are intended to decrease heart rate. Options B, C, and D describe expected or beneficial effects of medications, not adverse reactions. It is crucial for medical-surgical nurses to recognize adverse reactions promptly to ensure patient safety and provide appropriate interventions.

Question 106: Correct Answer: C) Monitoring vital signs every 4 hours

Rationale: Delegation is a crucial aspect of nursing teamwork and collaboration. In this scenario, monitoring vital signs is a task that can be delegated to a nursing assistant as it falls within their scope of practice and does not require specialized nursing knowledge. Assessing the wound for signs of infection (Option A) and changing the wound dressing using sterile technique (Option B) are tasks that should be performed by a licensed nurse due to the need for assessment skills and infection control knowledge. Providing patient education on wound care (Option D) involves critical thinking and should be done by a licensed nurse to ensure accurate information and individualized care.

Question 107: Correct Answer: A) Electronic Health Record (EHR) system

Rationale: The correct answer is A) Electronic Health Record (EHR) system. EHR systems are essential in promoting seamless communication and collaboration among healthcare team members by providing real-time access to patient information, care plans, medication records, and treatment updates. This technology ensures that all team members are well-informed and can coordinate care effectively. Option B) Social media platforms and Option C) Personal email communication are not secure or HIPAA-compliant methods for sharing patient information among healthcare professionals, posing risks to patient confidentiality. Option D) Fax machine, although used in the past, is now considered outdated and less efficient compared to electronic health records in promoting interprofessional care.

Question 108: Correct Answer: D) Step 4: Assign a Risk Priority Number (RPN) to each potential failure mode

Rationale: In FMEA, after identifying potential failure modes (Step 3), the next step is to assign a Risk Priority Number (RPN) to each potential failure mode. The RPN is calculated by multiplying the severity, occurrence, and detection ratings assigned to each failure mode. This step helps prioritize which failure modes require immediate attention based on their potential impact on patient safety. Options A, B, and C are important steps in the FMEA process but do not involve assigning the RPN, making them incorrect choices for this question.

Question 109: Correct Answer: C) Transformational Leadership

Rationale: Transformational leadership focuses on inspiring and motivating team members by creating a compelling vision, setting high expectations, and demonstrating strong personal values. This model encourages innovation, creativity, and individual growth within the team. In contrast, Transactional Leadership (Option A) involves a more traditional approach of rewarding or punishing team members based on performance. Servant Leadership (Option B) emphasizes serving others first and prioritizing their needs. Laissez-Faire Leadership (Option D) involves minimal interference from the leader, which can lead to lack of direction and accountability within the team. Therefore, Transformational Leadership stands out as the most suitable model for fostering teamwork and collaboration in nursing settings.

Question 110: Correct Answer: C) Primary Nursing

Rationale: Primary Nursing is a care delivery model where one nurse is responsible for coordinating and providing care to a group of patients throughout their stay. This system promotes continuity of care, enhances nurse-patient relationships, and ensures personalized care. In this scenario, Primary Nursing aligns with the goal of individualized care for Ms. Johnson. Option A, Team Nursing, involves a group of healthcare providers working collaboratively but does not assign one nurse to oversee all care aspects. Option B, Total Patient Care, assigns one nurse to care for all patient needs but does not involve coordination among multiple patients. Option D, Case Management, focuses on coordinating care across different healthcare settings rather than within a single unit.

Question 111: Correct Answer: B) Ensuring she has a follow-up appointment scheduled with her primary care physician.

Rationale: In the scenario provided, the most critical action for the CMSRN to take to facilitate a seamless transition and continuity of care for Ms. Johnson is to ensure she has a follow-up appointment scheduled with her primary care physician. This step is essential to monitor her recovery progress, address any post-operative concerns, and coordinate ongoing care. Option A is important but may not be as immediate as ensuring a follow-up appointment. Option C is crucial but should ideally be done in conjunction with scheduling a follow-up appointment. Option D, recommending a new diet plan, is important but not as urgent or directly related to continuity of care as ensuring a follow-up appointment with the primary care physician.

Question 112: Correct Answer: C) Initiating opioid therapy with morphine as per the WHO analgesic ladder

Rationale: In palliative care, the WHO analgesic ladder is a widely accepted guideline for managing cancer pain. Opioids, such as morphine, are the mainstay of treatment for moderate to severe pain in patients like Mrs. Smith. Non-opioid analgesics like acetaminophen are not sufficient for severe cancer pain. Regular pain assessments every 4 hours, not 12 hours, are crucial for prompt pain management. Distraction techniques alone are inadequate for managing severe cancer pain and should be used in conjunction with pharmacological interventions. Therefore, initiating opioid therapy with morphine aligns best with evidence-based practice for managing Mrs. Smith's pain effectively.

Question 113: Correct Answer: A) Education level

Rationale: Education level is a crucial social determinant of health that impacts patient safety assessments and reporting. Nurses need to consider a patient's level of education to ensure effective communication, understanding of medical instructions, and compliance with treatment plans. In contrast, blood type, favorite color, and shoe size do not directly influence patient safety assessments and reporting in the same way as education level.

Understanding and addressing social determinants like education level can lead to improved patient outcomes and overall quality of care.

Question 114: Correct Answer: B) Establishing mentorship with experienced nurses

Rationale: Career Development Relationships in nursing education emphasize the importance of establishing mentorship with experienced nurses to gain valuable insights, guidance, and support in professional growth. Building strong communication skills with patients, attending educational seminars, and participating in physical fitness programs are essential aspects of nursing practice but do not directly relate to Career Development Relationships. Mentorship provides a platform for knowledge exchange, skill development, and career advancement, making it a crucial component in fostering a successful nursing career.

Question 115: Correct Answer: C) Acupuncture is based on the concept of meridians and energy flow.

Rationale: Acupuncture is a traditional Chinese medicine practice that involves inserting thin needles into specific points on the body to stimulate energy flow along meridians. This technique is believed to help restore the balance of energy, known as Qi, within the body. Options A, B, and D are incorrect as acupuncture is not a form of massage therapy, does not involve herbal remedies, and is not primarily used for surgical procedures. By understanding the fundamental principle of acupuncture related to meridians and energy flow, healthcare providers can better incorporate this complementary therapy into patient care management strategies.

Question 116: Correct Answer: B) Notify the healthcare provider immediately

Rationale: In this scenario, the nurse should notify the healthcare provider immediately because severe abdominal pain localized to the right lower quadrant could indicate appendicitis, which requires prompt medical evaluation and possible surgical intervention. Administering pain medication without further assessment or consulting the healthcare provider could mask symptoms and delay appropriate treatment. Reassessing the pain level in 30 minutes may lead to a critical delay in care. Documenting the findings is important but should not take precedence over timely notification of the healthcare provider in this situation.

Question 117: Correct Answer: C) Collaborating with the patient

Rationale: Patient-centered care emphasizes the importance of collaborating with patients in setting health goals. This approach values the patient's preferences, values, and beliefs, ensuring that the goals set are realistic and meaningful to the individual. By involving the patient in decision-making, healthcare providers can tailor care plans to meet the unique needs of each patient, leading to better outcomes and patient satisfaction. Options A, B, and D are incorrect as they go against the principles of patient-centered care, which prioritize active involvement and partnership between healthcare providers and patients.

Question 118: Correct Answer: C) Communicating effectively with the interdisciplinary team to prioritize patient care

Rationale: Effective teamwork and collaboration are crucial during emergency procedures to ensure optimal patient outcomes. In a disaster scenario, communication among healthcare providers is essential to coordinate efforts, share information, and prioritize patient care efficiently. By engaging in open communication with the interdisciplinary team, the medical surgical registered nurse can facilitate a coordinated response, allocate resources effectively, and address the needs of patients in a timely manner. This approach enhances teamwork, promotes collaboration, and ultimately improves the overall management of emergency situations. Options A, B, and D highlight actions that are contrary to effective teamwork and collaboration, emphasizing the importance of communication and teamwork in emergency procedures.

Question 119: Correct Answer: C) Involving family members in care decisions and treatment planning.

Rationale: In the realm of patient-centered care, involving family members in care decisions and treatment planning is crucial for holistic patient care. This approach fosters a collaborative environment where the patient, healthcare team, and family work together to ensure the best possible outcomes. Options A and D limit family involvement, which can hinder communication and support. Option B, providing limited information, can lead to misunderstandings and lack of transparency. In contrast, option C promotes shared decision-making, enhances communication, and acknowledges the valuable role of family in the patient's care journey.

Question 120: Correct Answer: C) Emphasizing open communication and collaboration among healthcare team members

Rationale: In high accountable organizations, such as those focusing on patient safety culture and patient/care management, open communication and collaboration among healthcare team members are crucial. Option A is incorrect as prioritizing cost-cutting measures over patient safety goes against the principles of high accountability. Option B is incorrect as teamwork is essential in such organizations rather than focusing solely on individual performance. Option D is incorrect as neglecting patient preferences and feedback contradicts patient-centered care management. Therefore, the correct answer is C, as open communication and collaboration enhance patient safety and quality of care in high accountable organizations.

Question 121: Correct Answer: B) Consulting the latest clinical practice guidelines for heart failure

Rationale: Evidence-based practice in nursing involves integrating the best available evidence with clinical expertise and patient preferences. Consulting the latest clinical practice guidelines ensures that patient care is based on current research and recommendations, leading to improved outcomes. Options A, C, and D do not align with evidence-based practice principles as they involve outdated protocols, personal experience, and intuition, respectively, which may not reflect the most effective and up-to-date care practices.

Question 122: Correct Answer: B) Call a code blue and initiate CPR

Rationale: In this scenario, the patient is showing signs of respiratory distress and poor perfusion, indicated by cyanosis and low oxygen saturation. The priority action for the nurse is to recognize the deteriorating status of the patient and call for immediate assistance by activating a code blue and initiating CPR to address the life-threatening situation. Administering pain medication (Option A) is not appropriate as the patient's airway and breathing need immediate attention. Increasing IV fluids (Option C) may not address the acute respiratory compromise. Re-positioning the patient (Option D) is not the priority when faced with a patient in respiratory distress.

Question 123: Correct Answer: B) Emotional barriers

Rationale: Emotional barriers can hinder effective communication by causing individuals to be defensive, anxious, or upset, leading to misunderstandings and lack of cooperation. In this scenario, Mr. Smith's frustration and agitation suggest the presence of emotional barriers, as he may be experiencing fear, anxiety, or discomfort related to his surgery and hospitalization. While language, physical, and cultural barriers can also impact communication, the emotional state of the patient is the primary factor affecting the interaction in this case. It is essential for the nurse to address Mr. Smith's emotional concerns empathetically to establish trust and facilitate effective communication.

Question 124: Correct Answer: B) Write down the order and then inform the physician

Rationale: Verbal orders are a common occurrence in healthcare settings, but it is crucial for nurses to follow the correct procedure to ensure patient safety and legal compliance. The correct approach is to write down the order accurately, read it back to the physician for confirmation, and then document it appropriately.

Implementing the order without questioning (Option A) can lead to errors or misunderstandings. Ignoring the order (Option C) or disregarding it (Option D) are not appropriate actions and can compromise patient care. Therefore, the best practice is to document and verify verbal orders to maintain clear communication and accountability in patient management.

Question 125: Correct Answer: B) Using alcohol-based hand sanitizer before and after tracheostomy care.

Rationale: The correct answer is B because using alcohol-based hand sanitizer before and after tracheostomy care is a crucial step in preventing the spread of infection. Alcohol-based hand sanitizers are effective in reducing the number of microorganisms on the hands. Option A is incorrect as gloves should be worn throughout the entire tracheostomy care procedure, not just during certain parts. Option C is incorrect as tap water and soap are not recommended for cleaning inner cannulas; sterile technique and appropriate solutions should be used. Option D is incorrect as reusing the same tracheostomy tube inner cannula can increase the risk of infection transmission.

Question 126: Correct Answer: C) Collecting comprehensive and accurate patient data

Rationale: The correct answer is C) Collecting comprehensive and accurate patient data. During the assessment phase of the nursing process, it is crucial for the nurse to gather all relevant information about the patient's health status, including physical, emotional, social, and spiritual aspects. This data forms the foundation for the subsequent steps of diagnosis, planning, implementation, and evaluation. Options A, B, and D are incorrect as they undermine the importance of a thorough assessment in providing quality patient care. Implementing interventions without proper evaluation, formulating diagnoses based on assumptions, or skipping the assessment phase can lead to ineffective or harmful outcomes for the patient.

Question 127: Correct Answer: A) Offering reassurance and empathy while actively listening to Mr. Smith's concerns.

Rationale: Option A is the correct answer as it demonstrates the essential communication skills required in mediating a patient's anxiety. By offering reassurance and empathy, the nurse can establish a therapeutic relationship with Mr. Smith, showing understanding and support for his concerns. Actively listening to his worries allows the nurse to address them effectively and provide emotional support. In contrast, options B, C, and D are incorrect as they do not prioritize the patient's emotional needs or promote effective communication. Option B focuses on quick fixes rather than addressing the underlying anxiety, while options C and D disregard Mr. Smith's feelings, which can lead to increased distress and hinder the nurse-patient relationship.

Question 128: Correct Answer: B) Limit phosphorus-rich foods

Rationale: In chronic kidney disease (CKD), the kidneys are unable to effectively filter waste products, leading to a buildup of phosphorus in the blood. Limiting phosphorus-rich foods such as dairy products, nuts, and whole grains is crucial to prevent further complications like bone and heart problems. Increasing protein intake (Option A) is not recommended in CKD as it can burden the kidneys. Encouraging high potassium foods (Option C) is also contraindicated as elevated potassium levels can be harmful in CKD. While promoting fluid intake is generally important, in CKD, fluid intake needs to be monitored and restricted based on individualized needs, making Option D incorrect.

Question 129: Correct Answer: A) Percutaneous endoscopic gastrostomy (PEG) tube

Rationale: Percutaneous endoscopic gastrostomy (PEG) tube is a common resource for alternate nutrition administration in patients who are unable to tolerate oral intake due to various medical conditions. PEG tubes are inserted directly into the stomach through the abdominal wall, providing a route for delivering liquid nutrition. Intravenous (IV) fluids are not typically used for long-term nutrition support and are mainly for hydration or medication administration. Nasogastric (NG) tubes are temporary solutions and are not ideal for long-term nutrition. Rectal suppositories are not used for nutrition administration but rather for medication delivery or bowel management. Therefore, the correct option is A) Percutaneous endoscopic gastrostomy (PEG) tube as it is the most suitable resource for alternate nutrition administration in such patients.

Question 130: Correct Answer: A) Offering competitive salary and benefits packages

Rationale: Offering competitive salary and benefits packages is a crucial strategy for improving recruitment and retention of medical-surgical nurses. Competitive compensation not only attracts top talent but also motivates existing staff to stay. In contrast, implementing mandatory overtime shifts (option B) can lead to burnout and decreased job satisfaction, negatively impacting retention. Providing limited opportunities for professional growth (option C) can deter nurses from staying long-term, as growth and development are essential for job satisfaction. Ignoring staff feedback and suggestions (option D) creates a negative work environment, leading to higher turnover rates. Therefore, option A is the most effective strategy for recruitment and retention in the nursing field.

Question 131: Correct Answer: A) To confirm and verify information exchanged during verbal communication.

Rationale: 'The correct answer is A) To confirm and verify information exchanged during verbal communication. 'Read-back' is a crucial communication technique where the receiver repeats back information received to ensure accuracy and understanding. This practice helps in reducing errors, enhancing clarity, and promoting patient safety. Option B is incorrect as 'read-back' focuses on accuracy rather than speed. Option C is incorrect as documentation is essential for maintaining a record of patient care. Option D is incorrect as relying solely on memory can lead to misunderstandings and mistakes in healthcare settings.'

Question 132: Correct Answer: A) Check the oxygen flow meter for proper settings.

Rationale: In this scenario, the correct action for the nurse to prioritize in troubleshooting the equipment is to check the oxygen flow meter for proper settings. This step ensures that the oxygen is being delivered at the prescribed rate. Option B is incorrect as increasing the oxygen flow rate without verifying the settings can lead to potential harm. Option C is incorrect as disconnecting and reconnecting the tubing may disrupt the oxygen supply further. Option D is incorrect as switching the patient to a different oxygen delivery device should only be considered after confirming the malfunction in the current system. Checking the oxygen flow meter first allows for a systematic approach to equipment troubleshooting.

Question 133: Correct Answer: B) Attending team meetings regularly and actively participating in discussions

Rationale: Effective teamwork within an interdisciplinary team involves active participation and collaboration. Attending team meetings regularly and actively engaging in discussions allows the CMSRN to contribute their expertise, share insights, and work collectively towards optimal patient outcomes. Options A, C, and D are incorrect as they promote actions that hinder teamwork, such as working in isolation, disregarding input from others, and refusing collaboration, which are not aligned with the principles of interprofessional care.

Question 134: Correct Answer: B) To enhance collaboration and patient care

Rationale: In an interdisciplinary healthcare team, information sharing plays a crucial role in enhancing collaboration and improving patient care outcomes. By sharing relevant information among team members, healthcare professionals can work together cohesively, utilize their collective expertise, and make well-informed decisions for the benefit of the patient. Options A, C, and D are incorrect as they promote negative outcomes such as

barriers, individualistic decision-making, and limited communication, which are counterproductive to the collaborative nature of interdisciplinary teamwork.

Question 135: Correct Answer: C) De-escalating the antibiotic therapy to a narrower spectrum based on culture results.

Rationale: Antimicrobial stewardship aims to optimize antimicrobial use to improve patient outcomes while minimizing unintended consequences such as antibiotic resistance. In this scenario, de-escalating to a narrower spectrum antibiotic based on culture results is the best practice as it targets the specific organism, reduces the risk of resistance development, and prevents unnecessary broad-spectrum use. Continuing broad-spectrum antibiotics (Option A) may contribute to resistance, stopping all antibiotics (Option B) is not appropriate in active infections, and antibiotic rotation (Option D) is not as effective as targeted therapy based on culture sensitivity.

Question 136: Correct Answer: B) Providing smoking cessation counseling to prevent lung cancer

Rationale: Primary prevention aims to prevent the onset of disease or injury before it occurs. Providing smoking cessation counseling falls under primary prevention as it targets the modifiable risk factor of smoking to prevent the development of lung cancer. Administering antibiotics for an active infection (Option A) is a treatment intervention, not a preventive measure. Monitoring blood glucose levels in diabetic patients (Option C) is a form of secondary prevention to manage an existing condition. Performing physical therapy after a hip replacement surgery (Option D) is a rehabilitative intervention post-injury, not a preventive measure.

Question 137: Correct Answer: C) Bradycardia

Rationale: Bradycardia is a known potential complication of epidural analgesia due to sympathetic blockade leading to decreased heart rate. Hypertension is not a common side effect of epidurals; in fact, hypotension is more frequently observed. Hypoglycemia is not directly related to epidural analgesia. Hyperkalemia is not a typical complication associated with epidurals. Therefore, among the options provided, bradycardia is the most relevant complication to be mindful of when managing patients with epidural analgesia.

Question 138: Correct Answer: D) Certified patient education materials

Rationale: Certified patient education materials are the most reliable and accurate resources for patients and families seeking information on managing chronic conditions at home. These materials are developed by healthcare professionals, ensuring credibility and accuracy. In contrast, social media platforms and online support groups may provide anecdotal or inaccurate information, leading to confusion or misinformation. While a hospital library may contain valuable resources, certified patient education materials are specifically designed to educate patients and families on managing their conditions effectively, making them the most suitable choice for reliable information and guidance.

Question 139: Correct Answer: C) Open communication about errors and near misses

Rationale: A positive patient safety culture is characterized by open communication where healthcare staff feel comfortable discussing errors and near misses without fear of retribution. Option A is incorrect as blaming individuals for errors fosters a culture of fear and hinders reporting. Option B is incorrect as prioritizing speed over accuracy can compromise patient safety. Option D is incorrect as ignoring staff concerns undermines the importance of addressing potential safety issues proactively. In contrast, open communication promotes learning from mistakes and improving patient care outcomes.

Question 140: Correct Answer: C) Assigning tasks according to each team member's scope of practice

Rationale: Effective delegation and supervision involve assigning tasks based on each team member's scope of practice to ensure safe and efficient patient care. Option A is incorrect as completing all tasks independently may lead to burnout and inefficiency. Option B is incorrect as delegation should be based on competence and workload, not personal preference. Option D is incorrect as ignoring tasks can compromise patient safety. By delegating tasks according to scope of practice, the nurse promotes teamwork, collaboration, and optimal patient outcomes.

Question 141: Correct Answer: A) Ensuring the patient has signed the consent form

Rationale: Obtaining informed consent is a critical pre-procedural standard in surgical/procedural nursing management to ensure patient autonomy, understanding of the procedure, and acknowledgment of associated risks. Administering post-operative medications (option B) is a post-procedural task. Documenting vital signs post-procedure (option C) is important but not specific to pre-procedural standards. Allowing the patient to eat immediately before the procedure (option D) goes against fasting guidelines necessary for many procedures to prevent aspiration. Thus, option A is the correct choice as it aligns with pre-procedural unit standards and patient safety protocols.

Question 142: Correct Answer: A) Decrease sodium intake to 2,000 mg per day.

Rationale: The correct answer is A) Decrease sodium intake to 2,000 mg per day. This goal is specific to Ms. Johnson's condition of heart failure and aligns with patient-centered care by focusing on individualized needs. Option B focuses on a general health goal that may not be suitable for Ms. Johnson's condition. Option C is a good goal but may not be feasible for Ms. Johnson initially due to her medical condition. Option D, while beneficial, does not directly address Ms. Johnson's primary health concern of heart failure. Therefore, option A is the most appropriate and patient-centered goal for Ms. Johnson.

Question 143: Correct Answer: B) Providing emotional support and reassurance to address Mrs. Smith's fear and anxiety

Rationale: Holistic patient care involves addressing not only the physical symptoms but also the emotional, social, and spiritual needs of the patient. In this scenario, Mrs. Smith's fear and anxiety are impacting her overall well-being. Providing emotional support and reassurance can help alleviate her anxiety, improve her coping mechanisms, and enhance her overall experience during treatment. While administering diuretics, monitoring vital signs, and educating on dietary restrictions are essential aspects of care, addressing Mrs. Smith's emotional needs is crucial for holistic patient-centered care in this situation.

Question 144: Correct Answer: B) Ensuring the patient has signed the informed consent form

Rationale: In the preoperative phase, ensuring that the patient has signed the informed consent form is the highest priority as it confirms that the patient has been informed about the procedure, risks, benefits, and alternatives. Administering preoperative antibiotics (Option A) is important but not the highest priority. Verifying the patient's identification (Option C) is crucial but falls after obtaining informed consent. Confirming the surgical site (Option D) is essential to prevent wrong-site surgery but is not the highest priority in the preoperative phase.

Question 145: Correct Answer: C) Providing post-operative care and education to patients

Rationale: The correct option is C because as a CMSRN, the nurse's scope of practice primarily involves providing comprehensive post-operative care to patients, including monitoring their recovery, managing symptoms, administering medications, and educating them on self-care post-surgery. Options A, B, and D are incorrect as CMSRNs do not perform surgical procedures independently, prescribe medications without physician oversight, or make final diagnoses. It is essential for CMSRNs to work collaboratively with the healthcare team and adhere to professional standards and ethical guidelines in their practice.

Question 146: Correct Answer: B) Implementing evidence-based practice to reduce unnecessary costs

Rationale: Implementing evidence-based practice to reduce unnecessary costs is a key aspect of fiscal efficiency in nursing. By utilizing evidence-based practices, nurses can streamline processes, reduce waste, and optimize resource utilization, ultimately leading to cost savings without compromising patient care. Ordering excessive supplies, ignoring cost-saving suggestions, and overstaffing shifts are all examples of practices that can lead to unnecessary expenditures and inefficiencies, highlighting the importance of evidence-based decision-making in promoting fiscal responsibility within healthcare settings.

Question 147: Correct Answer: B) Midazolam

Rationale: Midazolam is a benzodiazepine commonly used for moderate/procedural sedation due to its anxiolytic, sedative, and amnestic properties. It acts quickly and has a short duration of action, making it ideal for procedures. Furosemide is a diuretic used for managing fluid overload, Metoprolol is a beta-blocker used for hypertension and cardiac conditions, and Omeprazole is a proton pump inhibitor used for gastric conditions. These medications are not indicated for sedation purposes and do not possess the sedative effects required for procedural sedation in a medical-surgical setting.

Question 148: Correct Answer: C) Smoking

Rationale: Smoking is a modifiable risk factor that directly impacts patient safety. It is associated with various health complications such as respiratory issues, cardiovascular diseases, and delayed wound healing, making patients more vulnerable to adverse outcomes during surgical procedures or hospital stays. Age and gender are non-modifiable risk factors that may influence patient outcomes but cannot be altered. Genetic predisposition, while significant, is also non-modifiable and does not fall under the category of risk factors that can be actively managed to improve patient safety. By addressing modifiable risk factors like smoking, healthcare providers can enhance patient safety and overall care management.

Question 149: Correct Answer: B) Instruct Mrs. Smith to call for help before getting out of bed.

Rationale: The correct answer is to instruct Mrs. Smith to call for help before getting out of bed. This intervention promotes patient safety by involving the patient in fall prevention measures and encouraging them to seek assistance when needed. Placing a bed alarm (Option A) can be helpful but may not always prevent falls if the patient attempts to get out of bed without assistance. Applying physical restraints (Option C) is not recommended as it can lead to complications and is considered a last resort. Encouraging independent walking (Option D) may not be safe for a patient at high risk for falls. Therefore, educating the patient to call for help is the most appropriate intervention to prevent falls in this scenario.

Question 150: Correct Answer: C) Tailoring care based on the patient's unique needs and preferences

Rationale: Individualizing care involves tailoring interventions to meet the specific needs and preferences of each patient. This approach ensures that care is patient-centered, promotes better outcomes, and enhances patient satisfaction. Options A and D are incorrect as they advocate for standardized or uniform care, which may not address the individuality of each patient. Option B is incorrect as ignoring patient preferences contradicts the principles of patient-centered care. Therefore, option C is the correct choice as it aligns with the core concept of individualizing care in the healthcare setting.

Made in the USA
Coppell, TX
30 May 2024

32947836R00085